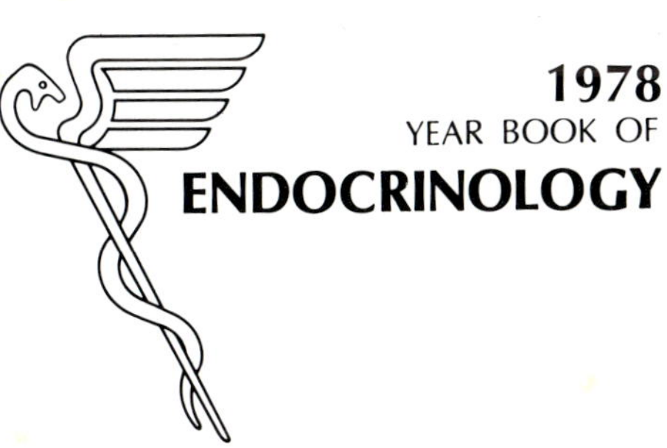

1978
YEAR BOOK OF
ENDOCRINOLOGY

THE 1978 YEAR BOOKS

The YEAR BOOK series provides in condensed form the essence of the best of the recent international medical literature. The material is selected by distinguished editors who critically review more than 500,000 journal articles each year.

Anesthesia
Drs. Eckenhoff, Bart, Brunner, Holley and Linde.

Cancer
Drs. Clark and Cumley.

Cardiology
Drs. Harvey, Kirkendall, Kirklin, Nadas, Paul and Sonnenblick.

Dentistry
Drs. Hale, Hazen, Moyers, Redig, Robinson and Silverman.

Dermatology
Drs. Malkinson and Pearson.

Diagnostic Radiology
Drs. Whitehouse, Bookstein, Gabrielsen, Holt, Martel, Silver and Thornbury.

Drug Therapy
Drs. Azarnoff, Hollister and Shand.

Endocrinology
Drs. Schwartz and Ryan.

Family Practice
Dr. Rakel.

Medicine
Drs. Rogers, Des Prez, Cline, Braunwald, Greenberger, Bondy and Epstein.

Neurology and Neurosurgery
Drs. De Jong and Sugar.

Nuclear Medicine
Drs. Quinn and Spies.

Obstetrics and Gynecology
Drs. Pitkin and Scott.

Ophthalmology
Dr. Hughes.

Orthopedics and Traumatic Surgery
Dr. Coventry.

Otolaryngology
Drs. Strong and Paparella.

Pathology and Clinical Pathology
Drs. Carone and Conn.

Pediatrics
Dr. Gellis.

Plastic and Reconstructive Surgery
Drs. McCoy, Dingman, Hanna, Haynes, Hoehn and Stephenson.

Psychiatry and Applied Mental Health
Drs. Romano, Freedman, Friedhoff, Kolb, Lourie and Nemiah.

Surgery
Drs. Schwartz, Najarian, Peacock, Shires, Silen and Spencer.

Urology
Dr. Grayhack.

The YEAR BOOK of
Endocrinology
1978

Editor

THEODORE B. SCHWARTZ, M.D.

Director, Section of Endocrinology and Metabolism, and Chairman, Department of Internal Medicine, Rush-Presbyterian-St. Luke's Medical Center; Professor and Chairman, Department of Internal Medicine, Rush Medical College

Associate Editor

WILL G. RYAN, M.D.

Associate Director, Section of Endocrinology and Metabolism, and Associate Professor of Internal Medicine, Rush Medical College, Rush-Presbyterian-St. Luke's Medical Center

YEAR BOOK MEDICAL PUBLISHERS, INC.
CHICAGO • LONDON

Printed in U.S.A.

Library of Congress Catalog Card Number: 47-1974

International Standard Book Number: 0-8151-7606-6

Table of Contents

The material covered in this volume represents literature reviewed up to November, 1977.

The Hypothalamus and Anterior Pituitary

General

MSH/ACTH 4–10 Influences Behavioral and Physiologic Measures of Attention. Recent evidence has clearly implicated attentional change as the predominant influence of MSH, ACTH and their analogues on behavior. Curt A. Sandman, Jack George, Thomas R. McCanne, J. Dennis Nolan, Jaques Kaswan and Abba J. Kastin[1] evaluated two critical aspects of attention, detection and discrimination, in 11 healthy men, aged 21–23, to evaluate the enhanced selective attention observed in both rats and human subjects with a visual discrimination procedure. Detection relates most specifically to perceptual threshold and discrimination assesses stimulus-processing capability. Subjects were given an infusion of MSH/ACTH 4–10 in a dose of 15 mg over 2 hours and a control infusion in a crossed and balanced procedure. Perception, attention and memory were tested in color identification tests under dark adaptation. A concept-learning procedure involving a two-choice discrimination problem was then introduced.

Treatment with MSH/ACTH 4–10 raised the subjects' perceptual threshold for detecting simple stimuli and facilitated perceptual integration of patterned information. The subjects' ability to discriminate tests of relevant from irrelevant information was improved by the heptapeptide. The heart rate deceleration response to the presentation of novel stimuli was augmented. There was no evidence of cortisol release by MSH/ACTH 4–10.

Presumably MSH/ACTH 4–10 has a predominant influence on attentional processes, and it may be uniquely coded for attentional-perceptual function. The heptapeptide may act to raise the absolute threshold for stimuli and may serve

---

(1) J. Clin. Endocrinol. Metab. 44:884–891, May, 1977.

as a filtering mechanism to protect the organism from distracting "perceptual noise." Once the detection threshold is reached, the processing or integration of patterned information is facilitated by the peptide. Disorders of attention or stimulus processing, as are evident in some forms of schizophrenia, psychopathy and mental deficiency, might be ameliorated by administration of MSH or ACTH fragments.

► [Some of you know that the initial draft of these comments are dictated. I have formed this habit not so much to flaunt my spontaneity and lucidity; rather, the habit grew out of necessity. When I attempt to write longhand, I can sit, pen poised, for eternities, debating, in a welter of indecision, which precisely is the *right* word to be selected. This sort of folly is greatly amplified when I am beginning a new year's set of comments. So, I open my mouth and begin.

The following are just a few of the points worth noting about this astonishing article. (1) The behavioral effects of the peptide fragment reported here in man represents an extension of animal studies with intact ACTH. Thus, we have an additional example of extra-adrenal effects of ACTH, effects which are demonstrable equally well in adrenalectomized animals. (2) The fragment tested here was identified by looking at the behavioral effects of smaller and smaller fragments of parent ACTH. Indeed, some effects are demonstrable with $ACTH_{4-7}$. (3) This fragment is present not only in ACTH and MSH but also in β-lipotropin, the pituitary prohormone for endorphins and enkephalins. (4) We endocrinologists of the old establishment have a new world before us. Either we enter it with our traditional rigor and vigor or we step aside and abdicate our claims to biochemists and psychometrists. I am delighted that this article was published in the *Journal of Clinical Endocrinology*. However, we cannot expect that the path into the new world will be wide and straight. For example, Small et al. (Acta Psychiatr. Scand. 55:241, 1977) found that ACTH 4-10 did not reverse the amnesia produced by electroconvulsive therapy in psychiatric patients. But, the authors, undismayed, are busily constructing experiments that might offer a better chance of yielding a positive result. —T.B.S.] ◄

► ↓ While the exploration of behavioral effects of hormones goes on apace, endocrinologic effects of "behavioral hormones" continue to be uncovered, as indicated below. — T.B.S. ◄

Stimulation In Vivo of Secretion of Prolactin and Growth Hormone by β-Endorphin. C. Rivier, W. Vale, N. Ling, M. Brown and R. Guillemin[2] (Salk Inst., La Jolla, Calif.) have attempted to isolate the endogenous ligand of the opiate receptors on the grounds that the opiate-like peptides might be involved in the release of pituitary hormones. The opiate alkaloids stimulate the secretion of prolactin and

---

(2)   Endocrinology 100:238–241, February, 1977.

growth hormone. The effects of three opioid peptides on prolactin and growth hormone secretion were examined with a cell culture assay of normal rat pituitary cells and a rat bioassay. Prolactin and growth hormone were measured by double antibody methods.

Morphine sulfate and the opioid peptide β-endorphin β-LPH-(61–91) stimulated prolactin and growth hormone release in both steroid-primed and untreated male rats when injected intravenously or intracisternally. On a molar basis, β-endorphin was at least 20 times more potent than morphine sulfate, whereas Met^5-enkephalin (β-LPH-[61–65]) and α-endorphin (β-LPH-[61–76]) were devoid of activity at the dosage used (300 μg). The in vivo stimulatory effects of β-endorphin on prolactin secretion were reserved by naloxone.

The absence of in vitro effects of morphine and β-endorphin on prolactin and growth hormone secretion by cultured rat pituitary cells suggests that they have a central nervous system site of action. The significance of opiate-like peptides in the physiologic control of prolactin and growth hormone secretion remains to be determined, but the present findings indicate one more biologic activity shared by morphine sulfate and the neurotropic brain peptides related to β-lipotropin.

▶ [So, β-endorphin and morphine stimulate the secretion of something that then stimulates the release of pituitary prolactin and growth hormone. In addition, Met-enkephalin, one of the active components of endorphin, does the same, and a synthetic analogue of Met-enkephalin (Kousan et al.: Nature 268:544, 1977) stimulates at a level of potency several orders of magnitude higher than that of the natural molecule. These studies fit with the notion that there is an opiate receptor in the hypothalamus that, when stimulated, trips off the appropriate hypothalamic hormone or hormones.

Similar results for growth hormone release have been reported by Dupont and associates (Proc. Natl. Acad. Sci. U.S.A. 74:358, 1977). β-Endorphin has this effect even in animals treated with an antiserum against somatostatin, so the effect is not due to somatostatin inhibition. The parallel activities of opiates and opioids are further documented by studies like those of Motomatsu et al. (Can. J. Neurol. Sci. 4:49, 1977), who showed that β-endorphin, like morphine, produced catalepsy in rats after intraventricular injection and that the effect was inhibited by naloxone, a known opiate inhibitor.

The hormonal effects of β-endorphin shown in this article suggest that, at least indirectly, there is autoregulation of the pituitary. Lipotropin secreted by the pituitary, with or without conversion to endorphin, could control the secretion of prolactin and growth hormone. This possibility becomes even more interesting when one considers the following article. —T.B.S.] ◄

β-Endorphin and Adrenocorticotropin Are Secreted Concomitantly by the Pituitary Gland. Adrenocorticotropin (ACTH) and β-endorphin are part of a much larger precursor glycoprotein synthesized by the cloned pituitary cells of the mouse cell line AtT-20/D-16v. ACTH, β-lipotropin and the biologically active peptides are all present in the same pituitary cells, raising the possibility that the active forms of ACTH and β-endorphin might normally be secreted concomitantly. Roger Guillemin, Therese Vargo, Jean Rossier, Scott Minick, Nicholas Ling, Catherine Rivier, Wylie Vale and Floyd Bloom[3] (Salk Inst., La Jolla, Calif.) have found this to be the case.

Male Holtzman rats had leg bones broken for studies of acute responses to stress and were given dexamethasone or were bilaterally adrenalectomized. Some rats were stressed 10 months after total hypophysectomy. Plasma and pituitary levels of ACTH and β-endorphin varied concomitantly and in remarkable parallelism in all experimental situations (table). In hypophysectomized rats, neither ACTH nor β-endorphin was detectable; hypophysectomy abolished the response to stress. Addition of purified corticotropin releasing factor and other secretagogues to cultures of adenohypophyseal cells also stimulated the concomitant secretion of

---

PLASMA AND PITUITARY CONCENTRATIONS OF ACTH AND β-ENDORPHIN AS MODIFIED BY ADRENALECTOMY, ADMINISTRATION OF DEXAMETHASONE AND, FOR PLASMA LEVELS, AS MODIFIED BY HYPOPHYSECTOMY

Treatment	Plasma (ng/ml)		Whole pituitary (μg/gland)		Adenohypophysis (μg/gland)	
	ACTH	β-Endorphin	ACTH	β-Endorphin	ACTH	β-Endorphin
None (controls)	0.8 ± 0.2 (3)*	1.5 ± 0.2 (9)	4.8 ± 0.3 (3)	2.6 ± 0.2 (11)	2.7 ± 0.5 (3)	1.1 ± 0.2 (3)
Adrenalectomy	8.8 ± 1.6 (3)	8.8 ± 1.0 (6)†	9.9 ± 1.1 (3)†	10.8 ± 1.5 (3)†	8.3 ± 1.1 (3)†	5.4 ± 0.7 (3)†
Dexamethasone	< 0.2 (6)‡	< 1 (7)‡	2.1 ± 0.1 (6)§	1.2 ± 0.1 (7)†		
Hypophysectomy	< 0.2 (3)‡	< 1 (3)‡				

*Numbers in parentheses represent number of replicates for that treatment; total of 40 rats were used in three separate experiments, results of which were pooled after demonstration of homogeneity of their variance (chi-square test); results were studied by analysis of variance in randomized (no block) design.

†P <0.01.

‡Indicates that content of each (plasma) sample was at or below lower limits of sensitivity of assay.

§P = 0.05 between experimental group and control group.

---

(3) Science 197:1367–1369, Sept. 30, 1977.

immunoactive ACTH and β-endorphin. Secretion of ACTH by fragments of the hyperplastic pituitary of a patient with Nelson's syndrome was accompanied by elevated secretion of β-endorphin.

It is concluded that where the pituitary secretes ACTH, it also secretes β-endorphin as part of a holistic response of the organism to stress. Profound changes in pituitary β-endorphin secretion are not, however, reflected in concomitant variations in brain β-endorphin levels. Peripheral targets for the β-endorphin secreted in response to stress must be sought.

▶ [That β-endorphin and ACTH should be secreted together under a wide variety of circumstances should come as no surprise when one learns that they are both chips off the same molecular block (Mains: Proc. Natl. Acad. Sci. U.S.A. 74:314, 1977). What's more, Pelletier et al. (Endocrinology 100:770, 1977) have shown by immunohistochemical techniques that ACTH and β-lipotropin are both stored and released in the same secretory granules, and Gilles et al. (Br. Med. J. 1:996, 1977) found elevated serum levels of both ACTH and lipotropin in Cushing's syndrome as well as Addison's disease.

The concordant release of β-endorphin and ACTH makes sense already. If ACTH and β-lipotropin enhance memory, detection and attention, this certainly is an appropriate additional response to stress. Furthermore, we may now have an explanation of why growth hormone is so bouncy and why levels of it and prolactin become elevated after nonspecific stressful stimuli.

Finally, the last sentence of this article is worth pondering. Where are the peripheral receptors for endorphin? If they exist, how do they help the organism? Are they related to true opiate addiction? Maybe we'll know next year but, in the meantime, back to the peptidurgic system. – T.B.S.]

Immunoreactive β-Melanocyte-Stimulating Hormone in Cerebrospinal Fluid and Plasma in Hypopituitarism: Evidence for an Extrapituitary Origin. Immunoreactive β-melanocyte-stimulating hormone (β-MSH) has been found in cerebrospinal fluid (CSF) in a concentration greater than in the plasma, and a physiologic role in the human central nervous system has been suggested. Sam Shuster, Andrew Smith, Norman Plummer, Anthony Thody and Frederick Clark[4] (Newcastle upon Tyne, England) examined the fate of β-MSH in the CSF when plasma levels are raised or depressed by studying 5 patients with severe panhypopituitarism, which followed craniotomy in 4 and was idiopathic in 1. Three patients had a chromophobe ad-

---

(4)   Br. Med. J. 1:1318–1319, May 21, 1977.

enoma and 1 had a craniopharyngioma. All had required replacement therapy with hydrocortisone and thyroxine; the 1 male also received testosterone. Hormone concentrations were also measured in the plasma of 14 other hypopituitary patients on replacement therapy.

The 5 chief study patients had higher β-MSH concentrations in CSF than those found previously, but they were not significantly higher. The plasma concentrations were higher than in normal subjects, but not significantly so. When plasma levels of β-MSH from all 19 patients were compared with normal levels, there was no significant difference; the overall mean plasma concentration was 94% of normal.

Both CSF and plasma concentrations of β-MSH are within the normal range in patients with hypopituitarism, with a CSF-plasma ratio of about 3:1. Possibly β-MSH is produced by and secreted from nervous tissue. Considerable amounts of immunoreactive β-MSH have been found in various brain regions, and comparable amounts of biologically active MSH have also been found. The finding of normal plasma β-MSH concentrations after complete surgical hypophysectomy suggests that the turnover of brain β-MSH is much faster than in the normal pituitary, since total brain β-MSH is only about 5% of that of the pituitary. It appears that MSH peptides are produced by the central nervous system as well as act on it.

▶ [It's clear. Unless the immunoassay used here is nonspecific, one must conclude that there is another source of β-MSH within or without the central nervous system leading to a concentration of this hormone in the cerebrospinal fluid. I mention the specificity of β-MSH because Bachelot et al. (J. Clin. Endocrinol. Metab. 44:949, 1977) have adduced telling evidence that what is measured in the β-MSH assay is really lipotropin. Enough oohing and aahing about the niceties of science; the immediacy of coarse clinical medicine calls! Look ahead. — T.B.S.] ◀

Clinical Features and Management of Pituitary Apoplexy. Acute massive infarction of a pituitary tumor is a rare condition which may be fatal or cause permanent visual impairment if not correctly diagnosed and appropriately treated. The clinical spectrum of pituitary apoplexy is wide. Margaret H. Lloyd and P. E. Belchetz[5] (London) report data on 3 patients with pituitary apoplexy who posed initial diagnostic problems.

(5) Postgrad. Med. J. 53:82–85, February, 1977.

CLINICOPATHOLOGIC FEATURES IN PITUITARY APOPLEXY

Pathological change	Clinical sequelae
Leakage of blood into subarachnoid space Leakage of necrotic tissue into subarachnoid space	Features of subarachnoid haemorrhage } (Adriano and Al-Mondhiry, Features of pyogenic meningitis ʃ 1967; Epstein *et al.*, 1971; Uihilein, Balfour and Donovan, 1957; List, Williams and Balyeat, 1952)
Destruction of pituitary tissue	Hypopituitarism (Adriano and Al-Mondhiry, 1967)
Pressure on: (a) Optic chiasm and tracts	Visual field defects, impaired visual acuity (Robinson, 1972)
(b) Cranial nerves 3, 4 and 6	Ocular palsies (Symonds, 1962)
(c) Internal carotid and its branches	Hemiplegia (Schnitker and Lehnert, 1952; Jefferson and Rosenthal, 1959)
(d) Hypothalamus	Hyperpyrexia, mental confusion, impaired water balance (Jefferson, 1940)

Woman, 29, had had severe headache and vomiting 4 days before and was febrile and drowsy with a rigid neck. She was clinically hypothyroid and lacked body hair. The right optic disc was pale and a right temporal field defect was present. Antibiotic therapy for presumed meningitis gave no improvement until hydrocortisone was added. A skull film showed an expanded pituitary fossa. The patient showed features of hypopituitarism. Craniotomy was done 24 days after the onset of illness and a large, suprasellar, necrotic tumor distorting the right optic nerve was aspirated. A small amount of solid tumor was present within the fossa and found to be part of a craniopharyngioma. The patient recovered uneventfully and had an improvement in visual acuity. The pituitary fossa was irradiated. Headache, vomiting and deteriorating vision led to readmission a month later. Dexamethasone resulted in some visual improvement. Gelatinous material was aspirated from the pituitary fossa at reexploration and the visual acuity then improved rapidly. Acquired diabetes insipidus was easily controlled by vasopressin. A right temporal field defect persisted 30 months after the first episode, but the patient was well on maintenance with thyroxine, cortisol and vasopressin.

The clinical features of pituitary apoplexy are summarized in the table. The most common features are sudden severe headache, altered state of consciousness and ocular symptoms. Pituitary apoplexy may resolve without serious sequelae on conservative management. Panhypopituitarism is not an inevitable sequel. Two of the present patients recovered spontaneously. A patient who presents with pituitary apoplexy requires corticoids and careful observation. Indications for surgery include deterioration in consciousness, visual acuity or the visual fields.

▶ [The table is helpful as a guide to what one might expect with this kind of catastrophe. The case briefly summarized here represents the first reported instance of pituitary apoplexy secondary to a craniopharyngioma.

I was brought up with the idea that apoplexy was more likely to occur in patients whose pituitaries were previously irradiated. This impression is strengthened by the observations of Weisberg (Am. J. Med. 63:109, 1977).

Among the many other causes of hypopituitarism, several were recently emphasized. Obstructive hydrocephalus has been incriminated (Weisberg: South. Med. J. 70:25, 1977), although the evidence would have been more convincing if more tests of pituitary function had been performed. Two groups (Dzur and Winternitz: ibid. 69:1377, 1976; and Weiss et al.: Am. J. Obstet. Gynecol. 127:678, 1977) describe patients with posttraumatic hypopituitarism, and Vessely et al. (Am. J. Med. 62:425, 1977) tell of a patient with the stigmas of hypopituitarism and sarcoidosis. Finally, Lawrence et al. (Arch. Intern. Med. 137:1134, 1977) tell of an acromegalic lady who suffered *hypothalamic* hypopituitarism after the advent of pituitary apoplexy. — T.B.S.] ◄

► ↓ The following article reminds us that not all patients with pituitary apoplexy have preexisting pituitary tumors. — T.B.S. ◄

Sheehan's Syndrome with Complete Bone Marrow Aplasia: Long-Term Results of Substitution Therapy with Hormones. A normochromic or hypochromic anemia is very often present in anterior pituitary insufficiency, but pancytopenia due to this cause is less common. E. Ferrari, E. Ascari, P. A. Bossolo and G. Barosi[6] (Univ. of Pavia) report a case of pancytopenia due to complete marrow aplasia associated with Sheehan's syndrome, in which the effects of substitution therapy were observed over 2 years.

Woman, 38, had had anemia for several years that had not responded to the usual treatment. Extremely severe hemorrhage from placenta previa had occurred at the end of her fourth pregnancy at age 32. Shortly afterward the patient noted fatigue, palpitations and effort dyspnea and a severe anemia was found which failed to respond to repeated treatment with transfusions, iron, liver extracts and vitamin B_{12}. Cold sensitivity, apathy, slow speech, slowed mentality, loss of libido, dry hair and loss of hair ensued. Well-marked genital atrophy was evident. Normochromic anemia was documented, along with leukopenia with lymphocytosis and thrombocytopenia. A marrow biopsy specimen showed total medullary aplasia (Fig 1). Ferrokinetic studies showed a prolonged plasma radioiron clearance rate and a reduction in red blood cell incorporation of ^{59}Fe. Urinary gonadotropins were below 5 mouse units/24 hours and there was no response to intravenous luteinizing hormone-releasing hormone. No somatotropin response to arginine infusion was observed and the blood cortisol did not respond to lysin-8-vasopressin. Weak and delayed water excretion followed a water load. Glucose administration yielded a flat curve.

---

(6) Br. J. Haematol. 33:575–582, August, 1976.

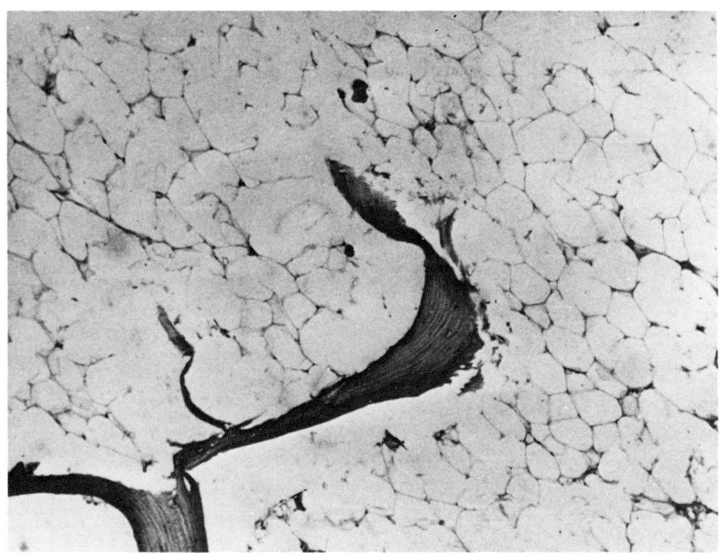

Fig 1.—Biopsy specimen of bone marrow from left posterior iliac crest; reduced from ×10. (Courtesy of Ferrari, E., et al.: Br. J. Haematol. 33:575–582, August, 1976.)

The patient was placed on polyhormonal substitution therapy without specific treatment of the anemia and very rapidly showed a good effect. No further blood transfusions were required and all the blood elements increased in the first few weeks of treatment. Her sex life was normal after 6 months and rhythmic pseudomenstrual bleeding was present. Blood values were normal at this time and sternal puncture yielded some hematopoietic marrow. Ferrokinetic studies indicated a recovery of erythropoiesis. After more than 2 years of polyhormonal therapy the patient is in good health and has normal hematologic findings.

There is no explanation as to how anterior pituitary insufficiency can lead to complete marrow aplasia. Correction of the hematologic disturbance depends on recognition of the endocrine illness that has interfered with hematopoiesis.

► [Figure 1 is included because it represents the kind of hematology an endocrinologist can understand. This striking complication of hypopituitarism is new to me and, I suspect, to many of you as well.—T.B.S.] ◄

► ↓ So what else is new? "This week's" surgical cure for microadenomas is shown below.—T.B.S. ◄

Transsphenoidal Microsurgery for Selective Removal of Functional Pituitary Microadenomas. Karl D.

Nielson, Clark Watts and Kemp Clark[7] have used trans-sphenoidal microsurgery to treat 29 patients with pituitary tumor in the past 3 years, including 10 with nonhormonally active chromophobe adenomas and 19 with functional adenomas. The latter included 15 growth hormone-secreting tumors, 3 prolactin-secreting neoplasms and 1 ACTH-secreting tumor. Transcranial surgery has been reserved for extremely large or eccentrically placed tumors in recent years. Operation (Fig 2) is performed with the patient semi-seated, under general endotracheal anesthesia.

Woman, 24, developed amenorrhea, obesity, moon facies, polyuria and polydipsia, striae, hypertension and hypothyroidism, and urinary 17-hydroxycorticosteroids and 17-ketosteroids were elevated. Dexamethasone suppression testing suggested an adrenal origin of Cushing's syndrome. Bilateral adrenalectomies were

Fig 2.—Transsphenoid approach to sella turcica. (Courtesy of Nielson, K. D., et al.: World J. Surg. 1:79–84, January, 1977.)

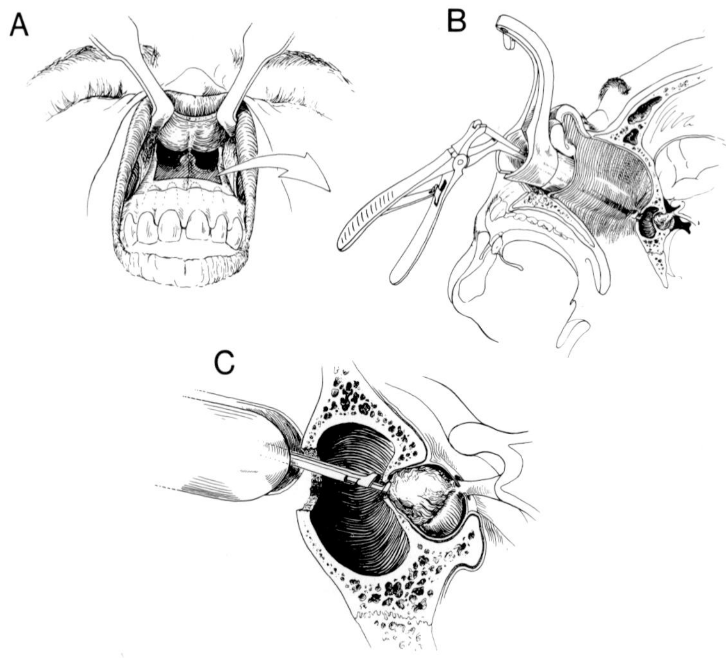

done, but only adrenal hyperplasia was discovered, and increasing skin pigmentation and postural hypotension developed within 2 months. The plasma cortisol concentration a year later was 2 μg/100 ml. An inferior incongruous quadrantanopsia for red objects was found. Serum ACTH values up to 4,750 pg were found and the patient had galactorrhea with a blood prolactin concentration of 43.5 ng/ml. Air study showed an "empty sella." A pituitary microadenoma was removed by transsphenoidal microsurgery. The patient did well postoperatively but required fluorocortisone for persistent polydipsia and polyuria. Prolactin concentrations were 24–28 ng/ml postoperatively.

Eleven of 15 acromegalics achieved normal growth hormone levels postoperatively, 2 had near-normal levels after reoperation and 2 had concentrations below 10 ng/ml. The other patients, with prolactin-secreting tumors, had decreasing prolactin levels and decreased galactorrhea postoperatively. Two patients transiently had nausea and low serum sodium and potassium levels after operation.

With familiarity with the oronasal-transsphenoidal approach and the availability of sophisticated operating equipment, the transsphenoidal approach to pituitary surgery is useful, safe and generally preferred.

▶ [This operation (let us all be properly impressed by Fig 2) is emerging as the favorite approach by neurosurgeons and endocrinologists alike. Correction! It is reemerging. First described in 1905, it was used extensively by Harvey Cushing and then abandoned.

In an invited commentary, Dr. Jules Hardy, of the University of Montreal, reported his experience with transsphenoidal removal of 225 hypersecreting pituitary adenomas. Fifty percent of these patients had normal-sized sella turcica and some of the lesions removed were smaller than 10 mm in diameter. "Clinical and biological cure" occurred after one operation in more than 80% of the cases.

In the present series no complications were reported but 1 patient "required fluorocortisone for persistent polydipsia and polyuria." To a paranoiac like me, this sounds like the patient had postoperative diabetes insipidus, a complication of pituitary surgery with which I am all too familiar. On the other hand, von Vild et al. (Acta Neurochir. (Wien) 35:5, 1976) report fairly extensive experience with both the transfrontal and transsphenoidal approaches in which hypophysectomy was total rather than selective. The results seem to me no worse than those reported here.

For a number of years now, I have been happy and relaxed in the company of neurosurgeons. It has not always been so. In medical school it was my view, shared widely with and by others, that the neurosurgeon had an ego unmatched by any other deity.

Recollected in tranquility is the following:

Neurosurgeon: "What is the best approach to the treatment of trigeminal neuralgia?"

Craven medical student: "Your posterior cerebellar approach, sir."
Neurosurgeon: "Correct. Is this a technically difficult approach?"
Craven medical student: "Not for a good neurosurgeon, sir."
Neurosurgeon: "That is correct. What is the cure rate?"
Craven medical student: "Dr. Wilder Penfield says. . ."
Neurosurgeon. "Next student!" — T.B.S.] ◄

GROWTH HORMONE

Characterization of Growth Hormone and Prolactin Produced by Human Pituitary in Culture. Human prolactin (hPRL) may be produced by the same subtype of pituitary cells that produce human growth hormone (hGH). Jay S. Skyler, Alan D. Rogol, Walter Lovenberg and Richard A. Knazek[8] (Natl. Inst. of Health) attempted to characterize both hGH and hPRL derived from a human pituitary tumor maintained in cell culture. The tumor was from an acromegalic patient. Levels of hGH and hPRL were determined by specific homologous double-antibody radioimmunoassay. Gel chromatography and analytic quantitative polyacrylamide gel electrophoresis (PAGE) were utilized.

The tumor secreted both GH and PRL, which were recovered in high concentrations. Tissue culture and pituitary-extracted hormones were eluted from Sephadex G-100 with the same partition coefficients. Growth hormone from the two sources showed parallel dose-response displacement curves, by logit-log transformation, both in specific immunoassay and in a specific lymphocyte binding assay. Parallel logit-log displacement curves were also seen with prolactin from both sources with one of three antiserums used, whereas the other two antiserums yielded nonparallel curves. With PAGE, tissue culture GH and PRL were indistinguishable from their pituitary-extracted counterparts.

Before purification, tissue culture-derived hormone can be characterized by multiple criteria and compared with a standard preparation. Structural differences can be detected, as in the case of PRL. When the hormones are indistinguishable, as in the case of GH, it becomes worthwhile to increase the scale of tissue culture production, with the prospect that tissue culture may serve as a source of hormone for both experimental and therapeutic purposes. The applica-

(8)   Endocrinology 100:283–291, February, 1977.

tion of mass culture techniques to increase the scale of hormone production holds much promise. With the use of one such technique, culture on an artificial capillary culture unit, prolactin secretion has been maintained at high levels for 4 months.

▶ [This article was included not to comment critically on logit-log displacement curves, but to remind you that biotic factories are on the horizon and they need not be stocked with recombinant DNA from *Escherichia coli.* — T.B.S.] ◀

Stimulation of DNA Synthesis in Isolated Chondrocytes by Somatomedin: II. Validation of Assay for Clinical Use and Comparison with Stimulation of Protein Synthesis. The effects of growth hormone (GH) on cartilage are thought to be mediated through somatomedins (SM). Stimulation of thymidine incorporation in isolated chick embryo chondrocytes by normal human serum has been described, exceeding that caused by serum from hypopituitary patients. John T. Garland, John Jennings, Lynne L. Levitsky and Fred Buchanan[9] (Chicago) compared SM activity as estimated by ^{3}H-thymidine incorporation with that estimated by ^{3}H-leucine incorporation in 46 serums from children with GH deficiency; short stature but normal GH responsiveness; or normal stature and normal GH responsiveness. Nine normal adults and 12 acromegalics were also evaluated.

Serum from children with GH deficiency had lower SM potency calculated from thymidine incorporation (SM_T) than did those from children with normal stature and normal GH responsiveness (Fig 3). Serum from children with short stature and normal GH responsiveness had higher than normal levels. Acromegalic adults had higher average SM_T activity than normal adults. Leucine incorporation was essentially the same in the different groups of children. Values in adults were somewhat higher, but the difference was not significant.

This study has validated use of thymidine incorporation into isolated chick embryo chondrocytes as an adjunct to the evaluation of children with short stature. Over 80% of samples from children gave results consistent with their status as determined by provocative tests for GH. The disparity between the results obtained with thymidine incorporation

(9)   J. Clin. Endocrinol. Metab. 43:847–851, October, 1976.

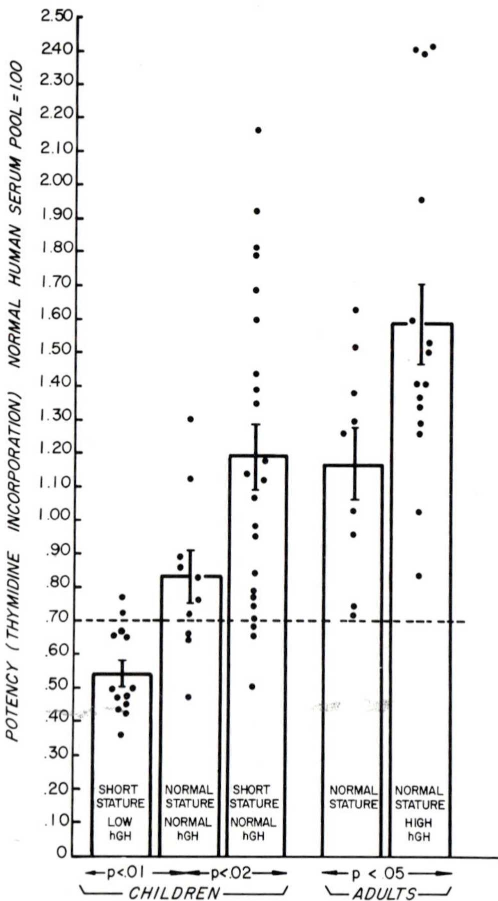

Fig 3. — Potency versus diagnosis for ³H-thymidine incorporation. Individual values for potency *(solid circles)* are indicated, besides mean ±SEM for each group. Nominal lower limit of normal (0.70) is indicated by broken line. Values for P are for 2-sided t tests between groups indicated. For these assays $\lambda = 0.24 \pm 0.4$ (SE), with range of 0.14–0.34. (Courtesy of Garland, J. T., et al.: J. Clin. Endocrinol. Metab. 43:847–851, October, 1976.)

and those obtained with leucine incorporation is unexplained.

▶ [Doctors Garland, Jennings and Buchanan function in the endocrinology section at Rush-Presbyterian-St. Luke's Medical Center. A glance at the title page of this YEAR BOOK will convince the reader that this group functions under a double handicap, saddled with the same individual as Section Director and Department Chairman. Despite this heavy burden, they are making steady progress in a very difficult field. The progression in Figure 3 makes biologic sense, but it would be nice if the variation about the means were smaller and we would appreciate suggestions from readers as to why results with thymidine incorporation are not comparable to those with labeled leucine. Similar results obtained with a different technique have been reported by D'Ercole et al. (J. Pediatr. 90:375, 1977) and Schwalde et al. (Br. Med. J. 1:679, 1977). Both groups find correlations between somatomedin levels and both growth rates and bone age. Somatomedin, therefore, emerges as the immediate stimulus for growth.

Since growth hormone stimulates somatomedin synthesis, serum concentrations of the two should be well correlated, right? Look ahead. —T.B.S.] ◄

Increasing Growth with Raised Circulating Somatomedin but Normal Immunoassayable Growth Hormone. Cases of active acromegaly with normal growth hormone (GH) levels have been described. R. Hoffenberg, A. Howell, S. Epstein, B. L. Pimstone, L. Fryklund, K. Hall,

---

GTT AND CPT DONE ON PATIENT IN (A) NOVEMBER, 1974, AND (B) JUNE, 1975*

A — GTT / CPT

Time (min)	Blood glucose (mmol/l)	GH (mu/l)	Blood glucose (mmol/l)	GH (mu/l)	Cortisol (nmol/l)	TSH (mu/l)	LH (u/l)	FSH (u/l)
0	5.1	1	5.0	3	550	4	4	4
30	8.2	1	2.1	16	–	15	15	6
60	6.8	–	3.7	5	472	8	12	5
90	6.2	5	4.9	1	500	–	–	–
120	6.4	19	5.0	1	898	–	–	–

B — GTT / CPT

Time (min)	Blood glucose (mmol/l)	GH (mu/l)	Blood glucose (mmol/l)	GH (mu/l)	Cortisol (nmol/l)	TSH (mu/l)	LH (u/l)	FSH (u/l)	SM-A (potency)[†]	SM-B (µg/ml)
0	4.4	19	4.7	16	268	4	3	2	2.4	11.9
30	5.9	4	2.0	27	–	19	13	4	–	11.6
60	5.9	4	3.1	50	702	14	11	4	1.8	12.1
90	5.0	3	3.8	48	789	–	–	–	–	–
120	5.0	3	4.3	30	813	–	–	–	5.6	–

*GTT, serial glucose tolerance tests with plasma growth hormone estimations. CPT, combined pituitary test, insulin 0.3 U/kg body weight, TRH 200 µg and LHRH 100 µg, all given intravenously at zero time with assay of blood glucose, GH, LH, FSH, TSH and cortisol.

†Potency is defined as $\dfrac{1,000}{\text{volume of serum } (\mu l) \text{ producing equivalent response to } 1,000\ \mu l \text{ standard serum}}$

S. Schwalbe and B. T. Rudd[1] recently encountered 2 young patients, 1 with clinical acromegaly and 1 with excessive growth, who had normal circulating GH levels but elevated somatomedin levels.

Girl, 15.6, had low backache radiating in a sciatic distribution and marked lumbar lordosis with dorsal scoliosis. The menses were regular. The patient was 195 cm tall and had an arm span of 197 cm and a lower segment of 105 cm. The 1st and 5th digits of both hands were deformed. The patient's shoe size was 11. Skull films were negative. A normal female karyotype was documented. The results of pituitary tests and glucose tolerance tests are given in the table. The serum somatomedin level by bioassay exceeded the mean for control children. Somatomedin A was elevated, but somatomedin B was within normal limits.

These 2 tall patients had high circulating levels of somatomedin but normal GH levels. The male patient had a classic acromegalic appearance. In both cases, a radioreceptor assay and a bioassay with use of chick embryo cartilage showed high somatomedin A concentrations. Somatomedin B, measured by radioimmunoassay, was within the normal range. The clinical syndrome appears to have resulted from the action of this growth factor, independent of immunoassayable growth hormone.

▶ [Here the relationship between somatomedin and growth hormone levels is discordant. Is somatomedin production in these patients hyperresponsive to normal growth hormone levels? Growth hormone administration here would be intellectually rewarding but morally questionable.

Research in this area will, it seems to me, stumble along until somebody holds the various somatomedins, pure, in eager, sweaty hands when laborious and error-prone bioassays will no longer have to suffice. —T.B.S.] ◀

Enhanced Peripheral Conversion of Thyroxine to Triiodothyronine during Human GH Therapy in GH-Deficient Children. Several alterations in thyroid function have been reported during human growth hormone (hGH) administration to GH-deficient children, and overt symptomatic hypothyroidism had developed. Tamotu Sato, Yukichi Suzuki, Tokuo Taketani, Kazumasa Ishiguro, Takeshi Masuyama, Ikuro Takata, Mieko Sano, Hiroko Kawashima, Shoichi Koizumi and Hironori Nakajima[2] (Kanazawa Univ.) studied changes in the hypothalamic-pituitary-thyroid axis

(1)   Clin. Endocrinol. (Oxf.) 6:443–448, June, 1977.
(2)   J. Clin. Endocrinol. Metab. 45:324–329, August, 1977.

during hGH therapy in 8 patients with idiopathic pituitary dwarfism. Growth hormone deficiency was diagnosed by a low or absent serum GH after arginine infusion and insulin-induced hypoglycemia, with a maximum GH below 5 ng/ml. Five patients were euthyroid (group I), whereas 3 (group II) had hypothalamic hypothyroidism with low serum thyroxine iodine levels and exaggerated and delayed thyrotropin responses to thyrotropin-releasing hormone (TRH). All group II patients also had ACTH deficiency and absent luteinizing hormone responses to luteinizing hormone-releasing hormone. Patients received 4–6 units of hGH intramuscularly twice weekly, and group II patients received L-thyroxine after 4–5 months of hGH therapy, as did 1 group I patient. The observation period was 6–14 months.

The findings are given in the table. All group I patients responded well to hGH but group II patients did not show a growth spurt until given 50 μg thyroxine daily in addition to hGH. Serum triiodothyronine rose immediately after hGH in group I patients but in group II patients it remained unchanged until thyroxine was administered. A marked increase in the serum T3-T4 level was observed. Acceleration of growth velocity was not related to the serum thyroxine iodine level but was associated with the elevation of serum T_3 in both groups. Abnormal thyrotropin responses to TRH were essentially unchanged by hGH therapy in group II and were completely inhibited by thyroxine replacement. No patient had clinical signs of hypothyroidism.

MEAN ±SD VALUE OF GROWTH VELOCITY, SERUM T_4-I AND T_3 CONCENTRATIONS DURING hGH TREATMENT

Patient's group	L-T$_4$ replacement	Growth rate (cm/M)		T$_4$-I (μg/100 ml)	T$_3$ (ng/100 ml)
		before GH	during GH		
I	(—)	0.23 ± 0.05	0.72 ± 0.13	3.4 ± 1.2 (23)*	178 ± 37 (21)*
II	(—)	0.13 ± 0.06	0.17 ± 0.07	1.6 ± 0.8 (8)	115 ± 21 (6)
	L-T$_4$ 50 μg		0.54 ± 0.15	3.3 ± 1.2 (15)	159 ± 37 (11)
P II *vs.* I	(—)	NS	*P* < 0.001	*P* < 0.01	*P* < 0.001
	L-T$_4$ 50 μg		NS	NS	*P* < 0.02
P I *vs.* the initial value			*P* < 0.001	*P* < 0.05	*P* < 0.001
II *vs.* the initial value	(L-T$_4$ −)		NS	*P* < 0.02	NS
	(L-T$_4$ +)		*P* < 0.01	*P* < 0.05	*P* < 0.01

*T_4-I and T_3 values of Case 2 after L-T$_4$ replacement were excluded. Number in parentheses equals number of samples.

These findings indicate that depression of the serum thyroxine level during hGH treatment is due not only to thyrotropin inhibition in the pituitary, but also to an altered thyroxine metabolism in peripheral tissues, in which conversion of thyroxine to triiodothyronine appears to be accelerated.

▶ [This article represents still another example of what I've come to call reversible secondary deficiency (RSD). While the changes described are complex, overall we have the phenomenon of overt hypothyroidism in patients with primary GH deficiency. With GH replacement alone, hypothyroidism disappears. Other examples of RSD are presented for the readers' edification in the table.

If the concept of RSD strikes you as strange, look ahead. – T.B.S.] ◀

Transitory Growth Hormone Deficiency Successfully Treated with Human Growth Hormone. Children with markedly delayed puberty may have reversible functional hypopituitarism, with reduced responsiveness to growth hormone (GH) stimulation tests, and they profit from human growth hormone (hGH) treatment. Olav Trygstad[3] (Rikshosp., Oslo) reports the successful treatment with hGH of 9 children who had transient GH deficiency and a comparison with the results obtained in 5 children of similar age who had an isolated GH deficiency. Thirteen prepuberal children, 8 boys and 5 girls, presented with severe growth retardation at chronological ages of 9.1–19.5 years and bone ages of 5.5–12 years. All had height velocities at or below the 3d percentile for more than a year of pretreatment observation. All but 2 had body weights within ±15% for height. Growth hormone deficiency was verified by at least two insulin tolerance tests. The standard dose of hGH was 2 mg twice weekly for children below 25 kg and 3 times weekly for taller children. One patient had received vasopressin and hydrochlorothiazide for diabetes insipidus. Another had developed severe anorexia nervosa at age 11.

No patient had a rise in hGH on vasopressin testing, despite a normal rise in serum cortisol. Increased sensitivity to insulin was observed. All children showed responses above 2 cm per year per year acceleration in the 1st year of treatment. The mean velocity in the 1st year was 7 cm, compared with 3.4 cm in the year before treatment, in patients with isolated GH deficiency. The respective figures for those with

---

(3) Acta Endocrinol. (Kbh.) 84:11–22, January, 1977.

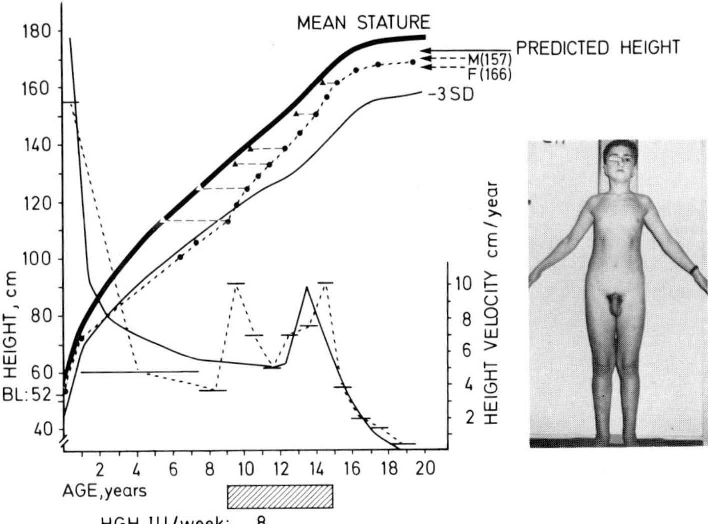

Fig 4.—Growth chart of patient with delay of growth and maturity with transient GH deficiency. He was successfully treated with hGH for 5.7 years. Triangles denote bone age; *BL*, birth length; *F* and *M* indicate heights of father and mother in SD; their heights in centimeters are given in parentheses. (Courtesy of Trygstad, O.: Acta Endocrinol. (Kbh.) 84:11–22, January, 1977.)

transient GH deficiency were 7.4 cm and 2.8 cm. The course of 1 patient is shown in Figure 4. Three boys with bone ages of 5.5–9.5 years showed definite effects of hGH therapy. The other patients, including those with true isolated GH deficiency, showed an initial spurt of growth and then a pubertal growth spurt. The girl with anorexia nervosa, who had transitory GH deficiency, showed an accelerated high velocity from 1.1 to 7.6 cm in the 1st year after hGH therapy.

Patients with transitory GH deficiency may benefit from hGH treatment. Repeated GH stimulation tests should be performed in children thought to have had hypopituitarism after they have entered puberty and terminated hGH therapy.

▶ [Readers, like myself, may well have difficulty in understanding this article. The addition of the following paragraph should help.

"Routinely the growth hormone stimulation tests have been repeated in patients treated with growth hormone some months after the end of treatment. The 9 patients considered to have transitory growth hormone deficiency, originally considered to have pituitary retardation of growth,

. . . responded very well." The author's thesis is that these patients had a reversible growth hormone deficiency that led in a number of them to secondary gonadal deficiency. Treatment with growth hormone permitted pubertal changes, even in some of the older patients, and subsequently the growth hormone deficiency disappeared. Whether or not the reversible growth hormone deficiency was secondary to growth hormone deficiency, I will leave for you to decide. — T.B.S.] ◄

Muscle Changes in Acromegaly. Enlarged muscles with weakness is a well-recognized finding in patients with acromegaly, but relatively few studies have been done on the myopathy of acromegaly. M. Nagulesparen, R. Trickey, M. J. Davies and J. S. Jenkins[4] (St. George's Hosp., London) used needle biopsy and histochemical techniques to study the muscle abnormalities in 18 patients with acromegaly of varying severity.

The 10 men and 8 women were aged 36–79 years. The probable duration of disease was 1–27 years. All patients but 2 were severely acromegalic; all but 1 were fully ambulatory. Only 1 patient had clinical diabetes. All patients but 2 had greatly elevated growth hormone levels at the time of diagnosis. Two patients were untreated, and 7 had normal growth hormone levels after 1–6 years of treatment. Quadriceps muscle specimens were obtained by needle biopsy.

Muscle abnormalities were found in all but 2 patients. Nine patients had hypertrophy of type 1 fibers, and 3 also showed hypertrophy of type 2A fibers. One patient had hypertrophy of type 2B fibers. In 1 untreated patient, hypertrophy was confined to type 2B fibers. Atrophy was most common in type 2A and type 2B fibers; in only 2 cases were type 1 fibers atrophied. Abnormal variation of fiber size within muscle types was observed in 8 cases.

The most common muscle abnormality in these acromegalic patients was hypertrophy of type 1 fibers and atrophy of type 2 fibers, particularly type 2A fibers. The atrophy was not that of simple disuse. Hypertrophy did not appear to be due to compensation for loss of function in the smaller atrophic fibers. Whether increased growth hormone levels are directly responsible for the atrophic appearances is not clear. The only patient in this series who died of heart failure from cardiomyopathy had skeletal muscle changes of atrophy with variation in type 1 fibers shortly before death.

---

(4) Br. Med. J. 2:914–915, Oct. 16, 1976.

There is no evidence that restoring normal growth hormone levels can reverse the muscle abnormalities. The relatively atraumatic needle biopsy technique is well suited for following the history of this condition.

► [The hypertrophy of type 1 fibers is to be expected; almost everything enlarges in acromegaly, including such tissues as kidneys and peripheral nerves. The associated muscle atrophy is more remarkable, and its cause is unknown.

How many of you know that acute acromegalic dyspnea, first described in 1896, was recently discussed by Dujovny et al. (Laryngoscope 86: 1397, 1976)? The patient had "inspiratory stridor that increased with exertion." He had diffuse laryngeal hypertrophy, still another site of acromegalic hypertrophy. Now, what may get smaller in acromegaly? You guessed wrong, it's the pituitary gland. Look ahead. – T.B.S.] ◄

Coexisting Primary Empty Sella Syndrome and Acromegaly. Most patients with the primary empty sella syndrome have normal pituitary function, whereas about 30% have varying degrees of hypopituitarism. It is not widely appreciated that the primary empty sella may harbor a pituitary tumor with resultant acromegaly. M. E. Molitch, G. B. Hieshima, S. Marcovitz, I. M. D. Jackson and S. Wolpert[5] report the records of 2 such patients who presented with active acromegaly.

Fig 5. – A, coronal and B, sagittal tomograms of the sella turcica obtained during pneumoencephalography. The subarachnoid air is shown within the confines of the sella turcica. Arrows indicate the air-soft tissue demarcation. (Courtesy of Molitch, M. E., et al.: Clin. Endocrinol. (Oxf.) 7:261–263, September, 1977.)

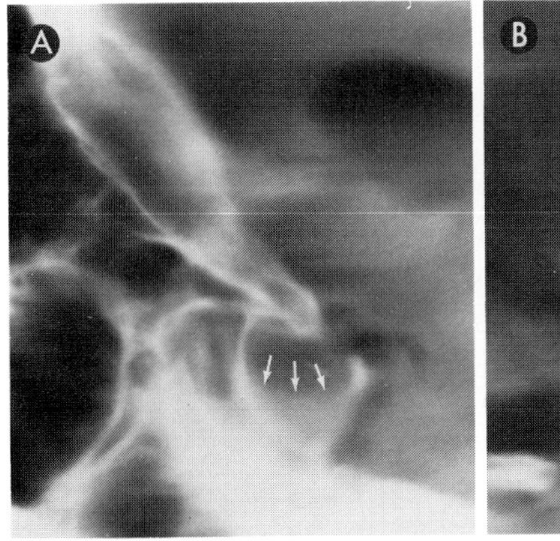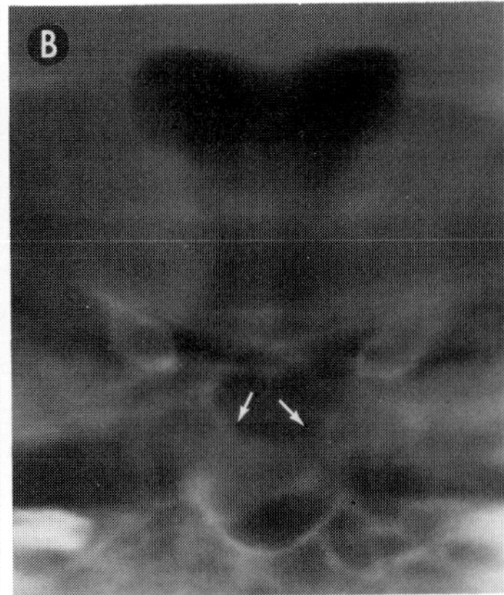

---

(5)   Clin. Endocrinol. (Oxf.) 7:261–263, September, 1977.

Woman, 52, had noted increasing head, hand and shoe sizes and increased perspiration for about 3 years. An isolated very severe headache had lasted several hours at age 50. Examination showed thickened, oily skin, hypertrophied gums, prognathism with malocclusion and broad hands and feet. The basal growth hormone was slightly elevated and there was a paradoxic elevation during oral glucose loading. Thyrotropin releasing hormone injection resulted in a normal rise of thyrotropin and a marked rise in growth hormone to 106 μg/L. The luteinizing hormone was appropriate for a postmenopausal woman. The sella was enlarged; pneumoencephalography showed a partially empty sella with subarachnoid air entering the structure (Fig 5).

The other patient, a man aged 60 with a history of acromegaly since his twenties and no recent size changes, had a markedly enlarged pituitary fossa which partially filled with air on pneumoencephalography.

These cases document the concurrence of active acromegaly and an "empty" sella in patients without previous treatment directed at the pituitary. This occurrence must be rare. The radiologic demonstration of an empty sella does not necessarily exclude the coexistence of hyperfunctioning pituitary tissue, and a complete endocrine evaluation is necessary to exclude hyperfunctioning tissue, since treatment directed at such tissue may be indicated.

▶ [The empty sella is nicely shown in Figure 5. Schaison and Metzger (Acta Endocrinol. (Kbh.) 83:483, 1976) enlarge on this association. In their 12 patients with empty sella, endocrine disturbances range from panhypopituitarism in 2 patients through no endocrine disturbance in 2 to proved prolactin-producing microadenomas in another 2.

Incidentally, pneumoencephalography has not become any more tolerable to patients; it hurts a lot. We find that the body CAT scanner may demonstrate an empty sella quite well. Which is preferable for our patients, the pain of expense or the expense of pain? As an "A.A.P.C." (active and practicing coward), I have no doubt. — T.B.S.] ◀

Treatment of Acromegaly by Transsphenoidal Microsurgery. Massimo A. Giovanelli, Enrico D. F. Motti, Alessandra Paracchi, Paolo Beck-Peccoz, Bruno Ambrosi and Giovanni Faglia[6] (Univ. of Milan) report the results of transsphenoidal microsurgery in 29 consecutive acromegalic patients. The 14 men and 15 women, aged 23–71, were seen in 1970–74 with active acromegaly. Seven patients had enlargement of the pituitary fossa with destructive

---

(6) J. Neurosurg. 44:677–686, June, 1976.

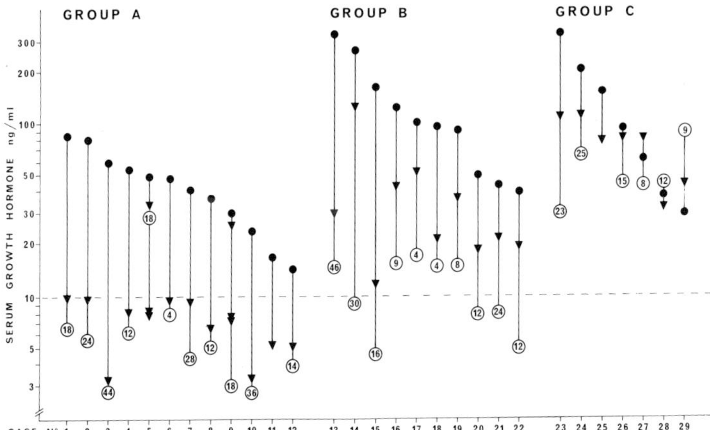

Fig 6.—Serum GH levels before surgery *(closed circles)*, after surgery *(closed triangles;* double triangles indicate a second operation) and after conventional radiotherapy *(open circles).* Figures enclosed in the circles indicate the time interval in months between surgery and the latest GH determinations. (Courtesy of Giovanelli, M. A., et al.: J. Neurosurg. 44:677–686, June, 1976.)

changes limited to part of the sellar floor and 2 had extensive sellar destruction. Seven patients had previously had conventional radiotherapy. Selective removal of an adenoma was possible in 7 patients. There were 24 eosinophilic and 5 mixed adenomas.

Serum growth hormone (GH) levels are shown in Figure 6. Serum GH levels fell below 10 ng/ml in 10 patients, to below 50% of basal levels in 10 patients with a further drop to below 20 ng/ml after radiotherapy, and did not fall below 30 ng/ml after either surgery or radiotherapy in 7 patients. Operation, sometimes repeated, and radiotherapy gave satisfactory results in 4 of 6 patients with suprasellar extension of the tumor. Transitory diabetes insipidus occurred in 5 patients and regressed spontaneously. Postoperative rhinorrhea resolved in 3 patients after repeated lumbar punctures.

These results clearly favor selective microsurgery in early diagnosed and operated tumors or microadenomas. A less than radical approach does not hold out much promise of functional normalization in patients with larger adenomas. Radiotherapy may be effective in nonnormalized cases. Results of thyrotropin releasing hormone tests are a good indication for radiotherapy even where the GH becomes normal after surgery by common assay methods. Transsphenoidal microsurgery resulted in improved visual acuity and visual fields in all but 1 of the present patients. No death or long-lasting complications have been reported in connection with this approach.

► [This is a reasonable report of the present status of the transsphenoidal surgery for acromegaly. Obviously, as the technical state of the art improves, results for the patients will improve as well. Figure 6 is interesting. Note that about one fourth of the patients (group C) had no significant reduction in GH levels after operation. These are mainly those patients with large adenomas often extending outside the pituitary. Note too, that group B patients showed further improvement after postoperative irradiation. Even with radiation, conclusions cannot be foregone ones. Gryzel (Arch. Intern. Med. 137:808, 1977) reported a patient responsive to external radiotherapy who, after a lapse of a year, had a recurrence of acromegaly, and Pistenma et al. (Int. J. Radiat. Oncol. Biol. Phys. 1:885, 1976) report their experience with megavoltage irradiation. Two patients required pituitary surgery 3 months postradiation because of failing vision. Furthermore, as mentioned in the 1977 YEAR BOOK (p. 24), the pituitary and hypothalamus may be damaged by radiation. An additional study (Shalet et al.: Acta Endocrinol. (Kbh.) 84:673, 1977) showed that radiation damage, as reflected by pituitary hormone deficiencies, is dose related.

Bromocriptine therapy in acromegaly was also discussed in the 1977 YEAR BOOK (p. 43). Subsequent reports give mixed reviews with divergent experiences at Hammersmith Hospital, London, and London Hospital. At the former, Cassar et al. concluded that bromocriptine treatment is "fully effective in only a minority of patients." At the latter, Wass et al. (Br. Med. J. 1:875, 1977) are more sanguine. They say, "bromocriptine offers a major advance in the medical management of acromegaly. . . ." The better results of the latter group may result from a greater total experience and a greater flexibility in amounts of drug given. — T.B.S.] ◄

"Somatostatinoma": Somatostatin-Containing Tumor of Endocrine Pancreas. The precise physiologic role of somatostatin is obscure, though it inhibits insulin and glucagon secretion when it is given exogenously. Om P. Ganda, Gordon C. Weir, J. Stuart Soeldner, Merle A. Legg, William L. Chick, Yogesh C. Patel, Amin M. Ebeid, Kenneth H. Gabbay and Seymour Reichlin[7] (Boston) studied a woman who had a pancreatic tumor containing an extremely high quantity of somatostatin, with no evidence of excessive production of several other hormones.

Woman, 46, presented with excessive urination and thirst and loss of 9 kg over 6 months. The urine contained 4^+ glucose, and a 2-

---

(7) N. Engl. J. Med. 296:963–967, Apr. 28, 1977.

hour postprandial blood glucose measurement was 488 mg/dl. She improved on dietary and tolbutamide and phenformin therapy. Gallbladder disease was diagnosed 7 years later, and a cholecystectomy was performed. A pancreatic mass was seen at operation, and biopsy was consistent with islet cell carcinoma. Insulin was necessary to control hyperglycemia after operation. Hepatic and splenic scintigraphy yielded normal findings, but angiography showed a vascular mass in the pancreaticoduodenal arcade, and a tumor was subsequently resected with the pancreatic head, duodenum, about half the stomach and all the regional nodes. Blood sugar concentrations were 68–108 mg/dl postoperatively without antidiabetes treatment. The patient was asymptomatic 20 months after operation and had no glycosuria or hyperglycemia.

The tumor had a distinctive endocrine morphological appearance, with cells containing particles resembling D granules. The tumor content of immunoreactive somatostatin was 301 ng/mg tissue (table). Tumor cells in culture released somatostatin into the medium. The patient has been euglycemic since resection of the tumor.

With respect to the possible role of somatostatin in pan-

| | HORMONAL CONTENTS OF VARIOUS TYPES OF ISLET TUMOR | | | |
PATIENT	SOMATO-STATIN	IMMUNO-REACTIVE INSULIN	IMMUNO-REACTIVE GLUCAGON	DIAGNOSIS
		ng/mg tissue		
A	0.18	760	12.3	Insulinoma
B	0.57	908	225	Insulinoma
C	0.12	3200	9.4	Insulinoma
D	0.05	9.48	†	Insulinoma
E	0.14	5.28	50.1	Insulinoma
F	0.07	320	*	Insulinoma
G	0.01	*	*	Insulinoma
H	0.005	0.9	120	Glucago-noma
I	†	0.4	100	Glucago-noma
Patient X	301	1.33	.011	Somatostati-noma
Normal pancreas‡	0.18±0.02[7] (rat)	104 ± 46[30] (man)	15.8±3.2[31] (man)	

*Not available.
†Not detectable.
‡Mean ± 1 SEM.

creatic hormone regulation, the most striking feature in this case was the remission of diabetes after removal of the tumor. The remission was probably induced by removal of a source of excessive somatostatin. Patients with diabetes and a "nonfunctioning" islet cell tumor may have a somatostatinoma.

▶ [It was inevitable — so inevitable that this is already the second patient described (see Lancet 1:666, 1977). This growth-inhibiting hormone has "evolved" into a pancreatic hormone, which, when secreted in excess, produces a form of diabetes. Nor is the pervasiveness of somatostatin fully explored. Kronheim (Clin. Endocrinol. (Oxf.) 6:411, 1977) found somatostatin in normal cerebrospinal fluid and Patel et al. (New Engl. J. Med. 296:529, 1977) found elevated somatostatin levels in patients with central nervous system damage.

You should know too that Griffiths et al. (Acta Endocrinol. (Kbh.) 85:1, 1977) suggest that levels of somatostatin (and other hypothalamic hormones) are modulated by the concentrations of peptidases that inactivate them. Finally, in this thumbnail review of what's new, I remind you that somatostatin's broad inhibitory propensities extend to intestinal glucagon-like hormone (J. Clin. Endocrinol. Metab. 44:695, 1977). — T.B.S.] ◀

Prolactin

Prolactin-Like Immunoreactivity: Localization in Nerve Terminals of Rat Hypothalamus. Thyrotropin- and somatostatin-containing nerve terminals have been demonstrated in various parts of the brain, particularly the median eminence of the hypothalamus, and these or closely related peptides may act as transmitters or modulators in the central nervous system (CNS). Kjell Fuxe, Tomas Hökfelt, Peter Eneroth, Jan-Åke Gustafsson and Paul Skett[8] (Stockholm) attempted to determine whether large proteins such as adenohypophyseal hormones can also be stored in nerve terminals in the CNS. The hypothalami of male albino Sprague-Dawley rats were analyzed for prolactin by the indirect immunofluorescence technique. Antibodies to rat prolactin were used in immunohistochemical studies of the hypothalamus and preoptic area.

Networks of varicose, fiber-like structures exhibiting prolactin-like immunoreactivity were observed in the anterior and particularly the posterior periventricular region of the hypothalamus and the preoptic area. Most varicose enlarge-

---

(8)   Science 196:899 – 900, May 20, 1977.

ments were $0.5-1.5$ μ in diameter and exhibited strong immunofluorescence. Networks of beaded fibers of medium density were also seen in the dorsomedial hypothalamic nucleus, arcuate nucleus, ventral hypothalamus, the subependymal and inner layers of the median eminence, the area ventral to the fornix, the premammillary nuclei, the preoptic suprachiasmatic nucleus, the area dorsal to the supraoptic nucleus and the area just dorsal to the roof of the 3d ventricle. Networks of medium density were also observed in the paraventricular rotundocellular thalamic nucleus, the supramammillary commissure and within Forel's field H_2. None of these terminals was observed after the treatment of prolactin antiserum with rat prolactin. The immunoreactive material was still present 1 month after hypophysectomy.

The findings are evidence for the existence of hypothalamic nerve terminals containing a prolactin-like protein. The close proximity of the terminal system to the ventricles makes it likely that part of the prolactin in the cerebrospinal fluid is derived from this neuronal pool of hypothalamic prolactin-like material. The initial data must be interpreted cautiously, since it is not known how other peptides react with the present antiserum.

▶ [So, is prolactin made not only in the pituitary, but in the central nervous system as well? The authors selected prolactin as an example of a large molecule to be sought in the central nervous system because of reports that it was present in normal cerebrospinal fluid. They suggest cerebrospinal fluid (CSF) prolactin may be secreted directly into the ventricles. This may be, but paraventricular prolactin-producing cells are probably not the only source of CSF prolactin. Schroeder et al. (J. Clin. Endocrinol. Metab. 43:1255, 1976) found CSF prolactin levels to be elevated in patients harboring pituitary tumors.

The cautionary note sounded in the last sentence of this article seems justified. Massive molecules like prolactin do not seem likely candidates as central nervous system neurotransmitters. Small molecules like histamine are more promising. Look below. —T.B.S.] ◀

H_1 and H_2 Histamine Receptor Participation in Brain Control of Prolactin Secretion in Lactating Rats. Histamine is present in the central nervous system with high concentration in the hypothalamus and appears to be involved in cerebral function. Histamine injected into the 3d cerebral ventricle increases serum prolactin titers in ovariectomized, estrogen-primed rats. M. C. Arakelian and C.

Libertun[9] (Buenos Aires, Argentina) examined the histaminergic control of prolactin secretion in the lactating rat and the possible involvement of H_1 and H_2 histamine receptors in this process. Prolactin was measured by radioimmunoassay in blood taken from lactating mothers 10 – 15 days after delivery. Test drugs were injected either systemically or intraventricularly just before the onset of suckling and after a basal sample was taken.

Suckling caused a 12- to 18-fold increase in serum prolactin within 10 minutes in saline-injected mothers. Systemic or intraventricular diphenhydramine and mepyramine, H_1 receptor antagonists, suppressed the rise in prolactin in suckled mothers. Intraventricular metiamide, an H_2 receptor antagonist, did not modify prolactin secretion in suckled mothers but markedly increased serum prolactin in nonsuckled mothers. Intraventricular histamine injection caused a small increase in prolactin in nonsuckled mothers. The H_2 agonist 4-methylhistamine was ineffective intraventricularly in nonsuckled mothers but suppressed prolactin enhancement in suckled mothers.

These findings support the view that the site of action of histamine in the central nervous system is on structures close to the 3d ventricle, probably the hypothalamus. It appears that H_1 and H_2 histamine receptors are operative in a neural area close to the 3d ventricle in controlling prolactin secretion. Brain histamine may have a dual control on prolactin secretion in lactating mothers. The H_2 receptors mediate events related to inhibition of prolactin release, whereas H_1 receptors appear related to a facilitatory mechanism.

▶ [For those of us who speak knowingly of H_1 and H_2 receptors but don't really *know,* here are a few facts. There are at least two receptors for histamine, and the tissue response depends on which receptor is filled. The H_1 receptors stimulate smooth muscle contraction and this effect is blocked by the earlier antihistamines. The H_2 receptors, when activated, stimulate gastric secretion and heart rate while inhibiting uterine contraction. The usual antihistamine drugs do not block H_2 receptors, but these have been shown to be blocked by a number of antagonists, including metiamide.

We may now add histamine to the increasingly bewildering array of neurotransmitters and, indeed, histamine receptors occur in other unexpected sites. There is, for instance, evidence (Endocrinology 100:61, 1977) that an H_2 receptor is present in the membranes of thyroid follicular cells and stimulates thyroid hormone secretion.

(9) Endocrinology 100:890–895, March, 1977.

Here we see evidence that both H_1 and H_2 histamine receptors may modulate prolactin secretion and partial confirmation is already upon us. Carlson and Ippoliti (J. Clin. Endocrinol. Metab. 45:367, 1977) obtained the same response using another H_2 receptor antagonist, cimetidine, in men. Again, the number of influences on prolactin secretion is unfairly large for an old school endocrinologist. Doctor Schally (Nobel Prize laureates are congratulated and are referred to henceforth as Doctor) et al. (Endocrinology 100:681, 1977) found that γ-aminobutyric acid (GABA) "can inhibit prolactin release by direct action on the pituitary gland. . . ." and Takahara (J. Clin. Endocrinol. Metab. 44:1014, 1977) found that γ-hydroxybutyric acid, a metabolite of GABA, injected intravenously in man, produces increases in both plasma growth hormone and prolactin. The specificity of the response may be questioned since a huge dose (2½ gm) was given. Evidence that serotonin also plays a role was adduced by Clemens et al. (Endocrinology 100:692, 1977). Finally, don't relax. Rivier et al. (ibid., p. 751) found that neurotensin and substance P also stimulate prolactin secretion. Whew! But, even this is not all, as shown in the following article. — T.B.S.] ◄

Effect of Dexamethasone on Prolactin and TSH Responses to TRH and Metoclopramide in Man. There is considerable evidence that the suppressive effects of glucocorticoids at the hypothalamic-pituitary level are not entirely specific to the adrenocorticotropic axis. James R. Sowers, Harold E. Carlson, Nachman Brautbar and Jerome M. Hershman[1] (Univ. of California, Los Angeles) determined the effects of short-term administration of high doses of glucocorticoids on thyrotropin and prolactin (PRL) secretion and the site of these effects by administering 8 mg dexamethasone daily for 5 days to 9 normal men aged 29–55 years. Subjects were fasted overnight and given 500 μg thyrotropin-releasing hormone (TRH) intravenously before and after dexamethasone administration. Seven normal subjects received 10 mg metoclopramide orally before and after 5 days of dexamethasone administration. Serum PRL was measured by radioimmunoassay and serum thyrotropin by a double-antibody method.

Dexamethasone reduced the mean baseline thyrotropin value and the thyrotropin response to TRH. The mean baseline serum PRL concentration was reduced by dexamethasone, as was the response to TRH. Dexamethasone also reduced the baseline serum triiodothyronine (T_3) concentration and the T_3 response to TRH. Serum PRL responses to metoclopramide are shown in Figure 7. The peak PRL re-

---

(1)   J. Clin. Endocrinol. Metab. 44:237–241, February, 1977.

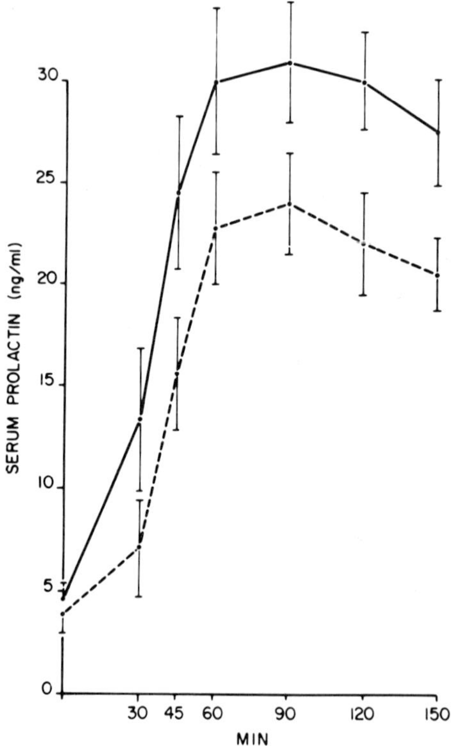

Fig 7.—Mean serum PRL responses to metoclopramide (given at 0 time) in 7 normal men before *(solid curve)* and after *(broken curve)* dexamethasone administration. Vertical bars denote SEM. (Courtesy of Sowers, J. R., et al.: J. Clin. Endocrinol. Metab. 44:237–241, February, 1977.)

sponse to metoclopramide was greater before than after dexamethasone administration.

Short-term, high-dose glucocorticoid administration decreases the baseline serum concentrations of PRL, thyrotropin and T_3 and blunts both the PRL and the thyrotropin responses to TRH in normal men. The decreased T_3 and thyroxine responses to TRH probably result from the inhibitory effect of glucocorticoid on thyrotropin secretion by the pituitary, but a direct inhibitory effect on thyroid release of the hormones cannot be excluded. The findings suggest that pharmacologic doses of glucocorticoids probably suppress both the basal secretion and the stimulated release of PRL at the pituitary level.

▶ [As you can see in Figure 7, metoclopramide, a dopamine antagonist, stimulates prolactin release from the pituitary, and this effect is blunted by dexamethasone administration. Metoclopramide works so well that Delitala et al. (Clin. Endocrinol. (Oxf.) 5:731, 1976) suggest its use as a function test for prolactin response. And, with similar logic, the same authors (Br. Med. J. 1:744, 1977) recommend metergoline, a serotonin antagonist as a potent inhibitor of puerperal lactation.

Thus far, we have cited a total of six distinct types of influences on prolactin secretions. Get set for two more. Intracellular glucopenia, induced by 2-deoxyglucose, (Woolf et al.: J. Clin. Endocrinol. Metab. 45:377, 1977) and monoamine oxidase inhibitors (Slater et al.: Lancet 2:275, 1977) also elevate serum prolactin levels. Whether all these modulators will be shown eventually to work through one or two final common pathways remains problematic. — T.B.S.] ◀

Evidence for a Role of Prolactin in Prostate and Seminal Vesicle Growth in Immature Male Rats. A pituitary factor may be involved in growth and maintenance of the prostate gland, and it has been proposed that prolactin may act synergistically with testicular androgens to bring about growth of the testes and accessory organs. A. Negro-Vilar, W. A. Saad and S. M. McCann[2] (Univ. of Texas, Dallas) attempted to clarify the condition under which prolactin acts on the sex accessory glands. Single anterior pituitary grafts were placed under the renal capsule in male rats, and control animals had grafts of a piece of muscle. Pituitary grafts were from adult female donors. Three weeks after transplantation the animals were killed. Serum prolactin and gonadotropins were measured by radioimmunoassay.

A single anterior pituitary transplant increased the weights of the seminal vesicles and the ventral and dorsal prostate. A small increase in adrenal weight was also noted. Serum prolactin levels rose significantly. The accessories increased significantly in weight in castrated rats given testosterone injections and pituitary transplants. No effect on adrenal weight was apparent. Prostatic weights increased in adrenalectomized animals given transplants, but no change in seminal vesicle weight was seen. Grafted hypophysectomized rats showed an increase in testicular, seminal vesicle and prostate weights. Prolactin levels were high

---

(2)   Endocrinology 100:729–737, March, 1977.

in these animals. Only in the hypophysectomized animals was a significant increase in body weight associated with pituitary grafting.

Prolactin secreted from anterior pituitary grafts stimulates growth of the sex accessory glands in intact, castrated, castrated-adrenalectomized and hypophysectomized rats. The effects are attributed to increased prolactin titers in the grafted rats. Prolactin may act directly at the organ level, by synergizing with circulating androgens or by increasing the output of androgens from the testes and/or adrenals. The findings in castrated-adrenalectomized animals suggest a direct effect of prolactin. Since the prolactin titers observed in grafted animals are within the range often seen in male rats after stress and with cannulation, the experiments further support the possibility that prolactin may play a physiologic role in the growth of the adrenals, testes and male accessory organs.

▶ [The editor promised constant readers that he would continue to provide modifications of the conclusions drawn when he wrote a review of prolactin some years ago (1973 YEAR BOOK, p. 7). In that YEAR BOOK, a possible role of prolactin in males was discussed briefly (p. 15). In this and the following article are confirmatory findings in an area where facts are difficult to come by.

Here we see that prolactin stimulates the prostate gland, a finding supported by earlier evidence. Also, Herbert et al. (Endocrinology 100:487, 1977) found that testosterone administration to rats leads to an increase in serum prolactin levels. What does this mean to the prostate? Presumably testosterone not only stimulates prostatic growth directly but also it conspires with prolactin for the two hormones to act synergistically.

Two corrections of data reported in the 1973 review are in order. First, the report that there are no changes in serum prolactin levels during the menstrual cycle has been refuted (Vekemans: J. Clin. Endocrinol. Metab. 44:989, 1977). The changes reported appear modest but convincing. Second, reports that prolactin has significant effects on water and electrolyte excretion have been challenged (Cary et al.: ibid., p. 850). Rather, these authors conclude that the effects are due to contamination of the hormone preparation with vasopressin. Does prolactin influence the adrenal cortex? Look below. — T.B.S.] ◀

Plasma Androgens in Women with Hyperprolactinemic Amenorrhea. Several androgens are secreted by the adrenal and ovary in women, but dehydroepiandrosterone seems to be secreted almost exclusively by the adrenal cortex. F. Bassi, G. Giusti, L. Borsi, S. Cattaneo, P. Giannotti, G. Forti, M. Pazzagli, C. Vigiani and M. Serio[3]

---

(3)   Clin. Endocrinol. (Oxf.) 6:5 – 10, January, 1977.

(Univ. of Florence) studied the effects of prolactin on the human adrenal cortex in 10 women who had amenorrhea with hyperprolactinemia and 11 who had secondary hypothalamic amenorrhea. None was hypothyroid. Twelve normal women were studied at the 2d day of the menstrual cycle. Nine of the hyperprolactinemic patients had galactorrhea when they were studied.

The findings are summarized in the table. Cortisol values did not differ significantly in the three groups. All patients with amenorrhea and hyperprolactinemia showed a clear increase in plasma dehydroepiandrosterone sulfate (DHAS). Dehydroepiandrosterone (DHA) was significantly increased in patients who had amenorrhea with hyperprolactinemia, but androstenedione and testosterone were comparable in the different groups. Total urinary DHA was significantly increased in hyperprolactinemic patients. Urinary 17-oxo-steroids and 17-hydroxycorticosteroids were comparable in the three groups. A clear decrease in plasma DHAS and a fall in plasma prolactin followed therapy with bromocriptine in all 3 hyperprolactinemic patients so treated.

Plasma DHAS, free DHA and urinary DHA are increased in women who have amenorrhea with hyperprolactinemia,

---

PLASMA CONCENTRATIONS OF PROLACTIN, GONADOTROPINS (LH AND FSH), ESTRADIOL, CORTISOL, DEHYDROEPIANDROSTERONE SULFATE (DHAS), FREE DEHYDROEPIANDROSTERONE (DHA), ANDROSTENEDIONE AND TESTOSTERONE IN NORMAL WOMEN (GROUP 1), WOMEN WITH SECONDARY HYPOTHALAMIC AMENORRHEA (GROUP 2) AND WOMEN AFFECTED BY AMENORRHEA AND HYPERPROLACTINEMIA (GROUP 3) (MEAN ± SEM)

	Group 1	Group 2	Group 3
No. of subjects	12	11	10
Age (years)	33 ± 3.2	28 ± 1.5	30 ± 1.6
Prolactin (μiu/ml)	360 ± 53	436 ± 66	18500 ± 7619†
FSH (ng/ml)	5.0 ± 0.5	2.3 ± 0.18	3.4 ± 0.4
LH (ng/ml)	3.0 ± 0.2	1.4 ± 0.2	2.6 ± 0.4
Oestradiol (ng/dl)	4.8 ± 1.3	2.6 ± 0.7	1.9 ± 0.6
Cortisol (μg/dl)	13.5 ± 1.1	15.6 ± 1.3	15.2 ± 1.4*
DHAS (μg/dl)	169 ± 17	141 ± 15	443 ± 30‡
DHA (ng/dl)	173 ± 27	196 ± 30	472 ± 133†
Androstenedione (ng/dl)	112 ± 12.4	120 ± 15	125 ± 16*
Testosterone (ng/dl)	24 ± 3.5	34 ± 3.3	29 ± 4.1*

*No significant differences among three groups.
†Significantly different from group 1 (P < 0.05) and group 2 (P < 0.05).
‡Significantly different from group 1 (P < 0.001) and group 2 (P < 0.001).

but not in amenorrheic women with normal prolactin levels. The findings strongly suggest that human prolactin can stimulate secretion of some androgens, especially DHAS, by the adrenal cortex. The specific increase in DHAS in hyperprolactinemic amenorrhea may be due to DHAS coming exclusively from the adrenal cortex or to a specific action of prolactin on the synthesis and secretion of steroid sulfates by the adrenal cortex. It may be of value to perform specific adrenal suppression and stimulation tests during plasma androgen studies in hyperprolactinemic amenorrhea.

▶ [This nice study suggests that prolactin can make distinctions that ACTH cannot; prolactin stimulates adrenal androgen but not glucocorticoid secretion. These findings have already been confirmed by Vermulen et al. (J. Clin. Endocrinol. Metab. 44:1222, 1977). These latter workers found increased plasma DHA and DHAS levels in hyperprolactinemic males as well.

I can't move on without cautioning the reader. The "significant" differences in the table between prolactin levels in group 3 and those in groups 2 and 1 are so *by definition*. They *have to be* different; otherwise the separate groups would not exist. — T.B.S.] ◀

Diminished Prolactin Reserve: Case Report. Isolated prolactin deficiency is an uncommon condition, having been described by Turkington in 2 cases. Irving M. Spitz, Heddy Landau, Uri Almaliach, Eli Rosen, Nachman Brautbar and Alex Russell[4] (Jerusalem) report data on a boy who presented with short stature, low basal prolactin levels and minimal prolactin response to dynamic stimuli, who fulfilled criteria for the diagnosis of diminished prolactin reserve.

Boy, 17, of Sephardic Jewish origin, was referred for short stature and delayed puberty. There was no consanguinity, and the parents and all siblings were healthy. Choroiditis had been diagnosed in infancy and toxoplasmosis excluded. Psychomotor development had been normal. The patient was 150 cm high (13 years) and weighed 44 kg (14 years); mild obesity was noted. Severe chorioretinal atrophy was seen in the blind left eye, and mild peripapillary atrophy in the right eye. The penis and testes were prepuberal and there were no signs of pubertal development. Urinary corticoid secretion was normal. The bone age was 10 years. There were no clinical or laboratory features of pseudohypoparathyroidism. The serum thyroxine and T_3 levels were normal.

The results of special investigations are given in the ta-

---

(4)   J. Clin. Endocrinol. Metab. 45:412–418, September, 1977.

Clinical Data

Test procedure	Parameter	Time (min)							
		−15	0	15	30	45	60	90	120
Insulin hypo-glycemia	Glucose (mg/100 ml)	77	76	27	30	46	57	74	82
	GH (ng/ml)	1.6	2.4	1.5	4.1	5.5	5.2	12.0	8.5
	Cortisol (μg/100 ml)		29				61		
	Prolactin (ng/ml)*	2.3	2.8	4.0	5.2	4.2	2.6	2.7	2.8
Arginine infu-sion	GH (ng/ml)		1.6	7.1	5.0	4.2	2.0	2.2	
	Insulin (μU/ml)		3	17	18	8	4	4	
	Prolactin (ng/ml)		5	5	5	5	5	5	
L-dopa	GH (ng/ml)		1.1			1.9	1.5	4.4	
	Prolactin (ng/ml)		5			6	3	3	
Chlorpromazine	Prolactin (ng/ml)	3.0		2.9	2.9	3.0	2.7	2.7	
Synacthen	Cortisol (μg/100 ml)		13				39		

*200 μg TRH administered together with insulin.

ble. The father, also of short stature, had normal hormone responses to LH-releasing factor, TSH-releasing hormone (TRH) and insulin.

Reduced prolactin reserve was documented in this patient. The prolactin deficiency is not absolute. The lesion could reside at or above the level of the hypothalamus, possibly resulting from secretion of prolactin-inhibiting factor or persistent dopaminergic stimulation. Alternately, there could be a deficiency of prolactin-releasing factor. The lesion could also be localized to the lactotrope of the pituitary. The patient has responded dramatically to treatment with chorionic gonadotropin but the prolactin response to TRH has been unchanged.

► [This patient, then, was normally responsive in terms of secretion of LH, FSH, GH, TSH and ACTH, while increases in plasma prolactin concentrations after multiple stimuli, including varying doses of TRH, were negligible.

Was this patient's delayed puberty due to an absence of synergism with testosterone for growth of internal and external genitalia? It's possible. The presence of prolactin is apparently not essential because the patient responded well to treatment with chorionic gonadotropin alone.

It would follow then, that hyperprolactinemia should lead to gonadal hyperresponsiveness. Right? Wrong! Look below. —T.B.S.] ◄

Ovarian Refractoriness to Gonadotropins in Cases of Inappropriate Lactation: Restoration of Ovarian Function with Bromocriptine. Induction of ovulation with clomiphene and human menopausal gonadotropins (hMG) has been successful in patients with ovulatory dysfunction, but not as successful when galactorrhea accompanies the amenorrhea. Hyperprolactinemia is a common feature in most of these patients.

A. M. Mroueh and T. M. Siler-Khodr[5] (American Univ. of Beirut) describe 10 patients with amenorrhea-galactorrhea who failed to respond to repeated courses of hMG, but responded to bromocriptine therapy. Sellar enlargement was suspected in 3 patients. Clomiphene therapy gave no response, except for scanty menstrual flow in 2 patients. Only 4 patients had scant anovulatory bleeding when given hMG and human chorionic gonadotropin.

Bromocriptine, 1.25 mg, was given twice daily. Four patients had nausea and dyspepsia. In 2 patients, treatment was withheld because of severe side effects. Serum hormone levels were determined by radioimmunoassay methods.

The results of bromocriptine therapy are summarized in the table. Galactorrhea ceased after 10–15 days of treatment in 7 of the 8 treated patients and decreased in 1 patient. Ovulation was noted in 7 patients, and 5 conceptions

RESPONSES TO BROMOCRIPTINE IN PATIENTS INSENSITIVE TO HUMAN MENOPAUSAL GONADOTROPIN

No	Suspected Diagnosis	Baseline Values*				During Treatment				Gonadal Effects Days from Start
		PRL	LH	FSH	TSH	PRL	LH	FSH	TSH	
	Pituitary					Pregnant 4th Ovul.				Menses D-41, Next
1	Tumor	450	4.9	9.0	7.6	29	8.7	8.9	4.0	Cycles Ovulatory
	Pituitary									No Bleeding, De-
2	Tumor	505	9.7	13.4	8.0	170	4.7	5.2	3.9	creased Lactation
	Pituitary									
3	Tumor	405	6.0	8.5	7.9	Pregnant 1st Ovul.				Ovulated D-36
	Pituitary									Stopped
4	Tumor	140	10.7	16.5	4.1	Could not tolerate				Medication Day 5
	Pituitary									Stopped
5	Tumor	270	4.2	9.0	7.0	Could not tolerate				Medication Day 5
	Pituitary									
6	Tumor	540	4.5	11.5	–	Pregnant 1st Ovul.				Ovulated D-22
	Pituitary					Pregnant 2nd Ovul.				Menses D-25, Next
7	Tumor	97	2.6	7.0	6.2	55	–	–	5.8	Cycles Ovulatory
	Idio-									Ovulated D-20
8	pathic	–	14.0	8.3	–	146	12.0	7.4	3.5	(Endometriosis)
	Hypo-									
9	thyroid	508	33.0	5.9	42.2	Pregnant 1st Ovul.				Ovulated D-20
	Hypo-									Ovulated D-21
10	thyroid	–	–	–	–	83	10.2	14.0	13.1	Husband Infertile

*PRL = ng/ml; LH-FSH = mIU/ml; TSH = μU/ml.

(5)   J. Clin. Endocrinol. Metab. 43:1398–1401, December, 1976.

occurred. Galactorrhea reappeared in 1 patient in the last trimester of pregnancy. Five normal infants were delivered. A pituitary tumor was confirmed in 1 of the 3 patients in whom sellar enlargement had been suspected. Two patients appeared to have hypothyroidism. During bromocriptine therapy, elevated prolactin (PRL) was reduced in all 8 treated patients, and normal ovarian function returned in 7. One patient had no menstrual bleeding despite a marked decrease in PRL.

Ovarian function may be restored by suppression of elevated PRL levels in most women with amenorrhea and galactorrhea. This suggests that elevated PRL may inhibit normal ovarian function. Since hyperprolactinemia may present without manifest galactorrhea, the possibility of PRL playing a role should be considered in any case of amenorrhea unresponsive to hMG therapy.

▶ [The table tells the tale quite nicely. The mechanism by which hyperprolactinemia inhibits gonadal function is the subject of considerable study and speculation. Van Campenhaut et al. (Am. J. Obstet. Gynecol. 127:723, 1977) looked at the effect of luteinizing hormone-releasing hormone (LH-RH) administration in these patients and found that responses were not uniform and, therefore, not interpretable. Glass et al. (Clin. Endocrinol. (Oxf.) 5:521, 1976) carried out a similar study except that they looked at the response to LH-RH after the patients were treated with estrogen and progesterone. The authors conclude tentatively, "failure of ovulation may be related to a failure of a positive feedback to estrogen. Estrogen negative feedback is unopposed, explaining the follicular development." A different view is taken by Lacherin et al. (J. Clin. Endocrinol. Metab. 44:1163, 1977). They suggest that perhaps the defect lies in the "pituitary lactotrope-hypothalamic dopamine system with aberrations resulting in hypoprolactinemia, acyclic gonadotropin secretion and pituitary microadenoma." A hypothalamic aberration certainly makes most intuitive sense. In a vague way, this conclusion is supported by the findings of van Der Steeg et al. (Lancet 1:502, 1977), who found that bromocriptine, which, as you remember, is a dopamine agonist, is effective in reversing postpill anovulation. —T.B.S.] ◀

Galactorrhea in a 12-Year-Old Boy with a Chromophobe Adenoma. Galactorrhea in males is rare at any age, particularly in prepuberal and adolescent boys. Quentin L. Van Meter, Frank J. Gareis, James W. Hayes (U.S. Naval Regional Med. Center, Oakland, Calif.) and Charles B. Wilson[6] (Univ. of California, San Francisco) describe a boy with galactorrhea and gynecomastia related to a pituitary adenoma.

---

(6)   J. Pediatr. 90:756–759, May, 1977.

Boy, aged 12 years 9 months, had noticed milk leaking from his breasts during exercise for 3 months. He had no other symptoms and was not using medications. Development had been appropriate. The boy had been obese since age 6. There was no family history of endocrinopathy, though all family members were somewhat obese. The boy was 162.5 cm tall and weighed 144.3 kg. He had symmetrically enlarged breasts with 3×3 cm glandular tissue palpable bilaterally. Milky substance flowed from the right nipple with slight pressure and less easily from the left (Fig 8). Growth of pubic hair was sparse. Skull films showed minimal sellar enlargement and asymmetric erosion of the sellar floor. Pneumoencephalography showed an intrasellar tumor, and a chromophobe adenoma was totally resected grossly by the transsphenoid approach.

This patient had elevated prolactin values preoperatively; prolactin was suppressed by L-dopa. Growth hormone and cortisol responses to insulin-induced hypoglycemia were

Fig 8.—Patient exhibiting spontaneous lactation. (Courtesy of Van Meter, Q. L., et al.: J. Pediatr. 90:756–759, May, 1977.)

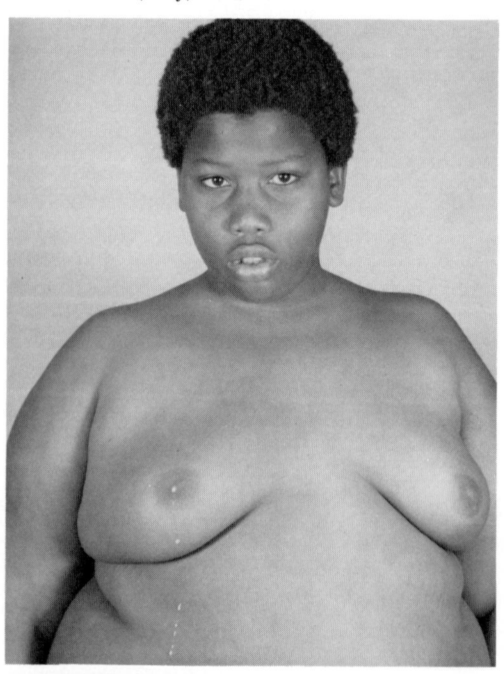

normal. A bolus dose of LH-releasing factor elicited a pubertal response of LH, and thyrotropin-releasing factor produced a physiologic release of thyrotropin. The prolactin level was normal postoperatively. Lactation ceased within a week of removal of the tumor and has not recurred.

Only 5 cases of galactorrhea in pediatric patients have been reported. Galactorrhea in males of any age is an indication for neurosurgical and endocrinologic evaluation once drug ingestion is excluded as a cause.

▶ [It's something of a relief to get back to a single, fairly clear-cut problem, as represented by this unfortunate boy. Figure 8 shows his confused and weary resignation. — T.B.S.] ◀

▶ ↓ Prolactin-producing tumors may be news to pediatricians, but they certainly are no longer to internists, as indicated by the following four articles. — T.B.S. ◀

Galactorrhea: Study of 235 Cases, Including 48 with Pituitary Tumors. David L. Kleinberg, Gordon L. Noel and Andrew G. Frantz[7] (New York) analyzed the records in a series of 235 patients seen in 1969–75 with galactorrhea, about three quarters of all galactorrheic patients presenting in this period. Serum prolactin was measured initially by mouse-breast bioassay and later by radioimmunoassay. Control values were obtained in 51 healthy subjects of each sex. The normal mean was 8 ng/ml for women and 4.7 ng/ml for men, a significant difference. The normal range was defined as 1–25 ng/ml for women and 1–20 ng/ml for men. The mean patient age was 30.9. Serum prolactin levels are shown in Figure 9.

Pituitary tumors were evident in 20% of patients. Most of the affected women were amenorrheic. These patients had the highest serum prolactin levels; the likelihood of pituitary tumor was directly correlated with the serum prolactin. Chlorpromazine did not produce a positive prolactin response in any of the 9 tumor patients studied or in 19 of 36 patients with other types of galactorrhea. Prolactin responses to thyrotropin-releasing hormone (TRH) were markedly blunted in the tumor patients. The L-dopa response was not of major differential diagnostic value. Eight tumor patients had clinical acromegaly, 6 had hypothyroidism and 1 had hypoadrenocorticism. About a third of all patients had idio-

---

(7)   N. Engl. J. Med. 296:589–600, Mar. 17, 1977.

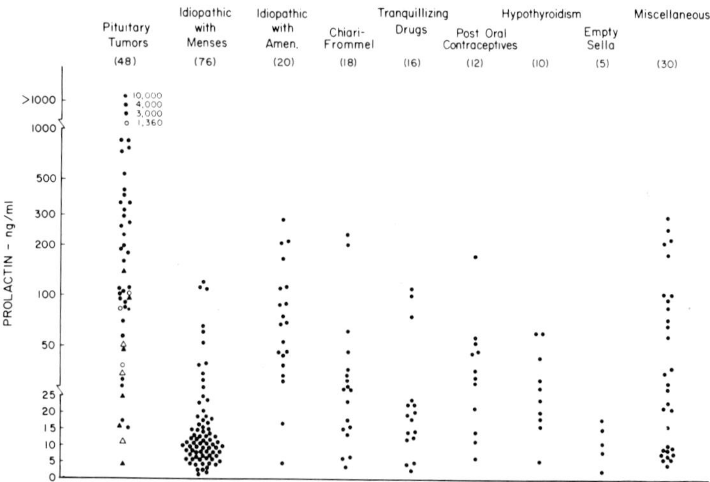

Fig 9.—Plasma prolactin in 235 patients with galactorrhea of varying causes. Among the patients with tumor, patients with acromegaly are denoted by closed triangles. Open circles or triangles denote patients studied only after radiotherapy or operation. (Courtesy of Kleinberg, D. L., et al.: N. Engl. J. Med. 296:589–600, Mar. 17, 1977.)

pathic galactorrhea with menses. The serum prolactin was normal in 65 of these 76 patients. In two thirds of patients, galactorrhea began with parturition and persisted despite the resumption of menses. Twenty patients had idiopathic galactorrhea with amenorrhea. Their mean prolactin was markedly elevated, in contrast to the patients with menses. Eighteen patients had the Chiari-Frommel syndrome, 23 were using oral contraception and 16 had galactorrhea in association with other drugs. Ten patients had primary hypothyroidism and 5 had the empty sella syndrome. Thirteen men, 6 of whom had pituitary tumors, presented with galactorrhea.

Both bromocriptine and lergotrile mesylate are effective in patients with idiopathic galactorrhea and amenorrhea. Lergotrile mesylate has given results in 4 tumor patients that were at least as good as those obtained by operation or radiotherapy.

► [There were 235 patients seen in 6 or 7 years. That's a lot of milk! But, even so, it is just, if you'll pardon the expression, a drop in the bucket. I have before me twelve articles that survived the initial literature survey and became candidate articles (see Introduction to 1977 YEAR BOOK, p. 10); they represent only a *sampling* of what has been published. Sounds like enough for an "instant" symposium," doesn't it? It might be worthwhile, but space does not permit it. Nonetheless, if one adds in the patients of twelve articles, one gets, at least, a rough measure of what is thought of as the "galactorrhea-amenorrhea syndrome." Extracting the pertinent data from each of the articles turns out to be a laborious task because, more often than not, they include cases extraneous to what I (and therefore most of you) want to know.

In the table presented below, an effort was made to exclude all known causes of galactorrhea-amenorrhea or of an elevated serum prolactin other than the "functionless" pituitary tumor. Thus, for example, males, patients with hypothyroidism and patients who had ingested drugs that stimulate prolactin secretion are excluded. What remains then, are females who have one or more of the following: galactorrhea, amenorrhea, elevated serum prolactin level or a pituitary tumor that secretes in excess no hormones other than prolactin. The statistics vary considerably, depending on what is taken as the point of entry. Thus, in this article by Kleinberg et al., the incidence of galactorrhea is 100% because galactorrhea was the basic requirement for inclusion of patients in the study. Similarly, if the presence of a pituitary tumor was the point of entry, results would be skewed appropriately. Disregarding, then, the point of entry, patients in the twelve study samples show the altered percentages seen in the table. The totals for the thirteen studies reveal that about three fourths of the patients with what I call the "GAPP syndrome" (for galactorrhea-amenorrhea-prolactin elevation-pituitary tumor) are likely to present with galactorrhea, amenorrhea and elevated serum prolactin levels. About one-third also harbor pituitary tumors.

Let us go on to review the efficacy of treatment. —T.B.S.] ◄

GAPP SYNDROME

Source	Total	Galactorrhea	Amenorrhea	Elevated Serum Prolactin	Pituitary Tumor
Kleinberg et al.	222	222	121	116	42
% of total		100	54	52	19
Sample	409	275	361	381	184
% of total		67	88	93	45
Sum of cases	631	497	482	497	226
% of total		79	77	79	36

Bromocriptine Therapy in Cases of Amenorrhea-Galactorrhea. Hyperprolactinemia is a common feature in most patients with amenorrhea-galactorrhea, and bromocriptine has been used successfully to suppress prolactin (PRL) in these patients. A. M. Mroueh and T. M. Siler-Khodr[8] (American Univ. of Beirut) reviewed the clinical and

---

(8) Am. J. Obstet. Gynecol. 127:291–298, Feb. 1, 1977.

CLINICAL AND CHEMICAL RESPONSES TO BROMOCRIPTINE IN PATIENTS WITH HYPOTHYROIDISM (GROUP I)

Pt. No.	Age	Amenor-rhea (yr.)	Galactor-rhea (yr.)	Basal value				During bromocryptine				Progesterone (ng./ml.)	Day of cycle	Total therapy (days)	First BBT shift	Comments
				PRL (ng./ml.)	LH (mI.U./ml.)	FSH (mI.U./ml.)	TSH (µU./ml.)	PRL (ng./ml.)	LH (mI.U./ml.)	FSH (mI.U./ml.)	TSH (µU./ml.)					
1	28	6	4	508	3.5	5.4	42.2	Pregnant, first ovulation				—	—	50	20	Delivered normal female
2	28	8	3	49	10.6	2.8	10.4	27	3.5	5.6	1.5	15.5	18	220	64	Currently pregnant
3	26	5	2	290	9.0	4.5	10.5	97	7.8	11.0	6.9	—	30	180	34	Currently pregnant
4	31	7	1	297	14.0	8.3	9.0	146	12.0	7.4	3.5	—	10	90	18	Has endometriosis
5	30	7	2	—	—	—	—	82	10.2	14.0	13.1	3.0	26	153	23	Husband is oligospermic
6	37	3	3	60	22.0	4.9	10.3	—	—	—	—	—	—	50	26	Had tubal ligation

biochemical responses to bromocriptine therapy in 28 patients aged 21–41 years with amenorrhea-galactorrhea. Thirteen patients presented after pregnancy. Eight patients had radiologic sellar enlargement. One patient was receiving a reserpine preparation for hypertension. No patient had evidence of hepatorenal disease or overt thyroid disease. Twenty-one patients wished to become pregnant. Treatment was begun with 2.5 mg bromocriptine twice daily.

Six patients had hypothyroidism (group I); their findings are summarized in the table. Thyroid-stimulating hormone (TSH) was usually normal in patients with pituitary tumors (group II), but PRL values were elevated. Findings were similar in the other 14 patients (group III). Treatment was well tolerated, except in 7 patients with nausea, dyspepsia and vertigo. In all group I women lactation ceased during treatment and they ovulated, and the 3 with no other apparent reproductive dysfunction conceived. In 5 of the 8 group II patients menses returned, and 3 had decreased lactation. Three patients in this group conceived. Most group III patients had a return of normal ovarian function. Lactation stopped after 1–3 weeks of therapy. After treatment was stopped or pregnancy was completed, group I and II patients reverted to their previous amenorrheic-galactorrheic state.

Bromocriptine is an effective, safe treatment for galactorrhea, and it reverses the associated hypogonadism. Where thyroid dysfunction is ruled out and pregnancy is not desired, bromocriptine may be used continuously without escape of PRL secretion. In patients desiring pregnancy, bromocriptine has been a superior means of inducing ovulation, and thereby ameliorating infertility.

► [The uniformly good results of treatment with bromocriptine is quite typical of a multitude of reports that have emerged since bromocriptine became available. Mighty unusual, however, is the finding that nearly a quarter of these patients, those shown in the table, are said to be hypothyroid. This is a considerably higher percentage than that found in other series. The reason for the discrepancy may be found in the authors' statement that the relative frequency of amenorrhea-galactorrhea found in hypothyroidism "demonstrates the sensitivity of TSH levels in defining these conditions, as triiodothyronine and thyroxine determinations were normal in some of these patients." In effect, some of these patients were thought to have what others would call "premyxedema." If so, we should be routinely measuring TSH in patients with GAPP syndrome who appear clinically to be euthyroid. – T.B.S.] ◄

Detection, Evaluation and Treatment of Pituitary Microadenomas in Patients with Galactorrhea and Amenorrhea. During 2½ years, R. Jeffrey Chang, William R. Keye, Jr., John R. Young, Charles B. Wilson and Robert B. Jaffe[9] (Univ. of California, San Francisco) performed transsphenoid microsurgical exploration of the sella in 34 women with galactorrhea or amenorrhea and abnormal sellar polytomograms. Selective removal of adenomas was performed in 25. Six patients had anterior pituitary biopsies when discrete adenomas were not seen. Three patients had cryosurgery when large dural venous sinuses precluded adequate exploration. Eighteen women had microadenomas 1 cm or less in diameter, 7 had macroadenomas and 5 had unidentified lesions. Only 1 had a normal pituitary.

The most common abnormality found at sellar polytomography was unilateral anteroinferior expansion of the sellar floor with cortical bone thinning. Plain films were interpreted as being normal in 11 of 19 cases. The serum prolactin value was elevated in all patients but 1 preoperatively; the mean concentration was 72 ng/ml in this group. Six patients had values below 50 ng/ml. All patients with macroadenomas had elevated levels, and a correlation with tumor size was evident. Baseline serum LH levels were abnormal in 6 patients and FSH levels in 5. The gonadotropin responses to gonadotropin-releasing hormone were not diagnostically contributory. Nine patients had blunted or absent growth hormone responses to insulin-induced hypoglycemia. Three patients had significant postoperative morbidity. Galactorrhea ceased postoperatively in 15 of 17 women with microadenomas and in 4 of 7 with macroadenomas. Menses resumed in all patients but 1 with microadenomas and in 2 of 7 with macroadenomas who presented with amenorrhea.

Sellar polytomography is useful for diagnosis of pituitary adenoma in women with hyperprolactinemia. Transsphenoid microresection of microadenomas is safe and effective. Twenty of 25 patients with adenomas in this series had used oral contraceptives. Further studies are needed to determine the mechanism of amenorrhea in these patients, whether all patients with microadenomas should be treated and what is the optimal therapy.

---

(9)   Am. J. Obstet. Gynecol. 128:356–363, June 15, 1977.

▶ [We have discussed pituitary microsurgery generally (see article by Nielson et al. in this chapter), in patients with acromegaly (see article by Giovanelli et al. in this chapter) and now, in what is emerging as the most common form of pituitary microadenoma, in those with the prolactin-producing variety. Again, it appears that this form of surgery is a highly effecttive form of treatment with little risk to the patient when performed by experienced operators. The question of when to operate remains knotty for those patients whose findings are equivocal, and medical management with continued observation may be the better part of valor. There are, for example, 3 patients already described (Check et al.: Am. J. Obstet. Gynecol. 128:688, 1977; and Bryner and Greenblatt: Obstet. Gynecol. 50: 375, 1977) who presented with the GAPP syndrome along with empty sellas. Do these sellas contain microadenomas, as have been found in a patient with Cushing's syndrome (1977 Year Book, p. 254)?

Another question of particular interest here arises in that four fifths of the patients had used oral contraceptives. Hmm. Estrogens are well-known stimulators of prolactin secretion. Do they also provoke microadenoma formation? — T.B.S.] ◀

Effect of 2-Br-α-Ergocryptin (CB 154) on Serum Prolactin and Clinical Picture in a Case of Progressive Gigantomastia in Pregnancy. Although mammary growth during pregnancy is natural, it is rarely excessive. The condition usually regresses after parturition, but tends to recur in later pregnancies. Attempts at endocrine therapy have failed. S. Kullander[1] (Univ. of Lund) evaluated CB 154, 2-Br-α-ergocryptin, in a patient using antiepileptics who developed gigantomastia during pregnancy. The treatment was based on the presumption that prolactin plays an important role in stimulating breast growth and function in pregnancy.

Woman, 23, with temporal epilepsy diagnosed at age 7 years, had been treated with Phenemal, Mesantoin, Tegretol and Valium. A pregnancy at age 19 had been uneventful, but a neonatal death occurred 2 years later and a spontaneous abortion followed. In the 3d month of a further pregnancy, both breasts were abnormally enlarged; penicillin therapy was unsuccessful and the woman aborted in the 3d month, after which mammary swelling regressed. At 14 weeks of a subsequent pregnancy the left breast in particular was swollen and engorged. Vaginal bleeding occurred at 16 weeks but soon ceased. The urinary human chorionic gonadotropin (hCG) then was 12,000 units/24 hours and the plasma prolactin was 16 ng/ml. At 23 weeks' gestation, the prolactin was 150 ng/ml and the hCG was 3,000 units/24 hours. Increasing breast enlargement was noted at 27 weeks, when the pregnancy test was nega-

---

(1)   Ann. Chir. Gynaecol. 65:227–233, 1976.

tive and clinically the pregnancy appeared to be retarded. Breast pain abated soon after the start of treatment with 2.5 mg CB 154 3 times daily. The dose was gradually reduced and the EEG abnormality decreased. Prolactin levels declined despite progression of the pregnancy. A normal infant was delivered by cesarean section at 36 weeks. Medication was discontinued from the day of delivery. The breasts were much smaller 5 months postpartum, but the patient requested mammaplasty. Severe fibrosis and lymphatic dilatation were observed. The same treatment was effective for breast enlargement recurring in a subsequent pregnancy.

No pathologic increase in plasma prolactin accompanied the extreme mammary growth during pregnancy in this patient. Probably at least the major part of circulating prolactin in the mother is of maternal pituitary origin. The cause of gigantomastia of pregnancy remains obscure but a change in hormonal balance that includes an increase in prolactin and steroids during pregnancy seems responsible for the development and duration of the symptoms.

The following review articles are recommended to the reader:

Cohen, K. L.: Metabolic, endocrine and drug-induced interference with pituitary function tests, Metabolism 26:1165, 1977.

Ettigi, P. G., and Brown, G. M.: Psychoneuroendocrinology of affective disorder: An overview, Am. J. Psychiatry 134:493, 1977.

Goldstein, A.: Opioid peptides (endorphins) in pituitary and brain, Science 193:1081, 1976.

Griffiths, E. C.: Peptidase inactivation of hypothalamic releasing hormones, Horm. Res. 1:179, 1976.

Snyder, S. H.: The brain's own opiates, Chem. Engineering News 55:26, 1977.

Wurfman, R. J. and Moskowitz, M. A.: The pineal organ, New Engl. J. Med. 296:1329, 1977.

The Neurohypophysis

Relationship of Aggregated Intramembranous Particles to Water Permeability in Vasopressin-Treated Toad Urinary Bladder. Freeze-fracture electron microscopy has shown that oxytocin stimulation of the isolated frog bladder induces a structural change in epithelial cell luminal membranes, with aggregation of intramembranous particles at multiple sites on the inner-membrane fracture face. Similar observations have been made in isolated toad bladder after vasopressin stimulation. William A. Kachadorian, Sherman D. Levine, James B. Wade, Vincent A. DiScala and Richard M. Hays[2] investigated the specific role of the vasopressin-induced alterations in membrane structure by inhibiting osmotic water transfer across toad bladder with methohexital; selectively inhibiting urea permeability with phloretin; and determining the extent to which the aggregation response is modified in each case. Studies were done on paired hemibladders from female Dominican toads *(Bufo marinus)*. Radionuclide permeability studies were done with $K_{trans}{}^{14}C$-urea.

Intramembranous particle aggregation is illustrated in Figure 10. Sites of aggregation were fewer in methohexital-treated bladders, and vasopressin-stimulated osmotic water flow was reduced by methohexital. The increase in short-circuit current after vasopressin was the same as in control bladders. The decrease in mean area of aggregates in methohexital-treated bladders was significant. Phloretin reduced vasopressin-stimulated urea movement by over 80% but did not affect hormonally induced osmotic water flow or the number of aggregates per area of granular cell luminal membrane.

The vasopressin-induced structural changes seen in granular cell luminal membranes of toad bladder correlate specifically with changes in osmotic water permeability. Vaso-

(2)   J. Clin. Invest. 59:576–581, March, 1977.

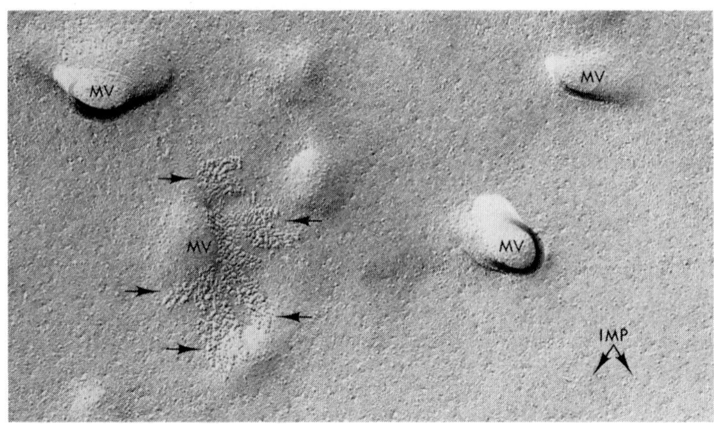

Fig 10.—Vasopressin-induced intramembranous particle aggregation on inner-membrane fracture face of control granular cell luminal membrane. Aggregates *(arrows)* are seen between and near bases of microvilli *(MV)*. Unaggregated intra-membranous particles *(IMP)* appear as small projections, which are randomly distributed; reduced from ×75,000. (Courtesy of Kachadorian, W. A., et al.: J. Clin. Invest. 59:576–581, March, 1977.)

pressin modifies the permeability of toad bladder by a mechanism involving mediation by intracellular cyclic adenosine monophosphate. The intramembranous particles aggregated by vasopressin may be actual sites of water transfer, since the water permeability barrier altered by vasopressin is specifically located in granular cell luminal membranes, and in the case of red blood cell membranes, intramembranous particles apparently can represent sites of water passage.

► [Figure 10 is a "Wow!" (abiding wonder) picture. My fascination with electron photomicrographs is well known to my family, and recently my oldest son and his wife made me a gift of a volume called Magnifications: *Photography with the Scanning Electron Microscope* by David Scharf (New York: Schocken Books, Inc., 1977). Apparently they didn't expect me to consult it very often, because, despite the fact that it contains many superb scanning electron photomicrographs, the salutation reads "To Dad, for the next time you're feeling small. . . ."

Well, the article here lies in an intriguing area that blurs the usually sharp distinctions between structure and function. It is becoming clear that, even for the biologist, Einstein is correct; mass and energy are becoming interchangeable.—T.B.S.] ◄

Physiologic Control of Two Neurophysins in Humans. Alan G. Robinson, Catherine Haluszczak, Julie A.

Wilkins, Alan B. Huellmantel and Charles G. Watson[3] (Univ. of Pittsburgh) examined events thought to be associated with oxytocin or vasopressin secretion because of evidence that neurophysin secretion is associated with hormone secretion.

Nicotine-stimulated neurophysin (NSN) and estrogen-stimulated neurophysin (ESN) were assayed during various physiologic maneuvers and pathologic states in human subjects. Blood was sampled at different times during pregnancy, labor and the postpartum period, and cord blood was sampled from infants. Amniotic fluid was sampled from women having therapeutic abortion at 3–5 months of pregnancy. Blood samples were also obtained from nursing mothers, patients with renal failure or alcoholic cirrhosis and evidence of feminization, patients with hypertension, patients with the syndrome of inappropriate secretion of antidiuretic hormone (ADH) and normal subjects before and after various maneuvers.

The maternal blood ESN was elevated in pregnancy without elevation of NSN. Cord blood and maternal values of ESN were similar, but the NSN value was much greater in cord blood than in maternal blood. The NSN value fell significantly in the first weeks of life. Neither neurophysin blood value was elevated in nursing women. The ESN value was significantly above normal in women using oral contraceptives.

Overnight dehydration did not alter the blood level of either neurophysin in normal subjects; neither was detected after an oral water load. No change in plasma ESN was seen after hypertonic saline infusion, but low levels of NSN were sometimes found. Only NSN was changed with acute volume depletion, and this not consistently. Elevated NSN levels were found during and after surgery.

The NSN level was elevated in 9 of 14 subjects with the inappropriate ADH level and the ESN level in only 2 (table). Both neurophysins were elevated in patients with renal failure, and ESN was significantly elevated in cirrhotic patients; prolonged exercise with water deprivation did not alter the level of either neurophysin.

The data suggest that neurophysins appear to be excreted

---

(3)   J. Clin. Endocrinol. Metab. 44:330–339, February, 1977.

NEUROPHYSIN IN THE INAPPROPRIATE ADH SYNDROME

Patient	Diagnosis	ESN	NSN
239	Head trauma	<0.5	0.9
257	Head trauma	0.5	1.3
998	Head trauma	<0.5	3.3*
258	Lung cancer	1.3	5.9*
301	Lung cancer	0.6	1.4
558	Lung cancer	0.8	10.4*
616	Lung cancer	0.5	3.9*
957	Lung cancer	1.2	5.6*
1126	Lung cancer	3.2*	3.6*
1070	Psychotic IADH	<0.5	1.3
1100	Psychotic IADH	6.4*	4.1*
1256	Tuberculosis	<0.5	<0.5
616	Idiopathic	<0.5	1.8*
1015	Idiopathic	<0.5	3.3*

*Greater than 2 SD from normal.

in the urine and/or catabolized by the kidneys. Secretion of NSN is seen in states in which secretion of vasopressin would be expected, but measurable changes in circulating NSN are seen only with potent stimuli for vasopressin secretion. With regard to ESN and oxytocin: They may be unrelated, related in the hypothalamus but not released together, or always released together. Evidence from anatomical studies support an association of ESN with oxytocin in the human being.

► [Doctor Robinson invented ESN and NSN (1976 YEAR BOOK, p. 49). Here, with his colleagues, he "markets" his invention. Fortunately, most of the present observations make physiologic sense; otherwise it would have been painful for him and for us. It is reassuring, for example, to find that ESN levels are increased in women using oral contraceptives.

Other physiologic relationships are beginning to emerge. It was reported a couple of years ago (ibid., p. 53) that angiotensin stimulates antidiuretic hormone (ADH) release. Malvin et al. (Science 197:171, 1977) find that angiotensin makes up for its water-retaining properties by inhibiting thirst in water-deprived rats, and Baylis and Heath (Lancet 2:248, 1977) suggest that insulin-induced hypoglycemia may provide the basis for a test of posterior pituitary responsiveness because it provokes an increase in plasma ADH. — T.B.S.] ◄

In Vivo Effect of Indomethacin to Potentiate Renal Medullary Cyclic AMP Response to Vasopressin. In vitro studies have indicated that prostaglandin E_1 (PGE_1) blunts the ability of vasopressin to increase water permeability of the distal nephron and impairs the ability of vasopressin to stimulate production of cyclic AMP. Gary M. Lum, Gary A. Aisenbrey, Michael J. Dunn, Tomas Berl, Robert W. Schrier and Keith M. McDonald[4] determined in intact rats whether drugs that block prostaglandin synthesis enhance the medullary cyclic AMP response to vasopressin. Study animals had water diuresis and then received 2 mg indomethacin per kg by slow intravenous injection along with 0.45% saline, or else 200 μU vasopressin. Some animals received vasopressin intravenously 30 minutes after indomethacin injection.

Indomethacin injection did not alter the mean control urinary osmolarity (U_{osm}) significantly and the medullary cyclic AMP content was unchanged. Medullary tissue contained markedly less PGE_1 than did control tissues. Both the U_{osm} and medullary tissue cyclic AMP increased significantly with vasopressin administration. The results of com-

Fig 11.—Comparison of medullary cyclic AMP values and U_{osm} in animals from control group, vasopressin group and indomethacin plus vasopressin group. Cyclic AMP determinations were done on 12 kidneys from 6 rats in each group. (Courtesy of Lum, G. M., et al.: J. Clin. Invest. 59:8–13, January, 1977.)

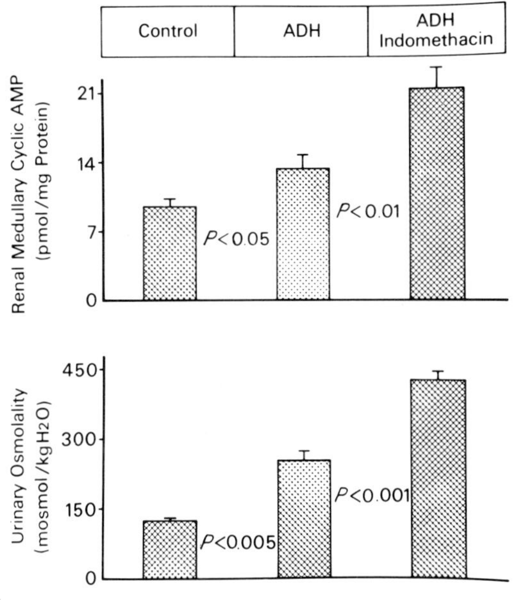

(4)   J. Clin. Invest. 59:8–13, January, 1977.

bined vasopressin-indomethacin therapy are shown in Figure 11. Combined treatment caused a significant rise in arterial pressure, but did not affect the glomerular filtration rate or para-aminohippuric acid clearance. Neither indomethacin nor indomethacin plus vasopressin had any effect on phosphodiesterase (PDE) activity, whereas aminophylline suppressed it to about one third of the control value.

It appears that indomethacin potentiates the in vivo hydro-osmotic effects of vasopressin by potentiating the ability of the hormone to stimulate cyclic AMP production. This effect is associated with suppression of the medullary PGE content, but not with demonstrable suppression of cyclic AMP PDE activity. Suppression of endogenous medullary PGE seems to constitute a pathway whereby indomethacin potentiates the action of vasopressin in vivo. Endogenous renomedullary prostaglandins may be physiologic and pathophysiologic modulators of the hydro-osmotic action of vasopressin.

► [An enlightening study! Figure 11 tells the story. Prostaglandins are becoming omnipresent and omnipotent.

Along the way, you should know of another nice study by Britton et al. (Post grad. Med. J. 53:374, 1977), who measured renal uptake of ^{131}I-labeled antidiuretic hormone (ADH). They found that normal persons and patients with diabetes insipidus have normal uptakes and therefore putative renal receptors for ADH. A patient with nephrogenic diabetes insipidus, on the other hand, did not and has not. — T.B.S.] ◄

Diabetes Insipidus Following Cardiorespiratory Arrest. Because diabetes insipidus may complicate the management of an already critically ill patient, it is important to recognize this potential sequel of hypoxemic encephalopathy. Martin Rothschild and Louis Shenkman[5] (New York Univ.) encountered 2 patients within 6 months in whom diabetes insipidus followed cardiac arrest and hypoxemic encephalopathy.

Case 1. — Woman, 32, was admitted with a 2-day history of cough, pleuritic chest pain and chills and was in moderate respiratory distress. Exophthalmos, diffuse thyromegaly, pretibial myxedema and pulmonary consolidation were evident. Thyroid storm precipitated by pneumococcal pneumonia was diagnosed, and the patient was given methimazole, sodium iodide, hydrocortisone,

---

(5) J.A.M.A. 238:620–621, Aug. 15, 1977.

propranolol, phenobarbital and antibiotics. Ventricular tachycardia and cardiorespiratory arrest occurred several hours after admission, and electric cardioversion was carried out. Diabetes insipidus followed resuscitation, and vasopressin therapy was begun on day 9. Terminal resistance to vasopressin developed, and the patient died after episodes of refractory hypotension, ventricular fibrillation and asystole.

CASE 2.—Woman, 30, with a history of poliomyelitis and pneumonectomy after recurrent aspiration pneumonias associated with surgery for bronchoesophageal fistula, had cardiorespiratory arrest after bronchoscopic cautery of the fistula. Hypothermia and diabetes insipidus developed, 3 days after resuscitation, which required cardiac massage, mechanical ventilation and vasopressors. The patient died after refractory hypotension and oliguria developed.

These patients exhibited features of diabetes insipidus within 3 days of cardiopulmonary arrest and hypoxemic encephalopathy. Both responded promptly to exogenous antidiuretic hormone. Both were comatose and required ventilatory assistance via tracheal tube when polyuria began. The hypothalamic injury was probably secondary to the hypoxemic encephalopathy and presumably reflected widespread neurologic damage. This disorder may be overlooked in critically ill patients who have several medical problems. It should be considered in any comatose patient in whom polyuria follows cardiorespiratory arrest.

▶ [Two points should be mentioned. (1) The associations of hypoxic shock and diabetes insipidus has been noted before (1976 YEAR BOOK, p. 57) in a reference to "nonpuerperal Sheehan's syndrome." (2) Have a care. We've seen twice in the past year what could be called "iatrogenic pseudodiabetes insipidus." These patients were monitored for shock with the use of central venous pressure measurements. Copious fluid administration was considered necessary and the patients obliged by increasing greatly their urinary volumes. The syndrome was transitory, and the patients recovering after the central venous line was removed. In one instance, we effected a "cure" by substituting serum albumin for isotonic saline and glucose solutions.—T.B.S.] ◀

Selective Osmoreceptor Dysfunction in Syndrome of Chronic Hypernatremia. An association of intracranial lesions of diverse etiology with impaired water regulation leading to chronic hyperosmolality of body fluids has been recognized. Patients often have extensive hypothalamic lesions with associated anterior pituitary dysfunction. Renal function is normal and clinical hypovolemia is absent. Jeffrey B. Halter, Andrew P. Goldberg, Gary L. Robertson and

Daniel Porte, Jr.[6] measured plasma arginine vasopressin (AVP) levels by a sensitive radioimmunoassay, in a patient with chronic hypernatremia and hypodipsia due to an iatrogenic lesion in the hypothalamic area, after independent stimulation of both osmoreceptor and baroreceptor mechanisms for AVP release.

Man, 46, was admitted with agitation, confusion, weakness and hallucinations that had been present for 1 week. Head trauma had been incurred twice, 18 and 3 years before admission. A carotid-cavernous sinus fistula had been treated surgically on the latter occasion by clipping of the left internal carotid artery at the level of the optic chiasm, embolization of muscle through the internal carotid and ligation of the left common and internal carotid arteries in the neck. Memory dysfunction and a fall in IQ were documented postoperatively. Laboratory data are given in the table. Myoglobin was present in the urine. The patient responded well to rehydration, though transient acute renal failure occurred. Thirst was not reported despite persistent plasma hyperosmolality. Trials of clofibrate and chlorpropamide therapy were unsuccessful.

Resting plasma AVP concentrations were inappropriately low for the degree of plasma hyperosmolality present (less than 0.5–2.1 pg/ml at over 300 mOsm/kg). Anterior pituitary function was normal on standard testing. Trimethaphan stimulation indicated adequate neurohypophyseal stores of AVP. Some residual osmotic regulation of AVP release was suggested by acute water-loading studies and hypertonic saline infusion. The osmotic threshold for AVP release was not above normal.

SERIAL LABORATORY DATA

	6/30/74	7/6	7/25	8/28	12/2	3/4/75
Weight (kgm)	72.3	78.6	—	—	84.0	84.7
Hematocrit (%)	50	32.8	31.4	35.5	41.4	42.2
Na (mEq/1)	184	145	156*	139	163*	155
SUN (mg/100 ml)	58	75	17	17	23	18
Creatinine (mg/100 ml)	3.5	6.9	1.9	1.2	1.3	1.7
Glucose (mg/100 ml)	170	155	119	103	104	110
Triglyceride (mg/100 ml)	—	—	630	220	288	314
Cholesterol (mg/100 ml)	—	—	200	209	196	221
Urine volume (ml/24 h)	750	3,500	3,000	1,150	800	950
24 h creatinine clearance (cc/min)	13	9	—	50	100	110
Urine osmolality (m osmol/kgm)	497	329	311*	369	934*	667

*After water deprivation for 15 hours.

(6)   J. Clin. Endocrinol. Metab. 44:609–616, April, 1977.

Presumably afferent input from the osmoreceptor-thirst area of the hypothalamus is selectively impaired in this patient. The findings demonstrate a dissociation of osmoreceptor function from the AVP secretory apparatus in man. The findings in other patients with the hypernatremia syndrome can be explained by a similar lesion, with clinical severity being related to the degree of reduced osmoreceptor input.

▶ [Okay. In this patient osmolality rises but the damaged osmoreceptor is not tripped off. Neither AVP release nor thirst is stimulated and the hypernatremia become established. Arginine vasopressin release is effected by induced hypotension; the effector limb is intact. A nice dissection!

Presumably, cigarette smoking would have served as well as the trimethaphan-induced hypotension, since Hayward and Pavasuthipaisit (Neuroendocrinology 21:120, 1976) demonstrated a striking elevation of plasma AVP after nicotine infusion in monkeys. — T.B.S.] ◀

Syndrome of Inappropriate Antidiuretic Hormone Secretion in Neonates with Pneumothorax or Atelectasis. Charles L. Paxson, Jr., Joan W. Stoerner, Susan E. Denson, Eugene W. Adcock III and Frank H. Morriss, Jr.[7] (Houston) describe the occurrence of nine episodes of the syndrome of inappropriate antidiuretic hormone (SIADH) secretion in 5 neonatal patients after pneumothorax or lobar atelectasis of the lung, two relatively common complications of modern respiratory disease management. The episodes were characterized by hyponatremia with serum hypo-osmolality, a urine osmolality greater than that of serum, the absence of volume depletion and dehydration, continued natriuresis and apparently normal renal and adrenal function. The findings in the 5 adequately documented cases are summarized in the table. Each patient was appropriately grown for gestational age. The patients were among 209 neonates with lung disease and 79 who required ventilatory assistance. Of the 209, 7 neonates had at least one episode of acute lobar atelectasis. Twenty-seven others had at least one episode of a form of air block, most often pneumothorax.

Each episode of SIADH followed an acute loss of lung volume, the result of either pneumothorax or lobar atelectasis. The occurrence of SIADH was significantly associated with pneumothorax, atelectasis and positive-pressure ventilation. Hypoxemia was not associated with SIADH. Hypona-

---

(7) J. Pediatr. 91:459–463, September, 1977.

CLINICAL FEATURES OF FIVE NEONATES WHO HAD EVIDENCE OF SIADH

Patient No.	Sex	Birth weight (gm)	Gestational age (wk)	Apgar scores (1 min/ 5 min)	Diagnoses	Apparent triggering event	Postnatal age at onset of SIADH (days)	Interval between triggering event and SIADH diagnosis (hr)	Duration of SIADH (days)	Outcome
1	M	980	28	7/8	IRDS*	Left pneumothoraces and shifting atelectasis	20	4	3	Died at age 61 days
							26	4	2	
							30	14	3	
							36	6	4	
							42	40	3	
2	M	1,340	31	7/8	IRDS	Left pneumothorax	19	12	1.5	Died at age 28 days
3	F	1,503	33	1/6	IRDS	Right upper, middle and lower lobar atelectasis	20	6	3.5	Survived
4	M	3,010	40	0/7	Pneu- monia	Right lower lobar atelec- tasis	3	22	4.2	Survived
5	M	1,820	32	7/8	IRDS; hydro- ceph- alus	Right pneumothorax	21	13	4.0	Survived
Mean (±SEM)		1,730 (±347)	32.8 (±2.0)				24.1 (±3.8)	13.4 (±3.9)	3.1 (±0.3)	

*Idiopathic respiratory distress syndrome.

tremia and serum hypo-osmolality occurred a mean of 13.4 hours after the triggering event and resolved in 1½–4 days with fluid restriction therapy and removal of the triggering event. Urine production was less in the first 24 hours of the episodes than before the triggering event. The SIADH was documented after 4 of 28 (14%) episodes of pneumothorax and after 5 of 16 (31%) episodes of lobar atelectasis.

This series included preterm infants; all were ventilated mechanically. The high incidence of SIADH after pneumothorax and atelectasis warrants close attention to fluid and electrolyte balance in susceptible neonates. Administration of a water load via the respiratory route should be avoided. If dilutional hyponatremia develops, water restriction rather than sodium infusion is the preferred treatment.

► [Other causes of lung volume loss or increased pulmonary pressure (Boyle's law still lives!) include consolidation from pneumonia, tuberculosis or cystic fibrosis (Cohen et al.: J. Pediatr. 90:574, 1977) and positive-pressure ventilation (1973 YEAR BOOK, p. 89).

It's bibliographic listing time again. The finding of SIADH has been documented after repair of a patent duct arteriosus (Weinberg et al.: J. Pediatr. 90:111, 1977), the ingestion of 50 chlorpropamide tablets (Piters: J. Clin. Endocrinol. Metab. 43:1065, 1976) and in patients with bacterial meningitis (Feigin and Kaplan: Am. J. Clin. Nutr. 30:1482, 1977) and Rocky

continued exposure of the metabolites to these enzyme systems results in the formation of other, less-iodinated metabolites, such as $3,3'T_2$, and studies have suggested that $3,3'T_2$ may have an extremely high metabolic clearance rate relative to the other iodothyronines. Kenneth D. Burman, Daniel Strum, Richard C. Dimond, Yin-Ying Djuh, Frances D. Wright, Jerry M. Earll and Leonard Wartofsky[9] (Walter Reed Army Med. Center, Washington, D. C.) devised a specific radioimmunoassay for $3,3'T_2$, which may be performed on unextracted serum.

A specific antiserum to $3,3'T_2$-bovine serum albumin conjugates was produced in rabbits. Cross-reactivity was less than 0.5% with T_3 and reverse T_3 and less than 0.01% with T_4. Intra-assay variation averaged 2.9%, and inter-assay variations were 7.8% and 18.5%, respectively, when serums with $3.3'T_2$ concentrations of 8 and 12 ng/dl were used. Assay sensitivity was considered to be 6 ng/dl by statistical criteria. Comparable values were obtained in unextracted samples with 8-anilino-1-naphthalene sulfonic acid used to inhibit $3,3'T_2$ binding to serum proteins and with samples extracted with ethanol before analysis. Exposure of serums to acid hydrolysis did not alter measured values of $3,3'T_2$. The mean serum $3,3'T_2$ concentration in 18 euthyroid subjects was 17 ± 1, ng/dl. Thyrotoxic patients generally had elevated values, whereas hypothyroid patients tended to have reduced concentrations. Eight normal thyroids had a mean tissue concentration of 0.4 μg/gm. Thyrotropin-releasing hormone (TRH) evoked no rise in serum $3,3'T_2$ in euthyroid subjects, but the values increased in 2 sheep given TRH.

The findings suggest that $3,3'T_2$ circulates in the serum of normal subjects and tends to parallel serum concentrations of T_4, T_3 and reverse T_3 in various states of thyroid function.

▶ [Another of the circulating, inactive thyroid hormone metabolites is discussed here. Burger and Sakoloff (J. Clin. Endocrinol. Metab. 45:384, 1977) have explored the behavior of T_2 further. They found it to rise in hypothyroid patients treated with T_3 and in euthyroid subjects treated with reverse T_3, thus supporting the idea that T_2 is a metabolite of these two substances. Old people have low T_2 values. – T.B.S.] ◀

Radioimmunoassay of Thyrotropin-Releasing Hormone in Human Serum and Its Clinical Application. Terunori Mitsuma, Yoshibumi Hirooka and Noriyuki

(9) J. Clin. Endocrinol. Metab. 45:339–352, August, 1977.

Nihei[1] (Nagoya Univ.) devised a thyrotropin-releasing hormone (TRH) radioimmunoassay system with a suitable inhibitor to prevent inactivation of TRH immunoreactivity by serum and evaluated it in patients with hypothalamic-pituitary-thyroid disorders. Inactivation of TRH immunoreactivity by serum was prevented by a mixture of 8 hydroxyquinoline sulfate and Tween 20; this persisted for a long period and did not affect TRH values. The TRH was extracted from serum with methanol. A tracer dose of ^{125}I-TRH was added to serum before the addition of activated charcoal.

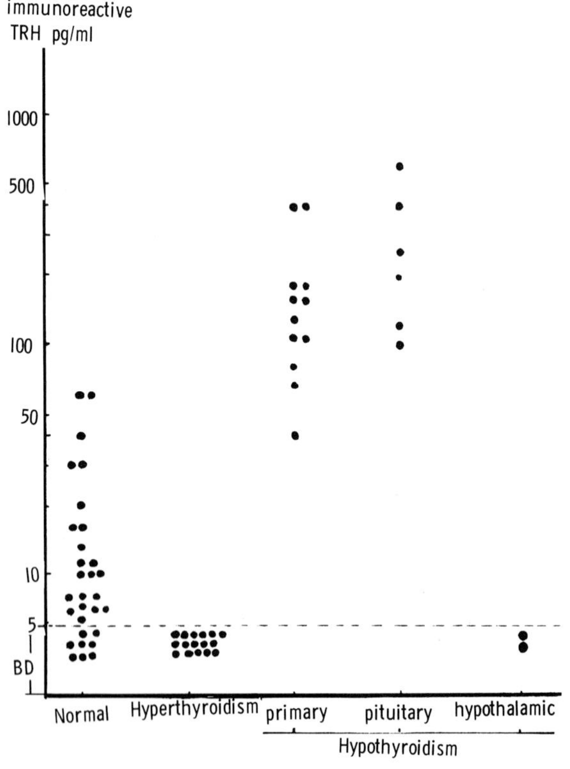

Fig 12.—Immunoreactive TRH concentrations in serum in various thyroid disorders. *BD*, serum concentrations of TRH below limit of detectability. (Courtesy of Mitsuma, T., et al.: Acta Endocrinol. (Kbh.) 83:225–235, October, 1976.)

(1)   Acta Endocrinol. (Kbh.) 83:225–235, October, 1976.

Studies were done in 30 normal subjects, 16 patients with hyperthyroidism, 12 with primary hypothyroidism, 6 with pituitary hypothyroidism and 2 with hypothalamic hypothyroidism.

Results of recovery studies, intra-assay reproducibility and interassay variation were quite satisfactory. The lowest detectable amount of TRH was 5 pg/ml. Immunoreactive TRH levels in serum were below 60 pg/ml in normal subjects, below the limit of detectability in hyperthyroid patients and 40–400 pg/ml in patients with primary hypothyroidism (Fig 12). Concentrations up to 600 pg/ml were found in pituitary hypothyroid patients, whereas hypothalamic hypothyroid patients had no detectable serum TRH. In primary hypothyroidism, TRH values fell to normal during thyroxine substitution. Most patients with hyperthyroidism had a rise to 5 pg/ml or above during antithyroid drug therapy, but a few continued to have undetectable amounts despite normal thyroid hormone values.

This assay system appears to be useful for study of the role of TRH in the hypothalamic-pituitary-thyroid axis in various clinical states.

► [My first reaction is that this is too good to be true. Everything falls so neatly into place. I am too suspicious, I guess. The authors apparently have solved the serious problem of TRH degradation by serum peptidases. Indeed, even the peptidase levels may vary physiologically. Kanigge et al. (Acta Endocrinol. (Kbh.) 83:449, 1976) show that hypophyseal portal plasma inactivates TRH at a much slower rate than does peripheral plasma, a nice protective effect.

Thyrotropin-releasing hormone is being used more and more frequently in the clinical arena, although it has been my view that it has been abused as a diagnostic test of things like hyperthyroidism. Dr. Jerome Hirschman's group (J. Clin. Endocrinol. Metab. 43:741, 1976; and ibid., p. 856) has examined a methylated TRH that is significantly more potent and long-lasting in its actions than is the naturally occurring hormone, and Berthezene et al. (Biomedicine 24:259, 1976) have found that several weeks of TRH administration can lead to the reemergence of TSH in patients in whom the hypothalamus and pituitary had long been inhibited by high ambient serum T_4 levels. —T.B.S.] ◄

Serum Thyroid Hormone and TSH Concentrations in Newborn Infants with Congenital Absence of Thyroxine-Binding Globulin. Familial absence of circulating thyroxine-binding globulin (TBG) is a well-known entity, J. H. Dussault, J. Letarte, H. Guyda and C. Laberge[2] (Laval

---

(2) J. Pediatr. 90:264–265, February, 1977.

SERUM TBG, T_4, T_3, R_{T_3} AND TSH* IN 10 INFANTS WITH
CONGENITAL HYPO-TBG-EMIA

	TBG	T_4	T_3	R_{T_3}	*TSH*
Mean	0.62	3.2	77	24.2	7.2
SEM	0.13	0.5	9	5.5	2.3

*Normal values 4–8 weeks: TBG 2–4 mg/dl; T_4 6–14 μg/dl; T_3 70–220 ng/dl; R_{T_3} 10–60 ng/dl; TSH < 20 μU/ml.

Univ.) measured filter paper spot thyroxine T_4 in 140,000 newborns and found 10 with absent TBG or hypo-TBG-emia. The incidence in Quebec province was 1 in 14,000 births. Nine of the infants were boys. The mean T_4 concentration in eluates of filter paper blood was similar to that found in hypothyroid infants (0.36 versus 0.39 ng/40 μl eluted blood). The mean filter paper spot thyrotropin (TSH) concentration was normal, in contrast to that of the hypothyroid infants. The mean serum TBG concentration was 0.62 mg/dl (table). The mean serum T_4 concentration, though subnormal, was higher than that in hypothyroid infants, and the mean serum triiodothyronine (T_3) concentration was also higher. The mean serum reverse T_3 (RT_3) concentration was lower than in normal neonates but similar to that in hypothyroid infants. The mean serum TSH concentration was 7.2 μU/ml.

Hypo-TBG-emia is a relatively frequent entity that can be detected through a screening program for neonatal hypothyroidism. The family should be alerted to the abnormality, since the low serum T_4 concentration characteristic of the condition might mislead a physician into diagnosing hypothyroidism.

▶ [I agree with the last statement in this article, but one should be careful not to mislead physicians into believing that absence of TBG is always innocuous. Barragry and Burr (Br. Med. J. 2:742, 1977) describe 2 siblings with growth retardation along with familial TBG deficiency. The authors are careful to point out that there is no good evidence that the TBG deficiency itself directly causes the retardation. And, from the same laboratory (Burr et al.: ibid. 1:485, 1977) comes a report that at high concentrations of TBG the true serum free T_4 is lower than one would calculate from a free thyroxine index. — T.B.S.] ◀

Extrathyroidal Conversion of Thyroxine to 3,3′, 5′-Triiodothyronine (Reverse T_3) and to 3,5,3′-Triiodothyronine (T_3) in Humans. L. Gavin, J. Castle, F. McMahon,

P. Martin, M. Hammond and R. R. Cavalieri[3] (Univ. of California, San Francisco) studied turnover rates of T_3 and reverse in T_3 (rT_3) adults with intact thyroids and hypothyroid patients on replacement doses of L-thyroxine to assess the relative contributions of thyroidal secretion and peripheral deiodination of thyroxine in the production of rT_3. Studies were done in 6 men without endocrine or hepatic dysfunction and in 4 males and 1 female who had received L-thyroxine for at least 2 years for clearly established hypothyroidism, either spontaneous or after thyroidectomy. The mean daily dosage of L-thyroxine was 0.19 mg. Studies were done with ^{131}I-labeled T_3 and ^{125}I-labeled thyroxine and rT_3. Serum T_3 and rT_3 were determined by radioimmunoassays. Metabolic clearance rates (MCRs) were computed by a noncompartmental method of analysis from the plasma disappearance of ^{125}I-rT_3 and ^{131}I-T_3 for 72 hours after simultaneous injection of the tracers.

The MCR of rT_3 averaged 97.1 L per day in hypothyroid subjects and the production rate, 34.3 μg per day. The respective figures for T_3 were 28.7 and 20.3, corrected to 70 kg body weight. The values were not significantly different from those in the control group. The proportions of total T_3 production accounted for by rT_3 averaged 62% in hypothyroid patients and 57% in the control group.

The findings in hypothyroid subjects indicate that production of rT_3 is a major route of thyroxine metabolism, equal to or exceeding that of T_3. Most if not all of the rT_3 produced in normal human beings is derived by extrathyroidal conversion from thyroxine. Production rates of T_3 and rT_3 are being studied in patients with thyroidal and nonthyroidal systemic illnesses.

▶ [This is a good study because it demonstrates more directly what everybody has been saying the past few years, namely that much of T_3 and most of rT_3 is produced by the deiodination of T_4 in tissues outside the thyroid gland. Chopra (Endocrinology 101:453, 1977) who has done much to open this field, studied the conversion of T_4 to T_3 in vitro using liver and kidney homogenates. Interestingly, rT_3 turns out to be "a very potent inhibitor of conversion of T_4 to T_3." Fishman et al. (ibid. 100:1055, 1977) studied the changes in liver T_3 aminotransferase activity with changes in thyroid function. Hypothyroid rats had low levels and these were raised to above normal with supraphysiologic doses of T_3. Interestingly, rT_3 was about as active as T_3 itself in enzyme induction. The biologic role of the

<hr>

(3) J. Clin. Endocrinol. Metab. 44:733–742, April, 1977.

enzyme itself is uncertain. It may be involved in the degradation of thyroid hormones. Herman et al. (J. Clin. Endocrinol. Metab. 44:660, 1977) looked at states which, predictably, would provoke changes in serum rT_3 levels. The responses in hypothyroid, hyperthyroid individuals and after TRH administration were, indeed, what you might expect, except that the increase in rT_3 after TRH was statistically significant but biologically very meager indeed. Ratcliffe et al. (Clin. Endocrinol. (Oxf.) 5:631, 1976) and Griffiths et al. (ibid., p. 679) both found more of the same. Finally, and the popularity of this entire subject is becoming inversely proportional to my patience, Westgren (Acta Endocrinol. (Kbh.) 84:281, 1977), among others, showed that levels of not only T_4 and T_3, but rT_3 as well, are higher in thyroid venous blood than in mixed venous blood. Thus, serum rT_3 is secreted by the thyroid, but mostly is converted from T_4 in the periphery and has very slight thyroid hormonal action. What does this mean at the bedside? Look below. — T.B.S.] ◄

Changes of Circulating Thyroxine, Triiodothyronine and Reverse Triiodothyronine after Radiographic Contrast Agents. It has been assumed that thyroid hormone secretion remains constant despite wide fluctuations in iodine supply, but recently thyrotoxicosis has been reported after radiographic contrast mediums. Hans Bürgi, Claus Wimpfheimer, Albert Burger, Wolfgang Zaunbauer, Helmut Rösler and Thérèse Lemarchand-Béraud[4], at three university centers in Switzerland, analyzed thyroid function prospectively after performance of three common radiographic studies involving iodinated substances.

The subjects were 58 patients, 28 of whom had euthyroid goiter. The studies were intravenous urography with diatrizoic acid, intravenous cholangiography with ioglycamic acid and oral cholecystography with sodium iopanoate. Four women with severe idiopathic myxedema and 4 healthy men were given sodium iopanoate, 2 gm.

Nonhormonal iodine remained elevated at 12 μg/100 ml 6 weeks after intravenous cholangiography.

After oral cholecystography, the serum thyroxine (T_4) rose significantly in 3–7 days in patients with and without goiter. The serum triiodothyronine (T_3) usually decreased within 3–7 days and rose again after 2 weeks. A rise in reverse T_3 was seen in patients who had had clear decreases in T_3 after oral cholecystography (table). Thyrotropin consistently increased.

After intravenous cholangiography, the serum T_4 in-

---

(4)   J. Clin. Endocrinol. Metab. 43:1203–1210, December, 1976.

Mean and Standard Error for T_3, Reverse T_3 and TSH
in Serum after Cholecystography with Na-Iopanoate

	T_3 (RIA) ng/100 ml (N = 7)	Reverse T_3 (RIA) ng/100 ml (N = 7)	TSH μU/ml (N = 9)
Day 0	194.0 ± 12.8	57.0 ± 7.8	5.5 ± 0.8
Day 3	142.6 ± 9.1***	121.0 ± 15.0***	12.2 ± 2.1**
Day 7	156.6 ± 17.9*	97.7 ± 12.5*	—

Asterisks give results of t tests for paired samples between day 0 and days 3 and 7: * = P < 0.02; ** = P < 0.01; *** = P < 0.005. Due to limited availability of serum, tests could not be done in all 22 study subjects.

---

creased slightly and the T_3 decreased; the response was highly variable between patients.

In hypothyroid patients on replacement therapy who were clinically euthyroid, sodium iopanoate produced a marked rise in thyrotropin, a significant fall in T_3 by radioimmunoassay and a rise in reverse T_3.

In normal subjects given L-thyroxine, sodium iopanoate produced a fall in serum T_3 and a rise in reverse T_3. Serum T_4 did not change significantly.

Cholecystography consistently produces changes in circulating thyroid hormones. It is not clear whether the fall in serum T_3 is due to decreased production or enhanced degradation of this hormone. A longer study is needed to assess the risk of hyperthyroidism occurring after use of radiographic contrast agents.

► [In the 1977 YEAR BOOK (pp. 116–122) an "instant symposium" delineating influences on the preferential conversion of peripheral T_4 to T_3 or rT_3 was presented.

Here we see an additional factor channeling T_4 to rT_3 rather than to T_3 itself. The increase in serum TSH shown in the table is presumably a compensatory response to the reduction in serum T_3.

The abiding notion is that the switch occurs to better the chances of survival in the face of stresses of various kinds, like inanition anorexia nervosa, old age, recent birth, acute illness and chronic illness. Some more specific examples have recently emerged. The same pattern holds in acute myocardial infarction (Westgren et al.: Acta Med. Scand. 201:269, 1977) and in malaria patients (Wartofsky: J. Clin. Endocrinol. Metab. 44: 85, 1977), as well as in severe chronic illness (Carter et al.: Clin. Endocrinol. (Oxf.) 5:587, 1976) and after surgery (Grant et al.: Lancet 2:1333, 1976).

In the 1977 YEAR BOOK (p. 120) it was shown that dexamethasone led to this kind of reversal and this glucocorticoid effect would make sense in terms of all the stresses enumerated. But there is more. The same reversal occurs with propylthiouracil administration (Westgren: Acta Endocrinol. (Kbh.) 85:345, 1977). Thus the diversion of T_4 to rT_3 rather than to T_3 can account in part for the salutary effect of propylthiouracil in hyperthyroidism. The same thing is found after propranolol therapy (Lotti: Clin. Endocrinol. (Oxf.) 6:405, 1977) although rT_3 was not specifically measured. Well, enough about the nonspecific factors that lower T_3! What raises it? Look ahead. — T.B.S.] ◄

Increase of Plasma Triiodothyronine Concentration in Man in a Cold Environment. There is much evidence of the important role of thyroid hormone in thermogenesis. The people of Kijimadaira, Nagano Prefecture, Japan, live in a cold environment for at least 5 months in winter without using adequate heating but enjoy a good temperature in summer. Hajime Nagata, Tomio Izumiyama, Kazuo Kamata, Shiro Kono, Yaichiro Yukimura, Masato Tawata, Toru Aizawa and Takashi Yamada[5] (Shinshu Univ.) assessed adaptive changes in endocrine function to cold in this population and also studied persons who worked for 3 hours in a cold environment culturing mushrooms and others working in air-conditioned rooms. The chronic effects of cold were assessed in 56 healthy men aged 20 – 44 who lived in Kijimadaira, both in the summer and the winter, when interior temperatures were 15 – 20 C and − 3 – 6 C, respectively.

Exposure to cold at 4 – 6 C for 3 hours did not alter the plasma T_3 level. Study subjects had slightly higher plasma T_4 levels in the summer as well as in the winter but the differences were not significant. Plasma T_3 levels rose significantly in the winter (table). Plasma TSH levels were comparable in study subjects and controls working in air-conditioned rooms. Acute exposure to cold did not affect the plasma TSH level. Even in winter, TSH was undetectable in 12% of the study population. Study subjects had comparable plasma cortisol levels in the summer and winter and the levels were similar to those of control subjects.

Despite marked seasonal variations in environmental temperature, these subjects showed no significant increase in plasma TSH levels in winter. No appreciable increase in plasma T_4 content was found, even after prolonged exposure to cold in winter. The precise nature of the role of the adre-

---

(5)　J. Clin. Endocrinol. Metab. 43:1153–1156, November, 1976.

PLASMA T_3, T_4 AND TSH CONCENTRATIONS IN CONTROLS AND
SUBJECTS EXPOSED TO COLD FOR SHORT OR PROLONGED TIME PERIODS

Group	T_3 concentration ng/100ml	T_4 concentration μg/100ml	TSH concentration μU/ml	
1. University employees				
summer	118.1 ± 4.5*(47)	8.6 ± 0.2 (47)	2.6 ± 0.2 (22)	Less than (4) 1.25 μU/ml
winter	119.1 ± 6.9 (45)	8.8 ± 0.1 (45)	2.5 ± 0.1 (23)	Less than (3) 1.25 μU/ml
2. People of Nakano City				
before cold	119.3 ± 10.9 (24)	8.4 ± 0.4 (24)	2.4 ± 0.3 (21)	Less than (3) 1.25 μU/ml
3 h after cold	122.9 ± 8.6 (24)	9.0 ± 0.4 (24)	2.8 ± 0.2 (22)	Less than (2) 1.25 μU/ml
3. People of Kijimadaira				
summer	127.8 ± 3.5 (56)	9.2 ± 0.5 (56)	3.1 ± 0.4 (48)	Less than (8) 1.25 μU/ml
winter	168.4 ± 6.8 (49)	9.6 ± 0.5 (49)	3.5 ± 0.3 (43)	Less than (6) 1.25 μU/ml

*Mean ± SE; number of subjects studied is in parentheses.

nal cortex in the body's defense against cold is not clear. Plasma cortisol levels were the same in summer and winter in the present subjects.

► [While we all have used a cold environment as the example, par excellence, for a physiologic increase in thyroid hormone secretion, as one can infer from this article, it is very difficult to document. A similar seasonal variation was shown in Montreal (1965–1966 YEAR BOOK, p. 70), but until now, clinical data have been very scant indeed. Similar seasonal curves for both T_4 and T_3 were adduced by Smals (J. Clin. Endocrinol. Metab. 44: 998, 1977), and Tuomisto et al. (Acta Endocrinol. (Kbh.) 83:522, 1976) demonstrated that going from what the Finnish authors call a "very moderately heated Finnish sauna bath" (Whew!) into a "relatively warm swimming pool" (Brr!) resulted in a slight but significant increase in serum TSH, without changes in serum T_3. The phenomenon is easier to demonstrate in rats, as shown by Krulich et al. (Isr. J. Med. Sci. 12:1090, 1976).—T.B.S.] ◄

Catecholamine Metabolism in Thyroid Disease: II. Norepinephrine Secretion Rate in Hyperthyroidism and Hypothyroidism. Blood and urine levels of catecholamines appear to be elevated in hyperthyroidism and reduced in hypothyroidism, but epinephrine metabolism is not significantly modified by thyroid status. Pierre Coulombe, Jean H. Dussault and Peter Walker[6] (Laval Univ.) determined plasma secretion rates of norepinephrine (NE) in 6 euthyroid subjects, 6 patients with untreated diffuse toxic goiter and 6 with untreated primary hypothyroidism. No patient had cardiac or renal disease or arterial hypertension. Norepinephrine was infused at a constant rate with tritiated NE, blood samples were collected at intervals of 1–24 hours and the plasma NE was measured fluorometrically.

Concentrations of epinephrine were similar in all three groups. Plasma NE was significantly elevated in hypothyroid patients. Plasma NE, corrected for age, was significantly elevated in the hypothyroid group (table). No significant differences in disappearance rates of labeled NE in plasma were noted. There were no significant differences in half-lives but the volume of distribution was significantly elevated in the hypothyroidism group. The calculated plasma secretion rate of NE and NE secretion rate were significantly higher in the hypothyroid group than in the hyperthyroid and control groups.

---

(6) J. Clin. Endocrinol. Metab. 44:1185–1189, June, 1977.

PLASMA CONCENTRATION, VOLUME OF DISTRIBUTION, FRACTIONAL RATE OF DISAPPEARANCE AND SECRETION RATE OF NOREPINEPHRINE IN NORMAL SUBJECTS AND IN PATIENTS WITH THYROID DISEASES*

Groups	No	Age (years)	NE_0 (ng/100 ml)	NE_c (ng/100 ml)	V.D. (liter)	K (day^{-1})	Weight (kg)	NES_p (μg/kg/day)
Control	6	29.0 ± 3.50	15.7 ± 3.3	18.3 ± 4.2	79.04 ± 5.48	5.33 ± 0.66	61.05 ± 5.58	1.46 ± 0.35
Hyperthyroid	6	35.8 ± 5.49	18.7 ± 2.8	17.5 ± 3.9	85.43 ± 2.60	6.19 ± 0.41	54.23 ± 3.25	1.74 ± 0.49
Hypothyroid	6	40.0 ± 4.11	33.7 ± 4.8§	30.3 ± 2.9†	153.46 ± 17.17§‖	6.57 ± 0.84	70.63 ± 8.23	4.62 ± 0.98†¶‡

*All results are expressed as mean ± SEM.
†P<0.05 hypo vs. control.
§P < 0.01 hypo vs. control.
‖P < 0.01 hypo vs. hyper.
¶P < 0.05 hypo vs. hyper.

These findings indicate that the plasma NE secretion rate is normal in hyperthyroidism and significantly elevated in hypothyroidism, explaining the higher plasma NE concentrations observed in hypothyroidism. The catabolism of NE appears to be unchanged in states of thyroid dysfunction. The higher plasma NE in hypothyroidism results from a higher plasma secretion rate of NE in this condition.

▶ [An interesting phenomenon is described. The fact that the elevated plasma norepinephrine levels in hypothyroid individuals are accompanied by an increased nonepinephrine secretion rate is interesting but not illuminating. Is this, too, a compensatory change to maintain blood pressure and other vital functions in these metabolically depressed patients?— T.B.S.] ◀

HYPERTHYROIDISM

Delayed Hypersensitivity in Graves' Disease and Exophthalmos: Identification of Thyroglobulin in Normal Human Orbital Muscle. The development of delayed hypersensitivity to thyroid and retro-orbital antigens may be important in the pathogenesis of Graves' disease and exophthalmos. Brian R. Mullin, Rachel E. Levinson, Adolph Friedman, Donald E. Henson, Roger J. Winand and Leonard D. Kohn[7] found that a partially purified retro-orbital antigen preparation contains thyroglobulin or a derivative of the thyroglobulin molecule that retains some of its immune determinants.

Inhibition of leukocyte migration was assayed, and the binding of ^{125}I-thyroglobulin to muscle membranes was investigated. The purified retro-orbital tissue antigen preparation exhibited a 50- to 150-fold higher specific activity than crude homogenates in its ability to act as an antigen in the migration inhibition factor (MIF) assay of exophthalmic patients. Immunodiffusion, ultracentrifugation and disk electrophoresis data indicated that the antigen preparation, obtained from normal human retro-orbital tissue, contained thyroglobulin or a derivative thereof. Immunofluorescence studies localized the antithyroglobulin reactive material to the plasma membranes of extraocular muscle fibers of normal subjects (Fig 13).

It is concluded that thyroglobulin or a derivative of the

---

(7)   Endocrinology 100:351–366, February, 1977.

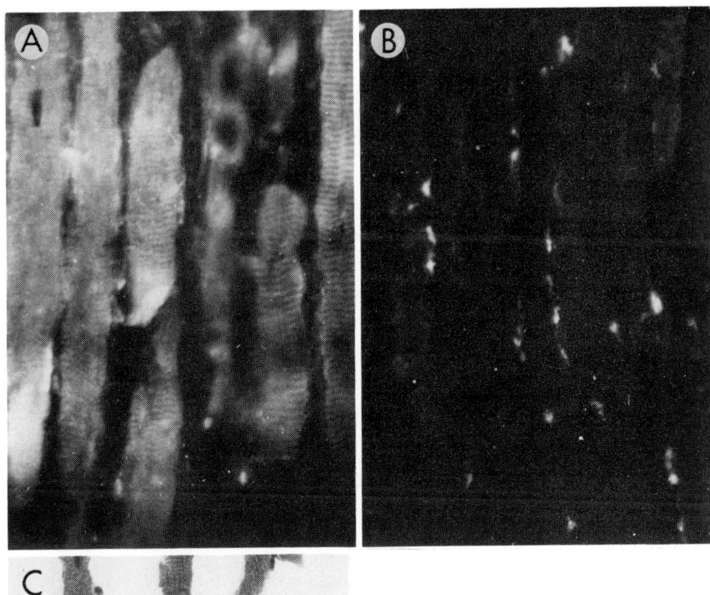

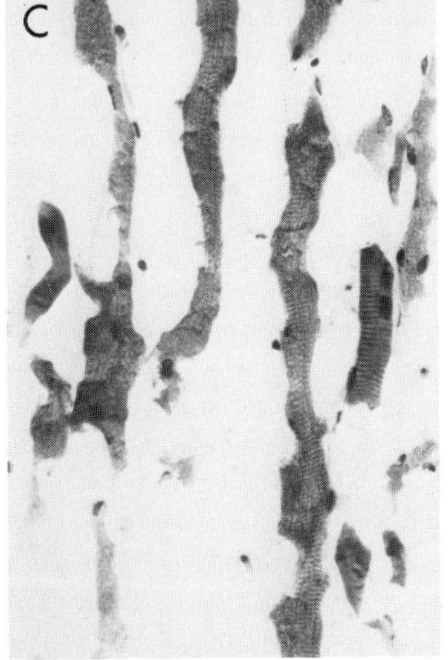

Fig 13. — Immunofluorescent staining of normal human extraocular muscle reacted with antiserum to human thyroglobulin (**A**) or preimmune serum from rabbit in which antihuman thyroglobulin was prepared (**B**). Immune serum preabsorbed with human thyroglobulin gave no reaction, similar to preimmune control. **C**, histologic section of this tissue stained with hematoxylin-eosin and magnified 300 times. (Courtesy of Mullin, B. R., et al.: Endocrinology 100:351–366, February, 1977.)

thyroglobulin molecule is present in the orbital muscle of normal subjects and is one of the antigens to which patients with Graves' disease and exophthalmos demonstrate delayed hypersensitivity. Possibly thyroglobulin-sensitized T lymphocytes interact with thyroglobulin already bound to the extraocular muscle membrane. Various lymphokines are elaborated by the T cells, including cytotoxins and leukocyte MIFs. Cytotoxins may cause orbital muscle fiber damage, whereas reduced leukocyte mobility due to MIF may explain round cell infiltration of the orbital connective tissue. Cell-mediated immunity may act with humoral immunity to cause tissue damage, and antigens other than thyroglobulin may be important in certain patients with Graves' disease.

Identification of Subgroups of Euthyroid Graves' Ophthalmopathy. Evidence of normal thyroid suppressibility in some patients with euthyroid Graves' ophthalmopathy suggested that this may be a heterogeneous group of disorders rather than a single entity. David H. Solomon,

Inder J. Chopra, Usha Chopra and Francoise J. Smith[8] (Univ. of California, Los Angeles) sought defining characteristics of Graves' thyroid disease, Hashimoto's disease and Graves' ophthalmopathy in 22 patients thought to have

DATA USED TO CLASSIFY PATIENTS WITH GRAVES' OPHTHALMOPATHY*

CASE No.	FREE T_4†	FREE T_3†	LATS-PROTECTOR ACTIVITY	THYROID RAIU	
				PRE-T_3	POST-T_3
	ng/dl	pg/dl		% administered dose	
Group H:					
1	2.0	849	+	23	20
2	4.2	704	+	45	NT
3	2.4	717	+	20	22
4	5.7	1,274	+	36	34
5	4.4	758	+	14	14
Group 1:					
6	2.1	548	+	25	22
7	2.0	543	+	43	47
8	1.9	322	+	34	NT
9	—‡	—	+	27	16
10	2.9	539	+	44	32
11	2.8	500	+	NT	38
Group 2:					
12	2.2	405	+	16	5
13	3.5	595	+	15	4
14	3.5	595	+	17	7
Group 3:					
15	3.2	457	UD	24	5
16	2.1	485	UD	18	7
17	2.9	380	UD	21	6
18	1.9	433	UD	15	6
19	2.9	575	UD	27	4
Group 4:					
20	2.6	362	UD	24	26
21	2.1	538	UD	30	29
22	3.2	410	UD	17	17

*T_4 = thyroxine; T_3 = triiodothyronine; LATS = long-acting thyroid stimulator; RAIU = uptake of radioactive iodine; NT = not tested; UD = undetectable— not significant at 5% level.

†Normal range of free T_4 is 1.8–4.2 ng/dl; that of free T_3 is 240–620 pg/dl.

‡Patient had free T_4 index of 7.8 (normal, 4.5–13) and free T_3 index of 175 (normal, 50–210).

(8) N. Engl. J. Med. 296:181–186, Jan. 27, 1977.

euthyroid Graves' disease. All had class 2–5 Graves' ophthalmopathy, and none had been treated for hyperthyroidism or complained of its symptoms. Five proved to have definite elevations of serum free triiodothyronine (T_3) and, in some cases, free thyroxine (T_4) as well. Serum specimens were also taken from 33 patients with untreated Graves' hyperthyroidism.

Antimicrosomal antibodies were more frequent in Graves' hyperthyroidism than in euthyroid Graves' ophthalmopathy, and long-acting thyroid-stimulator protector activity (LPA) was far more common in the former state. For analysis, the patients were classified into five groups: 6 patients with LPA and thyroid nonsuppressibility (group 1); 3 with positive LPA and normal suppressibility (group 2); 5 with undetectable LPA and normal suppressibility (group 3); 3 with undetectable LPA and nonsuppressibility (group 4) and 5 referred with a diagnosis of euthyroid Graves' ophthalmopathy who were found to be hyperthyroid (group H). The groups are compared in the table. Thyroid antibodies were present in high titer in most group 1 patients but were undetectable or insignificant in group 3 patients. Ophthalmopathy was less marked in group 3 than in the other groups.

Euthyroidism in Graves' ophthalmopathy may have more than one cause. Some patients have Hashimoto's thyroiditis, Graves' thyroid disease and Graves' ophthalmopathy, others have "isolated" Graves' ophthalmopathy without autoimmune thyroid disease, and still others are not yet classifiable.

▶ [The group 3 patients are the anomalous ones. The patients are euthyroidal, have no thyroid-stimulating immunoglobulins and the thyroid glands are normally suppressible. Whence, then, comes the Graves' ophthalmopathy? Is it the deposition of some unmeasured circulating immune complexes (Chano: Endocrin. Res. Commun. 3:307, 1976)?

Group 3 is one of nature's pigeons that has difficulty squeezing into one of man's pigeonholes. Another one is described by Teng and Yeo (Br. Med. J. 1:273, 1977), who found a subgroup of patients with ophthalmic Graves' disease with normal free thyroid hormone concentrations, but with impaired or absent TSH responses to TRH.

Would any of these categories change if we had more refined techniques for the clinical identification of Graves' ophthalmopathy? We don't have the answer, but we may be getting the techniques, as indicated below—T.B.S.] ◀

Dysthyroid Ophthalmopathy: Orbital Evaluation with B-Scan Ultrasonography. Ocular muscle swelling may be detectable by ultrasound scanning in cases of Graves' disease where clinical evidence of eye involvement is absent. J. V. Forrester, G. R. Sutherland and I. R. McDougall[9] (Univ. of Glasgow) determined the incidence of detectable orbital changes with use of B-scan ultrasonography in 41 patients with Graves' disease. Scans were made in three horizontal and vertical planes of both orbits with use of a scanner with a 5-mHz focused transducer. Six normal scans were used as controls and read with the study scans in a blind manner by one observer.

All patients with clinically evident ocular involvement showed an increase in muscle size by ultrasound study. This included patients with minimal signs of lid-lag and stare only and no proptosis. Patients with proptosis and clinical muscle impairment tended to have the greatest increases in muscle size, but the degree of muscle enlargement could not be predicted by the clinical class (table). Ultrasonic evidence of muscle enlargement was obtained in 63% of studies of patients without eye signs and over half these patients had marked muscle enlargement. Three quarters of patients with obvious muscle swelling on ultrasound study were euthyroid, whereas two thirds of those with neither ultrasonic nor clinical signs were frankly thyrotoxic.

This study confirms the value of diagnostic ultrasound in Graves' disease, especially in cases of unilateral proptosis

CLINICAL DATA

Clinical Class (Werner, 1969)

		0	1	2	3	4	Total
Number of orbits examined by ultrasound		32	10	3	19	18	82
Definite muscle enlargement on ultrasound		20 (63%)	10 (100%)	3 (100%)	19 (100%)	18 (100%)	70 (85%)
Degree of muscle enlargement	Mild	5	5	0	4	2	
	Moderate	3	3	1	7	6	
	Marked	12	2	2	8	10	

(9)   J. Clin. Endocrinol. Metab. 45:221–224, August, 1977.

and euthyroidism. The presence of subclinical muscle enlargement in the fellow eye supports a diagnosis of dysthyroid disease and differentiates it from local orbital disease.

► [Impressive numbers are presented in the table. — T.B.S.] ◄

HLA System and Graves' Disease. Studies since 1972 have suggested several associations between the HLA system and diseases of certain or probable autoimmune nature. These studies led C. Jaffiol, J. Seignalet, L. Baldet, M. Robin, H. Lapinski and J. Mirouze[1] (Montpellier, France) to study this system in Graves' disease in order to document the physiopathologic hypothesis advanced to explain the mechanism of this form of hyperthyroidism.

METHOD. — HLA typing was done in 100 patients with Graves' disease and 270 controls. In each patient, diagnosis was based on clinical and laboratory evidence of hyperthyroidism (plasma T_4) and Graves' disease (high radioiodine uptake by thyroid and accel-

HLA DISTRIBUTION IN PATIENTS AND CONTROLS

ANTIGENS	FREQUENCY % IN 100 PATIENTS	FREQUENCY % IN 270 CONTROLS	P NONCORRECTED	P CORRECTED
A 1	26	19,63	NS	
A 2	39	45,93	NS	
A 3	27	21,11	NS	
A 9	21	27,78	NS	
A 10	14	10,37	NS	
A 11	12	14,81	NS	
A 28	5	9,26	NS	
A 29	16	15,56	NS	
AW 32	7	7,41	NS	
Mo 26	16	12,59	NS	
B 5	21	14,07	NS	
B 7	11	15,56	NS	
B 8	35	16,30	0,0002	0,005
B 12	23	34,07	0,05	NS
B 13	3	5,19	NS	
B 14	6	8,52	NS	
B 18	15	12,22	NS	
B 27	5	8,52	NS	
BW 15	7	10	NS	
BW 17	6	4,44	NS	
BW 21	6	6,29	NS	
BW 22	7	4,07	NS	
BW 35	23	19,63	NS	
BW 38	5,08	2,59	NS	
BW 40	8	7,04	NS	

*NS = not significant. Mo 26 = patients with either Da25 or Fe55, specifications not differentiated in the study.

(1) Ann. Endocrinol. (Paris) 37:219 – 226, July – Aug., 1976.

erated hormonopoiesis, uncontrolled by T_3). By a lymphocytotoxicity microtechnique, 25 HLA antigens were characterized, 10 on locus A and 15 on locus B. All were studied in every patient, with the exception of BW 38, which was tested in only 59 patients.

HLA grouping was carried out with 136 selected immunoserums containing monospecific or paucispecific antibodies. Each HLA antigen was tested with at least three immunoserums for better grouping accuracy. A difference in corrected P ($\times 25$) of less than 0.05 was considered significant.

Results indicated an increased incidence of HLA B8 antigen in patients with Graves' disease (35%) as compared to controls (16.3%) (table). The difference was highly significant. Variations in distribution of other antigens were slight and insignificant.

The main symptoms and evolutionary features of Graves' disease were compared in carriers and noncarriers of the B8 antigen. There was a higher incidence of male patients with hereditary thyroid disease and of goiter and exophthalmos in HLA B8 carriers, but these variations were not significant.

The pathogenic hypothesis seems justified by the familial character of Graves' disease and the relationship between the HLA system and immunity. The HLA genes are part of the major histocompatibility complex (MHC) which also includes the mixed lymphocyte culture (MLC) genes. The role of the HLA genes is still unclear. The MLC genes seems to direct the initial phase of the immune reaction in identifying antigens by T lymphocytes, followed by activation and multiplication of these cells. The possible presence of Ir genes in man has been suggested by animal experiments. They are thought to control the intensity of immunologic responses.

Presence of Graves' disease implies presence of thyrostimulating factors other than TSH and having the structure of immunoglobulins. The etiology and mechanism of hyperthyroidism seem to include genetic and nongenetic factors. The latter could be explained by the existence of one or several Ir-IgG loci, situated near the HLA B locus. In genetically predisposed individuals, an imbalance could exist in the relationship between the Ir-IgG and HLA B8 alleles. The contact between T lymphocytes and the antigens of the causal agent would induce an immunologic reaction. Antibodies with thyroid-stimulating and exophthalmos affinities explain the principal symptoms of Graves' disease.

▶ [The table provides a nice perspective of how these kinds of relationships are adduced. The eye is caught by the B8 line where frequency of this HLA antigen is twice as great in patients with Graves' disease as in normal subjects. The corrected P value, that is, the P value multiplied by 25, remains "significant." My guess is that the multiplication is done because a total of twenty-five antigens were measured and the interpreter is at risk of finding a "significant" difference in one of these by chance alone. These results have already been confirmed by Ford et al. (Aust. N.Z. J. Med. 6:297, 1976) and Farid et al. Tissue Antigens 8:181, 1976). However, Chopra et al. (J. Clin. Endocrinol. Metab. 45:45, 1977) carried the studies one step further by looking for a variety of laboratory abnormalities of Graves' disease as well as HLA antigens in the relatives of patients with Graves' disease and Hashimoto's thyroiditis. They confirm the excess of HLA B8 in Grave's disease but found, surprisingly, that there was no correlation with the HLA B8 antigen and the occurrence of Graves' disease abnormalities in the relatives of patients with Graves' disease.

Once again we await future developments with the pious hope that the truth shall make us free. — T.B.S.] ◀

Thyrotoxic Vomiting. Increased appetite with weight loss is one of the cardinal symptoms of thyrotoxicosis; only infrequently do patients complain of anorexia and, under modern conditions, nausea and vomiting appear to be rare complications. F. D. Rosenthal, C. Jones and S. I. Lewis[2] (Leicester, England) report the findings in 7 patients with vomiting in thyrotoxicosis. Two patients presented with prolonged intermittent vomiting, and thyrotoxicosis was not suspected until late in the course of the disease.

Woman, 41, presented with anorexia, nausea, vomiting and faintness, as well as continuous epigastric pain. She vomited blood three times in the next 3 weeks, and passed melena stools on the 3 days before admission. The pulse was 120 on admission. The blood urea was 9 mM/L, but later fell to normal. The serum bilirubin was 1.5 mg/100 ml, and the serum aspartate and alanine transferase levels were elevated. The patient had taken an aspirin-containing compound for the epigastric distress. Symptoms resolved, but the patient was admitted twice in the next 6 months for abdominal pain, vomiting, diarrhea and depression. An elevated protein-bound iodine level was attributed to contamination. Examination showed the patient to be warm, sweaty and tremulous. She had lost 20 kg in weight. The 4-hour ^{131}I uptake was 83%, and the 48-hour protein-bound ^{131}I was 2.88%. Fluorescent antibodies to thyroid cytoplasm were present. Carbimazole was given, and symptoms

---

(2) Br. Med. J. 2:209–211, July 24, 1976.

resolved over the next 4 months as the patient became euthyroid. Liver function test results returned to normal.

Vomiting appears to have been partially forgotten as a symptom of thyrotoxicosis. Five of the present 7 patients were thought to have moderately severe thyroid disease, but they were certainly not in crisis. Two patients had prolonged intermittent vomiting without other symptoms of thyrotoxicosis. There was no evidence of hypermetabolism of the central nervous system in these cases. Only 3 patients had diarrhea. There was no evidence of any serious metabolic disorder other than thyrotoxicosis.

At times, vomiting may be the only presenting feature of thyrotoxicosis, leading to considerable difficulty in making the diagnosis.

▶ [I feel somewhat at a loss, not for a comment (you all know me better than that), but for a comment that does justice to the authors. The workups of the 7 patients were eminently acceptable. In their discussion, the authors state, "there was no evidence of serious metabolic disorder other than thyrotoxicosis in our patients," yet nowhere in the patient workups or in the discussion is there mention of the possibility that these patients suffered from hypercalcemia with attendant anorexia, nausea and vomiting. That hyperthyroidism may provoke hypercalcemia is hardly a secret (Parfitt and Dent: Q. J. Med. 39:171, 1970). Some hypercalcemic patients have associated primary hyperparathyroidism and may respond to calcitonin administration (Woodhouse et al.: Horm. Res. 7:238, 1976). Other associations include psychosis (Pehling and Mork: Minn. Med. 60:169, 1977) and hyperviscosity syndrome (Bussman et al.: J. Pediatr. 90:266, 1977).

Sometimes vomiting is salutary, as was the case in a woman who swallowed about 100 tablets of thyroxine (Von Hofe and Young: J.A.M.A. 237: 1361, 1977).

I mention for completeness, and apropos of practically nothing, that Reschini et al. (J. Clin. Endocrinol. Metab. 43:924, 1976) report a rare occurrence. Theirs is only the eleventh instance of a TSH-producing tumor that provoked hyperthyroidism. Speaking of rarities, look ahead. — T.B.S.]

Graves' Disease Associated with Familial Deficiency of Thyroxine-Binding Globulin. Decreased serum levels of thyroxine-binding globulin (TBG) are often found in thyrotoxicosis, but the levels are generally not markedly reduced and return to normal with return of euthyroidism after treatment. David L. Horwitz and Samuel Refetoff[3] (Univ. of Chicago) encountered 5 patients with symptoms of Graves' disease who had marked reductions in TBG capacity

---

(3)   J. Clin. Endocrinol. Metab. 44:242–247, February, 1977.

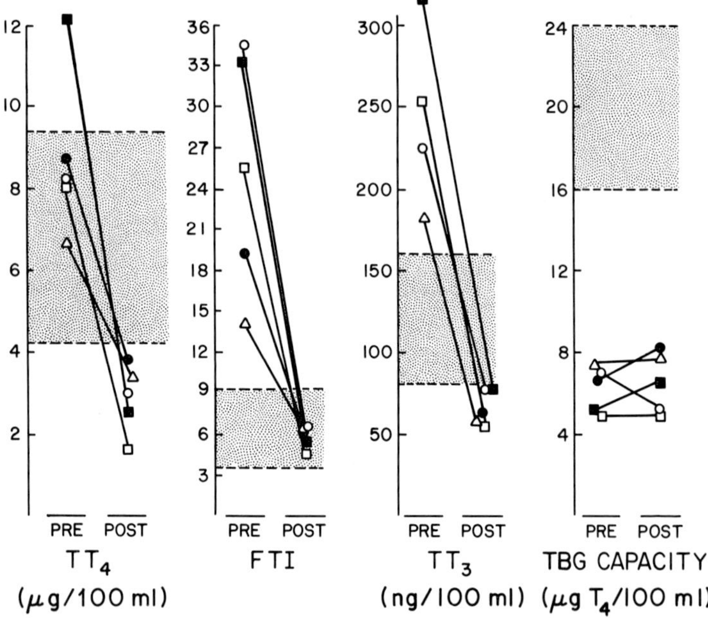

Fig 14. — Serum TT$_4$, FTI, TT$_3$ and TBG capacity in 5 patients with thyrotoxicosis before *(pre)* and at least 1 month after achievement of euthyroidism *(post)*. Stippled area is normal range (mean ± 2 SD). *Solid squares,* Case 1; *open squares,* Case 2; *open circles,* Case 3; *solid circles,* Case 4; *open triangles,* Case 5. (Courtesy of Horwitz, D. L., and Refetoff, S.: J. Clin. Endocrinol. Metab. 44:242–247, February, 1977.)

that failed to resolve after treatment. These patients and their available relatives were evaluated to uncover a possible inherited TBG abnormality.

While thyrotoxic, the patients had a mean total serum thyroxine (TT$_4$) of 8.8 μg/100 ml, a TBG capacity of 6.1 μg thyroxine (T$_4$) per 100 ml, a free T$_4$ index (FTI) of 25.3 and a total serum triiodothyronine (TT$_3$) of 244 ng/100 ml (Fig 14). When euthyroid, both TT$_4$ and TT$_3$ were below the normal range, and the FTI was normal. All patients were men and family studies showed decreased TBG capacity in blood relatives consistent with X chromosome-linked inheritance. All relatives of the propositi were euthyroid. Seven other patients who were euthyroid but had decreased TBG capacity were seen in the same period.

The occurrence of thyrotoxicosis in 5 of 12 patients with

inherited TBG deficiency suggests an association. It is important to determine TT_3 and the FTI in patients who are clinically thyrotoxic but have normal TT_4 values. It seems most likely that the genes predisposing to Graves' disease and TBG deficiency are on separate chromosomes. Since the complexity of the genetics of Graves' disease suggests a possible multifactorial inheritance, however, at least part of the genetic "background" necessary for the development of Graves' disease may be linked with TBG deficiency.

► [Unfair! Figure 14 tells the story nicely. We have enough trouble without being hit with this kind of "biologic artifact."—T.B.S.] ◄

Hyperthyroidism from Autonomous Metastases of a Thyroid Cancer. M. Daumont, R. Mornex, G. Pousset, J. Brière, G. Maret, P. Charleux and J. C. Paffoy[4] (Lyons, France) present the twelfth reported case in which hyperthyroidism is associated with autonomous metastases of thyroid cancer.

Woman, 64, had undergone thyroidectomy 8 years previously. At operation, a hard, turgescent, hypervascularized left lobe and a soft right lobe containing opaque fluid were revealed, and total left and subtotal right lobectomy was performed. Pathologic examination had shown a benign microfollicular thyroid adenoma in the right lobe and a thyroid tumor with colloid-free vesicles in the left lobe. Between the cells, there were large capillaries with wall distortions caused by thyroid tissue but no evidence of invasion: a picture typical of trabeculovesicular adenocarcinoma.

The patient remained well without treatment for 8 years postoperatively. Then an osseous tumor of the 3d right rib was excised. The pathologist reported epithelial proliferation of papillovesicular type, with sporadic eosinophilic deposits resembling thyroid colloid. There was significant tumoral vascularization but no clear cytonuclear abnormality, all of which pointed to a glandular epithelioma of thyroid origin.

Clinical signs of hyperthyroidism had coexisted for a year with tachycardia, weight loss of 20 lb, moist skin and tremors; there were no ocular signs. Pelvic radiography showed increased density in the right supracoxal area. Whole body scintigraphy demonstrated radioiodine uptake at the hepatic level, in the areas of the right coxal bone and the sternal manubrium and in the periumbilical and paravertebral zones (Fig 15).

After treatment with TSH (100 units/day) for 6 days and lithium (9.92 mEq/day) for 3 days, the patient absorbed 120

---

(4)   Ann. Endocrinol. (Paris) 38:125–135, Mar.–Apr., 1977.

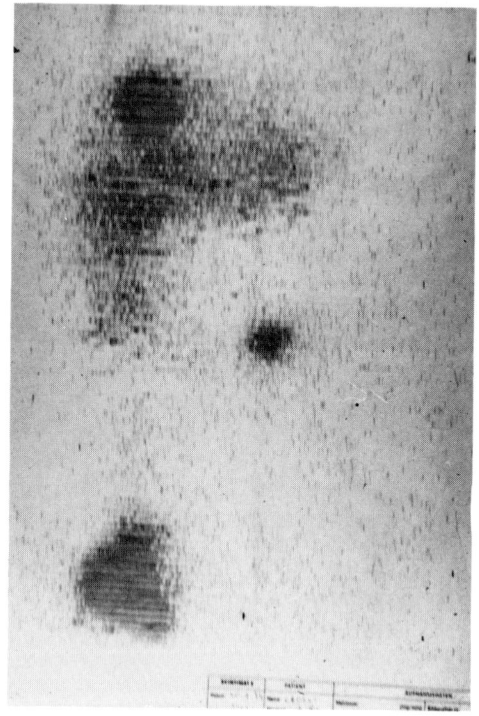

Fig 15. — Abdominal scintigraphy. The active zones correspond to the hepatic mass, the right supracoxal area and the paraumbilical region. (Courtesy of Daumont, M., et al.: Ann. Endocrinol. (Paris) 38:125 – 135, Mar. – Apr., 1977.)

mCi ^{131}I. Three months later, clinical and laboratory hypothyroidism was noted; isotopic exploration showed persistence of hepatic and coxal uptake. Another dose of 120 mCi ^{131}I was administered after treatment with lithium (9.92 mEq/day) for 5 days. Daily treatment with T3 (75 μg) was instituted. Nine months later, hypothyroidism persisted; the liver was not palpable, but coxal condensation was unchanged. Body scintigraphy showed total absence of fixation of iodine.

Eleven reported cases of thyroid cancer with hyperthyroidism are briefly summarized. The similarities in these cases and the present case combine to form a general picture of this rare disease, in which hyperthyroidism is severe, with occasional cardiac complications, ocular signs are absent, and significant hyperhormonemia is noted. The main features of hypersecreting, autonomous metastases in thyroid cancer are the superior uptake capability and an unusual iodoprotein structure.

► [I have seen 1 such patient, not previously described, who had metastases in the right humerus and left scapula. The hyperthyroidism responded well to massive ^{131}I therapy. Survival was lengthy.

I mention in passing that it is worthwhile to reduce the iodide pool with lithium or diuretics, if feasible. — T.B.S.] ◄

Attempted Prevention of Neonatal Thyrotoxicosis. The mortality of untreated neonatal thyrotoxicosis is 12%. Ian Ramsay[5] (London) reports a case in which the fetus was recognized as being at risk when the mother was 5 months' pregnant and in which carbimazole was given to the mother in an attempt to control the fetal thyroid.

Woman, 29, had had a partial thyroidectomy at age 11 for Graves' disease and became hypothyroid at age 16 and was started on thyroxine in a dosage of 0.3 mg daily. At age 21 she aborted a macerated female fetus at 28 weeks; a goiter was found at autopsy. At age 23 she gave birth to a 36-week boy who developed exophthalmos and died neonatally with an enlarged, slightly nodular thyroid and increased heart weight. At 5 months' gestation of the current pregnancy, the patient was euthyroid but had bilateral exophthalmos and diplopia. She was given 5 mg carbimazole 3 times daily with 0.4 mg thyroxine daily and remained euthyroid. A healthy girl was delivered at 37 weeks. Cord blood total T_4 and total T_3 levels were 209 and 0.8 nM/L, respectively, and the thyrotropin concentration was less than 0.5 mU/L. Tachycardia developed the day after delivery, when the infant was sweating, fed voraciously and had prominent eyes. The thyroid was palpable. Carbimazole was given in decreasing doses for 3 weeks. After 14 months the mother's blood level of long-acting thyroid stimulator protector (27 units/ml) was consistent with that associated with the development of neonatal thyrotoxicosis. The child was normal at age 2½ years.

This is the first report of an attempt to protect a fetal thyroid against maternal thyroid-stimulating immunoglobulins. Carbimazole crosses the placenta more readily than thyroid hormones. The treatment succeeded in keeping the

---

(5) Br. Med. J. 2:1110, Nov. 6, 1976.

fetus euthyroid in utero. Clinical thyrotoxicosis became apparent a day after birth as the transplacentally administered carbimazole lost its effect.

▶ [Suppose you had a patient, similar to the one described here, whom you treated with an antithyroid drug (more likely methimazole in the United States); at birth, her infant was premature but otherwise normal, but showed alarming symptoms of neonatal thyrotoxicosis on the 5th day. What would you do? Well, Pearl and Chambers (Br. Med. J. 2:738, 1977) treated the infant with propranalol, starting at 2 mg/day and increasing dosages to 24 mg/day in the 7th week. The child did well. I mentioned earlier that a child with neonatal Graves' disease was found to have hyperviscosity syndrome with an hematocrit of 73% (Bussman et al.: J. Pediatr. 90: 266, 1977). — T.B.S.] ◀

Painless Thyroiditis and Transient Hyperthyroidism without Goiter. Recently a number of patients with painless thyroiditis and transient thyrotoxicosis have been reported. Most have had a goiter, and all have followed the course of subacute thyroiditis. Steven G. Dorfman, Michael T. Cooperman, Roger L. Nelson, Harstry Depuy, Robert L. Peake and Robert L. Young[6] (Wilford Hall USAF Med. Center, San Antonio, Texas) made serial observations on 8 women with this syndrome in the past year. The patients, who had had no palpable thyroid abnormality at any time, constituted 15% of all thyrotoxicosis seen during the preceding year. The average patient age was 40 years. All had low radioiodine uptakes. None had a history of thyroid pain, viral syndrome or recent iodine contamination. All denied a family history of thyroid disease.

The thyrotoxic features, which lasted 1–3 months, were controlled by propranolol therapy. Thyroid function test results are given in the table. All patients became euthyroid or hypothyroid within 3 months. Three went through transient hypothyroid phases, which did not require treatment. Complement fixation titer elevations resolved within 3 months. Fluorescent antibody was detected in 4 patients. All patients had elevated antithyroglobulin antibodies. The titers fell in the 5 patients followed for over 4 months, although not to normal levels. The sedimentation rate was slightly elevated in 3 of 4 patients. No patient had thyroid tenderness or a goiter during the follow-up period of 4–13 months. All have become euthyroid.

---

(6) Ann. Intern. Med. 86:24–28, January, 1977.

MEAN VALUE AND RANGE OF THYROID FUNCTION TESTS IN PATIENTS WITH
PAINLESS THYROIDITIS AND TRANSIENT HYPERTHYROIDISM*

Time	FT$_4$ Index	T$_3$ (RIA)	TSH	RAIU
months		*ng/dl*	*μU/ml*	*%*
0-1	28 (12-48)†	410 (253-431)	1.5 (<1.3-3.0)	0.9 (0.3-1.7)
2-3	5.5 (2-10)	140 (51-204)	34 (4.9-129)	32 (20-35)
9-13	8 (6-10)	160 (96-185)	5 (<1.3-10)	21 (14-28)
Normal values	[4.5-12]	[80-250]	[<6]	[5-30]

*FT$_4$ index = free thyroxine index; T$_3$ (RIA) = serum triiodothyronine by radioimmuno-
assay; TSH = serum thyrotropin; RAIU = 24-hour radioactive iodine uptake.
†Mean value, with range in parentheses.

The exact pathophysiology of this syndrome is unclear, but most cases have occurred in a circumscribed period, and all reported biopsies have shown lymphocytic thyroiditis. If the syndrome is subacute thyroiditis, it is a new form, possibly due to a virus or representing a variable response to a previously described virus. It is also possible that the syndrome is a rare form of early chronic lymphocytic thyroiditis. The thyrotoxic phase is uniformly short and requires only symptomatic therapy.

▶ [This "outbreak" of transient hyperthyroidism with painless thyroiditis is paralleled by others (1976 YEAR BOOK, pp. 128–130), with a total of 7 patients being described with the same syndrome. I have made a mistake (those who wish to reproduce this last sentence have permission to do so). He should have selected one of three articles (Nobuiuki et al.: J. Clin. Endocrinol. Metab. 44:130, 1977; Ginsberg and Walfish: Lancet 1:1125, 1977; and Ginsberg and Walfish: Ann. Intern. Med. 87:155, 1977) that deal with postpartum transient and self-limited thyroidism. In all, 23 patients are described and they probably all had thyroiditis, mainly autoimmune. Now having rectified my error of omission and cleared the air, I will remind you that some patients with thyroiditis become transiently *hypothyroid* postpartum (1977 YEAR BOOK, p. 149).

As usual, once you read about these episodes, the heightened awareness leads to identification of more patients. I am currently treating a hyperthyroid young lady, 2 months post partum, who also had had an episode of transient hyperthyroidism with a previous pregnancy. Despite sizable doses of propranolol she remained quite hyperthyroid and I felt forced to add antithyroid drug therapy. It is possible, after all, that she will not have transient disease and that more definitive therapy may be necessary.

Speaking of treatment, look below. — T.B.S.] ◀

Short-Term Antithyroid Drug Therapy for the Thyrotoxicosis of Graves' Disease. Nearly all patients with thyrotoxicosis can be brought into remission by antithyroid drug therapy, but treatment for a year or longer involves considerable delay and expense if radioiodine or surgery will eventually be necessary. Monte A. Greer, Huldrick Kammer and Donald J. Bouma[7] found that 2 patients who ran out of their medication at about the time they became euthyroid remained in remission after 1 or 2 months. A study was then begun in which all patients with thyrotoxic Graves' disease were treated only until euthyroidism returned. Thirty-one previously untreated patients with diffuse toxic goiter were included in the study, as were 9 patients who had previously had at least 1 full-year course of antithyroid drugs or subtotal thyroidectomy. Treatment was begun with 30 mg methimazole daily in a single dose, and if severe toxicity persisted at 6 weeks, 60 mg daily was given. Methimazole was stopped when the patient became euthyroid by both clinical and laboratory criteria.

The patients became euthyroid in a mean of 3.7 months, and the mean total length of treatment was 4.7 months. Twelve have remained in remission after a mean follow-up of 29 months, whereas 19 patients relapsed a mean of 2.3 months after discontinuance of methimazole. Three of 9 patients given a subsequent 1-year course of drug therapy had a second relapse. The 6 other patients were followed for a mean of 1 year. Patients with small glands initially had a greater rate of lasting remission. Only 1 of the 5 patients with triiodothyronine toxicosis relapsed. The 9 previously treated patients attained euthyroidism in a mean of 4 months, and 4 remained in remission for a mean of 13 months. One of 3 patients given a 1-year course after relapse had a further relapse.

Why some patients with Graves' disease remain in lasting remission after antithyroid drug therapy is discontinued is unclear. This may be due to underlying cyclic fluctuations of the disease, but many patients have only one attack in their lifetimes. This empirical approach is advantageous at present, especially in avoiding the expense and inconvenience of months of unnecessary treatment.

(7)   N. Engl. J. Med. 297:173–176, July 28, 1977.

▶ [First, here is a diversion. Some of you may know that I am a hopelessly addicted handball player. I receive a number of benefits from my addiction. After finishing a strenuous session, I experience two noble emotions: (1) the triumph and relief of the survivor (no treadmill nonsense for me!) and (2) I feel that I have extended myself, including all the contractile elements of my body, resulting in a set of sensations that approaches exaltation, what I call "blessed fatigue." Another form of healthy release occurs in short bursts on the court as well. It is the sadistic joy of beating the hell out of a little black ball, and for a number of years I was content. But recently, I have found an additional bonus. Instead of setting my lips in a tight line and fuming inwardly when I miss an easy "kill" shot, I now startle one and all by releasing a howl of mingled anguish and fury while vigorously jumping up and down in frustration. I relate this to you because you should visualize me at this moment with teeth bared in a snarl, legs apart, hips and knees both flexed at about 90 degrees and about 3 feet in the air. The reason for this primitive response is that I have just learned that it will be necessary for me to repeat the dictation of a series of comments completed last week. For unfathomable reasons, the tape recorder did not function properly. So, back to work with an abiding conviction that the repeat comments generated will not approach the quality of the lost originals!

We have here an excellent example of the exploitation of what was a serendipitous observation. "Two patients who had run out of their antithyroid medications at about the time they became euthyroid failed to return until 1 or 2 months later. We thought it would be interesting to see whether the remissions might be long-lasting. To our surprise, they were." The observations therefore, do not rest on any hypothesis; they are nonetheless interesting and helpful and we intend to take advantage of them.

I had the pleasure, some months ago, to visit with Doctor Greer and his colleagues for a few days. It's a small world. Did you know that Dr. Don Bouma married Judy Cooke, the daughter of friends who live across the street from the Schwartzes? Anyway, a good time was had by me, if not by all . . . .

You should be aware that Davies (Lancet 1:1181, 1977) used a somewhat different marker to distinguish the patients who run a high risk of relapse. They found that patients with high levels of serum thyroid-stimulating antibodies at the time of drug withdrawal relapsed within 2 months of discontinuing therapy, while the patients with low levels remained in remission. Before moving on, I feel impelled to tell you that Barnes and Blizzard (J. Pediatr. 91:313, 1977) describe their experience with antithyroid drug therapy in children over a 30-year period. Also, Scazziga (Schweiz. Med. Wochenschr. 107:423, 1977) followed 302 patients with Graves' disease over a 2- to 15-year period with 71% showing a prolonged remission, a far better record than any other study I know. Finally, agranulocytosis secondary to antithyroid drug treatment is discussed by Luther et al. (South. Med. J. 69:1356, 1976) and Rossab (West. J. Med. 126:339, 1977). — T.B.S.] ◀

Propranolol in Treatment of Thyrotoxicosis by Subtotal Thyroidectomy. Propranolol relieves many peripheral manifestations of thyrotoxicosis, and use of this agent

did quite well: no deaths, no bilateral nerve injuries and less than 1% permanent hypoparathyroidism. Wesley et al. (Surg. Gynecol. Obstet. 145: 343, 1977) treated 43 children surgically. Again, there were no deaths, no recurrent laryngeal nerve injury and no permanent hypoparathyroidism. Only 1 patient had recurrent hyperthyroidism, but 25 patients are hypothyroid, and transient hypocalcemia developed in 22. Unintimidated, they state, "effectiveness and safety of the surgical treatment for hyperthyroidism in children are reaffirmed," and Perzik (Am. J. Surg. 132:480, 1976) indicates in no uncertain terms, after a review of 909 total thyroidectomies, "nothing less than total thyroidectomy should be performed." —T.B.S.] ◄

Successful Treatment of Thyrotoxic Crisis by Continuous Plasmapheresis with Blood Cell Separator is described by K. Horn, G. Brehm, J. Habermann, C. R. Pickardt and P. C. Scriba[9] (Univ. of Munich). At the time of a clinical diagnosis of thyrotoxic crisis 13 hours after thyroid surgery, the patient, aged 26, had increased serum thyroid hormone levels. Progressively deepening coma led to the choice of continuous plasmapheresis with an IBM blood cell separator in an attempt to eliminate circulating thyroid hormone. Five liters of plasma were exchanged, removing a total of 633 μg T_4 and 13.6 μg T_3; the patient regained consciousness during the procedure. Because the replacement plasma contained 280 μg T_4 and 5.7 μg T_3, the actual amounts of hormone removed were 353 μg T_4 and 7.9 μg T_3. No fall in total T_4 and T_3 levels in the serum was observed, most likely due to the rapid reflux of thyroid hormones from the tissue into the intravascular space. The T_3-uptake test, and thus the index of free thyroid hormone, did show a fall as proof of diminished circulation of free thyroid hormone. This decrease of serum T_4 and T_3 was evident in the diminished urinary excretion of both hormones during the plasmapheresis. These findings are explained on the basis of a new supply of binding sites for thyroid hormone with the donor plasma and the increased serum level of the T_4-binding globulin. With continued antithyroid treatment total thyroid hormones in the serum diminished surprisingly rapidly during the next 24 hours. Clinical data are presented in the table.

The present observation confirms the value of plasmapheresis with a cell separator for management of a thyrotoxic crisis. A practical advantage is the easy and nontraumatic

(9) Klin. Wochenschr. 54:983–986, Oct. 15, 1976.

CLINICAL DATA FROM PATIENT IN THYROTOXIC CRISIS TREATED BY PLASMAPHERESIS*

Date	Time	Serum T$_4$ (μg)	T$_3$ (ng)	T$_3$-uptake (%)	Index of Free Thyroid Hormone (μg)	TBG (mg)	Urine T$_4$ (ng/hr)	T$_3$ (ng/hr)
6/24/75	7:30 PM	18.5	271	74.8	13.8	0.93}	516	567
6/25	12:10 AM	16.0	266	76.0	12.2	0.90	173	178
	3:45 AM	15.5	285	68.6	10.6	1.37}		82
	9:00 AM	14.4	239	67.8	9.8	1.12}	126	79
	6:00 PM	–	–	–	–	– }	105	36
6/26	9:00 AM	8.9	147	57.4	5.0	1.20}	56	50
	7:00 PM	–	–	–	–	– }	71	78
							79	
6/27	9:00 AM	8.3	162	50.9	4.2	1.52	–	–
6/28	9:00 AM	7.3	105	46.9	3.4	1.29	–	–
Normal Range		4.5–10	85–150	32–42	2–3.8	1.5–3.3	40–100	40–100

*Fall of total T$_4$ and T$_3$ in serum and urine, alteration of thyroid hormone binding to serum albumin (T$_3$-uptake test, index of free thyroid hormone) and increase of circulating levels of T$_4$-binding globulin in serum (TBG) during plasmapheresis and 3 following days under continued antithyroid treatment. Period of plasmapheresis is delineated by interrupted line and normal range of procedures is listed in last row.

technique; the only disadvantages are the immediate need of large amounts of fresh plasma and the risk of hepatitis. The increased supply of thyroid hormone binding sites is even more important for management of the crisis than is the removal of thyroid hormones.

▶ [A novel idea whose time may well have come is presented here. Dr. John Verrier Jones in our department of medicine is a strong advocate of plasmapheresis for the treatment of a variety of disorders, including a number of immunogenic diseases. We, therefore, have access to a busy cell separator and, should the occasion arise, we will see how well this technique works. Certainly, there is no certain form of treatment of thyroid storm. Erikson et al. (N. Engl. J. Med. 296:263, 1977) report a failure with propranolol. — T.B.S.] ◀

HYPOTHYROIDISM

Isolated Thyrotropin Deficiency with Thyrotropin-Releasing Hormone-Induced TSH Secretion and Thyroidal Release. It seems plausible that a spectrum of partial to complete thyrotropin deficiency may exist among patients with isolated thyrotropin (TSH) deficiency. Timothy M. Boehm, Richard C. Dimond and Leonard Wartofsky[1] (Walter Reed Army Med. Center, Washington, D. C.) report the findings in a patient with isolated TSH deficiency in whom thyrotropin-releasing hormone (TRH) administration produced measurable secretion of immunoassayable TSH, which was shown to possess biologic activity.

Man, 41, presented with dry skin and increasing fatigue and received TRH both by bolus injection and by continuous infusion. The patient's serum thyroxine was 1.9 μg/100 ml, the T_3 resin uptake was 24% and the 24-hour radioiodine uptake was 9%. The serum cholesterol was 305 mg/100 ml. The radioiodine uptake rose to 26% after stimulation with 10 units TSH for 3 days. Anterior pituitary function was normal after 2 weeks of treatment with 0.1 mg L-thyroxine daily. The patient was restudied 6 months later, after thyroxine had been discontinued for 8 weeks. Initially serum TSH was not measurable. A level of 1.8 μU/ml was present basally after 5 months of thyroxine therapy; TRH produced no rise in serum TSH but a normal rise in plasma prolactin level before treatment. On reevaluation, TRH produced small increments in serum TSH. Changes of increased thyroidal iodine secretion were observed on studies with ^{125}I and ^{131}I-thyroxine, although the serum T_3 and thyroxine did not change.

---

(1) J. Clin. Endocrinol. Metab. 43:1041–1046, November, 1976.

Isolated TSH deficiency need not be complete and may be associated with detectable immunoassayable TSH. The TSH released by the present patient possessed in vivo biologic activity. Treatment with thyroid hormone may have facilitated TSH release. Once isolated TSH deficiency is diagnosed, patients should be observed for the possible development of a pituitary tumor. The criteria for diagnosing isolated TSH deficiency include clinical and biochemical evidence of hypothyroidism, a decreased or absent TSH response to TRH and documented integrity of function of other anterior pituitary hormones.

▶ [An interesting patient! The authors' observations suggest that this patient, in addition to his other troubles, had "myxedema of the pituitary." Initially, there was no TSH response to TRH administration but, after initiation of thyroxin treatment, a rise in serum TSH did follow TRH stimulation, a change that suggests that the T_4 had a salutary effect on pituitary function. Further evidence of such a phenomenon is provided by Hood et al. (J. Clin. Endocrinol. Metab. 43:1360, 1976), who found a "paradoxical" rise in serum TSH after thyroxine therapy in a patient with primary hypothyroidism.

The authors' caution that one should look for a pituitary tumor in a patient with isolated TSH deficiency has merit. Lee and Faiman (Can. Med. Assoc. J. 116:520, 1977) report the finding in such a patient. And, to complete the gradation, Berthezène (Nouv. Presse Med. 5:2138, 1976) describes patients with low pituitary thyrotropin reserve, that is, patients with serum TSH levels in the normal range, but who are unresponsive to TRH. Most had either diabetes or acromegaly. – T.B.S.] ◀

Hypothyroidism due to Thyroid Hormone-Binding Antibodies. F. Anders Karlsson, Lars Wibell and Leif Wide[2] (Univ. of Uppsala) describe a hypothyroid patient with normal thyroid tissue function, in whom the hypothyroid state was probably due to abnormal binding of triiodothyronine to circulating antibodies of high amount and affinity.

Woman, 26, had low serum thyroxine and resin uptake values and had preferred warm rooms for 5–10 years. She increasingly felt the cold after a pregnancy, sleep requirements increased and mental ability was impaired. Myxedematous swelling of the face and limbs and cool, dry skin were present. The thyroid was slightly enlarged but of normal consistency. Persistent slight blood eosinophilia was present. The serum thyrotropin value was 18 mU/L. Total thyroxine was normal, but the serum T_3 value was over 50 nM/L. Thyroid ^{131}I uptake was normal. Repeated thyroid biopsies showed normal thyroid cells and showed no increase in lymphoid

---

(2)   N. Engl. J. Med. 296:1146–1148, May 19, 1977.

RESULTS OF LABORATORY TESTS ON PATIENT BEFORE AND DURING THERAPY*

Test	Reference Value†	Apr, 1975	Nov, 1975	Jan, 1976	3/2/76	3/23/76	4/21/76	5/5/76
TSH (mU/liter)	<5	3.9		18	2.8	5.0	7.1	2.2
T_4 (nmol/liter)	60–125		22	82	94	67	122	
T_3 (nmol/liter)‡	1.4–3.2	7.5		12	34	29	37	35
T_3 resin uptake (%)	75–115		29	31	43	34	29	
[131]I uptake (%):								
At 4 hr	10–30			16				6
At 24 hr	25–50			41				18
TRH test (nmol/liter)§				18–102				
ATT	<1/100			1/100				1/100
ATA	<1/10			1/100				1/100
Hormone therapy						T_3 (2/9-4/16)		L-T_4(4/23)

*TSH, thyrotropin; T_4, thyroxine; T_3, triiodothyronine; TRH, thyrotropin-releasing hormone; ATT, antithyroglobulin titer; and ATA, anticytoplasmic thyroid antigen.
†Mean ± 2 SD in healthy subjects.
‡Total T_3 determined by radioimmunoassay after dissociation of antibody-bound T_4.
§TSH response.

cells. Immunofluorescence to cytoplasmic thyroid antigen was found. After hormone-binding antibody was found in the serum, T_3 was given in a dosage of 20 μg twice daily and later 4 times daily, until clinical euthyroidism returned. Subsequently levothyroxine was used in a dosage of 0.15 mg daily.

Laboratory findings in this case are summarized in the table. The calculated free triiodothyronine concentration was 85–90% of the euthyroid level a year before euthyroidism returned and 30–40% several months before this time.

The mechanism behind the development of thyroid hormone antibodies is obscure. Possibly the patient previously passed through a state of subclinical thyroiditis during which intracellular material, including thyroglobulin in immunogenic amounts, was released. Disturbed plasma transport of hormone influenced the outcome of diagnostic tests in this case and contributed to a clinical picture of hypothyroidism.

▶ [This patient was carefully studied, but I remain puzzled. The TSH levels were elevated but not to astronomical levels, and one wonders why there was not enough negative feedback to increase TSH secretion with resultant increased thyroid stimulation, with resultant increased thyroid hormone levels, of both T_4 and T_3, to maintain the euthyroid state. In any event, I doubt that this will prove to be a common cause of hypothyroidism. — T.B.S.] ◀

Myeloneuropathy Associated with Hypothyroidism. Polyneuropathy is a rare complication of hypothyroidism. P. D. Mohr and H. Reid[3] (Manchester, England) describe a patient who had a myeloneuropathy, which improved on treatment with thyroxine.

Man, 61, had had progressive dragging of the feet, hand weakness and finger and toe paresthesias for 2 years. The skin was dry and there was distal weakness and wasting of the calf, peroneal and intrinsic hand muscles. Sensation was impaired in a globe-and-stocking pattern. The tendon reflexes were reduced in the arms and absent at the ankles; plantar responses were extensor. Hypothyroidism was confirmed. The serum thyroxine concentration was 2 μg/100 ml and 24-hour radioiodine uptake was 12%. Electromyography showed denervation. Nerve conduction velocities were reduced, and no sensory potential could be evoked at 200v. Sural nerve biopsy showed considerable demyelination and increased perineural connective tissue. Muscle biopsy showed group atrophy combined with scattered eosinophilic fibers, which had an

---

(3)   Br. Med. J. 1:1005–1006, Apr. 16, 1977.

increased number of internal nuclei. The patient was given 0.2 mg thyroxine daily and was euthyroid after 4 months, with a serum thyroxine concentration of 8.2 μg/100 ml. The serum thyrotropin value fell from 100 to 1 mU/L. The patient's neurologic state improved over 1 year, leaving him free from symptoms. The conduction velocity of the ulnar nerve increased from 45.6 to 62 m per second and a small sensory potential was evoked.

Nerve biopsies of patients with myxedema polyneuropathy have shown segmental demyelination and remyelination of nerve fibers with Schwann cell proliferation. Muscle biopsies have shown a denervation pattern and a more diffuse myopathic change. This patient had a neurologic syndrome that resembled myeloneuropathy rather than simple polyneuropathy. Damage to the brain and the cranial and peripheral nerves is well documented in hypothyroidism, and it would seem unlikely that the spinal cord is necessarily exempt from the metabolic effects of this condition.

▶ [The authors have shown that this is more than the usual carpal tunnel syndrome.

This associated finding of hypothyroidism permits us to bring to your attention briefly other associated findings. First, you should know that a similar patient, similarly treated with similar salutary results, has been described by Potton (Lyon Med. 15:217, 1976). Next, reversible also is the hyperlipemia of hypothyroidism, as shown by Mishkel and Crowther (Clin. Chim. Acta 74:139, 1977), and the lipoprotein composition in hypothyroidism was discussed by Wahlqvist et al. (ibid. 77:269, 1977). McDaniel et al. (Metabolism 26:867, 1977) discussed abnormalities in the muscle of patients with hypothyroid myopathy. Then Turner and Rapoport (Postgrad. Med. J. 53:343, 1977) and Chipurt (Am. J. Dig. Dis. 21:807, 1976) tell us of patients with treatment-resistant ascites who responded to thyroid replacement therapy. Next, Guinet (Lyon Med. 236:549, 1976) reminds us that the pituitary gland not only hyperfunctions but enlarges in patients with primary hypothyroidism. Finally, Christ and Morris (Am. J. Med. 62:239, 1977) and I both want to remind you that there exists such an entity in patients as hypothyroid Graves' disease, that is, patients without a prior history of hyperthyroidism who present with Graves' ophthalmopathy in the hypothyroid state. A former medical student and myself were among the first to emphasize this association (Fox and Schwartz: Ann. Intern. Med. 67:377, 1967).—T.B.S.] ◀

Impaired Renal Concentrating Ability in Hypothyroid Man. There is much evidence suggesting abnormal sodium and water handling in myxedema. Carlos A. Vaamonde, Ulrich F. Michael, James R. Oster, Mario J. Sebastianelli, Liliana S. Vaamonde, Eugene L. Klingler, Jr., and Solomon Papper[4] observed decreased maximum urinary

---

(4) Nephron 17:382–395, 1976.

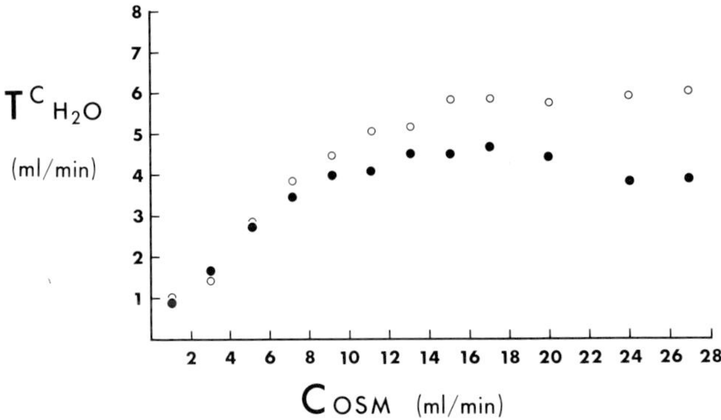

Fig 17.—Average relationship between T^{c}H$_2$O and C$_{osm}$ in myxedema and control patients. All C$_{osm}$ and corresponding T^{c}H$_2$O values are grouped at about 2-ml increments in C$_{osm}$ and represent the mean values for each group. Above a C$_{osm}$ of 10 ml per minute there were statistically significant differences in T^{c}H$_2$O between the groups ($P < 0.05$ to <0.005); *open circles,* controls (5); *closed circles,* myxedema (10). (Courtesy of Vaamonde, C. A., et al.: Nephron 17:382–395, 1976.)

osmolality (U$_{osm}$ max) and solute-free water reabsorption (T^{c}H$_2$O) in hypothyroid patients. Ten patients with untreated myxedema, 7 men and 3 women with a mean age of 43 were studied. Eight had primary myxedema; 3 were severely hypothyroid at the time of study. Fifteen euthyroid men with a mean age of 34, 6 of them hospitalized, were also studied.

The U$_{osm}$ max was lower in myxedema patients than in control subjects (792 versus 921 mOsm/kg H$_2$O) and the maximal urine-to-plasma osmotic ratio was significantly lower in the study patients. There were no significant differences in the minimal urine volume and serum osmolality attained after hydropenia. Urea concentration in maximally concentrated urine was lower in the study patients. The mean rate of urea excretion during hydropenia was 41% lower in the hypothyroid group. The relationship between T^{c}H$_2$O and osmolal clearance is shown in Figure 17. Clearances of inulin and para-aminohippurate were 30% and 34% lower in hypothyroid patients, respectively. Filtration fraction was not different in the two groups. The fraction of the filtered load of sodium excreted in the urine was significantly higher in the patients than the control subjects. No consistent changes in concentrating ability followed treatment of 3 patients with desiccated thyroid. There was a gross inverse correlation between the clinical severity of myxedema and the U_{osm} max in these patients.

The renal concentrating mechanism is abnormal in hypothyroid patients. The results may be best explained by a decrease in NaCl reabsorption in the ascending limb of Henle's loop or a decreased permeability of the distal nephron, or both.

► [Clear-cut observations are presented here. Myxedematous patients cannot concentrate osmols in the urine as well as do normal individuals and the patients tend to secrete more sodium. It is possible that this is due in part to augmented secretion of vasopressin in the myxedematous state. At least Skowsky and Fisher (Endocrinology 100:1022, 1977) think so. Certainly this state strongly resembles innappropriate antidiuretic hormone secretion clinically, and there is a report of a patient with inappropriate antidiuretic hormone secretion syndrome along with myxedema coma (Pasquiei et al.: Sem. Hop. Paris 53:1144, 1977).

Thyroid function in chronic renal failure has been studied by Lim et al. (J. Clin. Invest. 60:522, 1977), Spector et al. (Ann. Intern. Med. 85:724, 1976) and Dandona et al. (Br. Med. J. 1:34, 1977). In capsule summary, there is a low serum T_3 probably from diversion of peripheral metabolism of T_4 to reverse T_3, a relative unresponsiveness of pituitary TSH secretion to TRH, and, with long-term dialysis, a subnormal thyroid response to TSH stimulation. Despite all this, the patients are not clinically hypothyroid. —T.B.S.] ◄

Endocrine Studies in Cystinosis: Compensated Primary Hypothyroidism. Anne W. Lucky, Peter M. Howley, Klara Megyesi, Stephen P. Spielberg and Joseph D. Schulman[5] (Natl. Inst. of Health) evaluated the possibility of the occurrence of potentially treatable endocrine failures in cystinosis, because modern medical therapy and renal transplantation may prolong the lives of children with cystinosis. Stimulatory tests of hormone secretion were carried out and thyroid function evaluated in 7 patients with nephropathic cystinosis. The pathologic findings were reviewed in 4 additional cases that had come to autopsy and review was made of the records of 24 patients with cystinosis. All 7 study patients had clinically and biochemically proved nephropathic cystinosis.

One patient was frankly hypothyroid at presentation. Two others had serum thyrotropin levels at or just over the upper limit of normal and 2 had clearly elevated levels. Ten of 11 patients whose records were reviewed had retarded

---

(5)　J. Pediatr. 91:204–210, August, 1977.

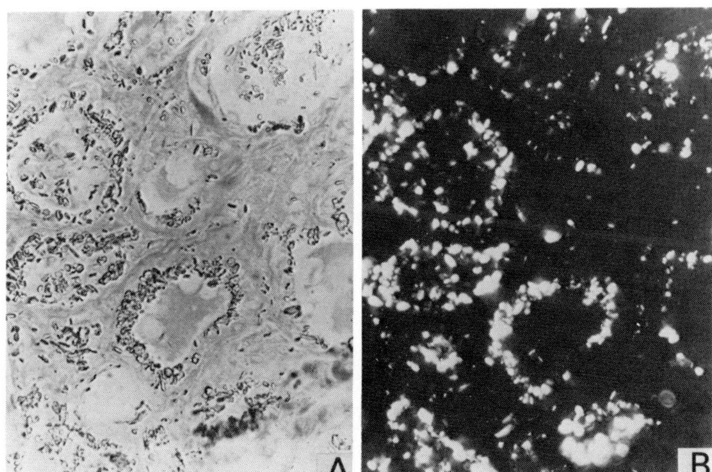

Fig 18.—**A,** section demonstrating cystine crystals within follicular epithelial lining cells and within follicles. Alcohol-fixed section, Fast Green FCF stain; reduced from ×400. **B,** same field visualized with polarized illumination to demonstrate cystine crystals. (Courtesy of Lucky, A. W., et al.: J. Pediatr. 91:204–210, August, 1977.)

bone ages; most had not had thyroid function assessed. All study patients responded normally to intravenous ACTH and had at least one positive response to a growth hormone stimulation test. Levels of nonsuppressible insulin-like activity (NSILA-s) were normal. The oldest patient had an elevated serum LH but a normal FSH level. Autopsy study of thyroid glands showed extensive destruction and infiltration of the epithelium with cystine crystals (Fig 18). Other glands showed cystine crystals in the stroma but no epithelial destruction. The parathyroids were uniformly hypercellular secondary to renal failure.

In nephropathic cystinosis, "compensated" primary hypothyroidism occurs frequently and early and may be diagnosed by measuring serum thyrotropin concentrations. In light of the finding of elevated serum LH in the oldest boy in this series, the possibility of overproduction of gonadotropins as well as of thyrotropin should be considered.

▶ [Studies like these I find to be both satisfying and unsettling. It is satisfying because it shows that there are still some new things under the clinical sun. The combination of hypothyroidism and cystinosis was first noted in 1953 (Jackson and Clark: Am. J. Dis. Child 85:531, 1953) and reported in

16 patients by Chan et al. (Am. J. Med. 48:678, 1970) and, in the same issue in which the article by Lucky et al. appears, there are two other reports (J. Pediatr. 91:340, 1977; and ibid., p. 341). In one, myxedema coma supervened. In addition, Grünebaum and Lebowitz (Am. J. Roentgenol. 129:629, 1977) make a neat point. When the child with cystinosis is rickety, the retarded bone age of hypothyroidism is not demonstrable roentgenographically. With vitamin D treatment, the retarded bone age becomes overt.

I was unsettled because I didn't know about cystinosis as a cause of myxedema. "Hoo! The old boy's arrogance is getting out of hand," the constant reader says. Well, no. I have just completed writing a 60-page review of hypothyroidism in which cystinosis as a cause of myxedema was not mentioned. Bad.

Why a treatise on hypothyroidism? It was undertaken as a diversion for me, and hearing a little about it might be a diversion for you. I have become increasingly distressed by the "bad press" that American medicine is receiving, with malpractice suits, the Laetrile legitimatizing of quackery and the general condemnation of soaring medical costs. Everyone has been urged to learn about medicine, so that our democratic decisions will be informed. Indeed, everyone, it appears, has become an expert *about* medicine, but no one seems to know much about *medicine*. I had the bright notion that I should write an article for the layman in which I would impart in my inimitable, witty fashion everything worth knowing about a single disease, hypothyroidism. The reader, then, would be in a position to knowledgeably approach problems that the physician faces in the decision-making process that takes place, in case finding, diagnosis and management. I showed an early draft to a number of intelligent layfolk, including my wife, my brother, several children and close friends. My wife, a loving and dutiful soul, laboriously read and conscientiously made notes, but was mostly sympathetically silent. My brother, a dentist, began to read with interest but was soon scanning pages cursorily and ended up by saying that nobody, intelligent or otherwise, would ever plow through the damned thing. One friend, who has had editorial experience, began his critique with an uplifting comment. "Don't be discouraged," he said. Well, I want you and them to know that I am *not* discouraged and I still hold visions of a meteoric rise as a medical interpreter to the world.— T.B.S.] ◄

Primary Hypothyroidism and Galactorrhea. Over 25 cases of primary hypothyroidism with galactorrhea have been reported since 1956. Toshio Onishi, Kiyoshi Miyai, Toshihiro Aono, Takenori Shioji, Toshihide Yamamoto, Yoshiaki Okada and Yuichi Kumahara[6] (Osaka, Japan) compared 5 patients who had this combination of conditions with 11 who had primary hypothyroidism without galactorrhea. The patients, all women, were evaluated with 16 clinically normal women. None was on medications when the diagnosis was first made. The galactorrhea started post par-

---

(6)   Am. J. Med. 63:373–378, September, 1977.

tum and had been present for 4–8 years. Three patients were amenorrheic and 2, oligomenorrheic. Two patients without galactorrhea had oligomenorrhea. One patient without galactorrhea had an enlarged sella.

The serum prolactin concentration was above normal in 10 hypothyroid patients, including all those with galactorrhea. Basal thyrotropin and prolactin concentrations were correlated, and a correlation was found between the maximum increases after thyrotropin releasing hormone (TRH) injection. No significant group differences in thyroid hormone values were observed. Galactorrhea disappeared on triiodothyronine therapy, as the serum prolactin and thyrotropin concentrations fell to normal. Responses to TRH also became normal during treatment. Galactorrhea reappeared when the medication was stopped in 1 patient and disappeared when the medication was resumed. Basal and post-TRH concentrations of thyrotropin and prolactin were also reduced by thyroid or triiodothyronine in the patients without galactorrhea.

Elevated prolactin levels in patients with primary hypothyroidism are presumably mediated by feedback-induced TRH secretion or an enhanced response to endogenous TRH. The combination of delivery and prolactin excess may induce persistent galactorrhea in patients with primary hypothyroidism.

▶ [Points of interest: (1) Not all myxedematous patients have hyperprolactinemia; (2) not all hypothyroid patients with hyperprolactinemia have galactorrhea; and (3) the galactorrhea of hypothyroidism may present as typical Chiari-Frommel syndrome, lending weight to the recent suggestion of Frantz (N. Engl. J. Med. 298:201, 1978), "Once lactation has been initiated by childbirth or some other hormonal disturbance" breast tissue "acquires the ability to continue secreting with essentially normal levels of circulating prolactin." To that I would add the possibility that once lactation is initiated in the presence of high prolactin levels, the same perseverative behavior would tend to be even more obvious.

From the group that wrote this article by Onishi et al. comes another (Aono et al.: Fertil. Steril. 28:878, 1977) in which a galactorrheic hypothyroid patient treated with T_3 successfully became pregnant. Two other patients with galactorrhea and hypothyroidism described by Pillosi et al. (Obstet. Gynecol. 50:392, 1977) also had increased gonadotropin secretion, in contrast to most hypothyroid patients in whom LH and FSH secretion is diminished. Anything new about treatment? Look ahead.—T.B.S.]

Reassessment of Daily Dose of Oral Thyroxine for Replacement Therapy in Hypothyroid Children. The optimal daily dosage of sodium L-thyroxine $(L\text{-}T_4)$ replacement therapy has been debated. Iraj Rezvani and Angelo M. DiGeorge[7] (Philadelphia) reevaluated daily requirements for L-T_4 in children with primary hypothyroidism. The minimal dose of oral L-T_4 needed to suppress the serum concentration of thyroid-stimulating hormone (TSH) to normal was determined in 11 children aged 1–14 years, and growth rates were followed for up to 12 months of therapy. Patients initially were on 100–200 μg synthetic L-T_4 daily. The daily dosage was reduced at a rate of 25–50 μg per month.

Serum TSH concentration is related to the oral dose of L-T_4 in Figure 19. The dose was inversely related to the serum TSH concentration. The fall in the latter to normal was abrupt in all cases when the dosage approached 3 μg/kg or

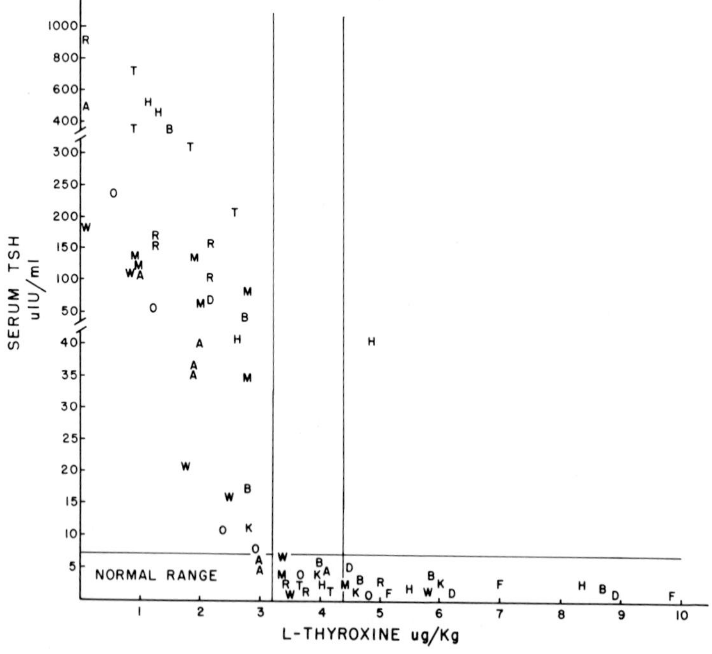

Fig 19.—Serum concentrations of TSH as function of daily dosage of L-T_4. Dose is calculated as micrograms per kilogram body weight. Each letter represents initial of patient. Perpendicular lines depict 95% confidence limit (±2 SD) of optimal dose of L-T_4. (Courtesy of Rezvani, I., and DiGeorge, A. M.: J. Pediatr. 90:291–297, February, 1977.)

(7) J. Pediatr. 90:291–297, February, 1977.

100 μg/sq m. The mean "suppressive" dosage was 3.78 μg/kg or 104.6 μg/sq m. The dosage of L-T$_4$ was strongly correlated with serum T$_4$ concentration, but the adequacy of therapy could not be confidently established in this way, and the same was true for serum total triiodothyronine. All 7 patients followed for 5–12 months were clinically euthyroid. Height velocities were normal in all children, and 2 appeared to have an acceleration of growth, possibly due to previous growth deceleration during suboptimal L-T$_4$ therapy.

The mean "optimal" dosage of L-T$_4$ in this study, 3.78 μg/kg, was considerably lower than the dosages generally recommended. All patients appeared to be euthyroid and grow normally during treatment with the optimal dosage of L-T$_4$. Close monitoring of the serum TSH concentration is indicated if administration of the optimal dosage of L-T$_4$ is planned. Further experience with this regimen is needed before it can be ascertained that it is clearly better than previously recommended dosages derived from years of empirical experience.

▶ [This laborious work, carefully performed, resulted in the striking figure 19. As the authors indicate, whether precise dosing, as monitored by serum TSH levels, makes a clinical difference, is unknown. Recall that the liver takes up thyroid hormone very rapidly (1970 YEAR BOOK, p. 126) and I have wondered whether the liver could, by releasing thyroid hormone, serve as a functional reservoir to compensate for the ineptness of physicians. If so, the kind of precise titering found here would be more a demonstration of physician virtuosity than patient value.

The careful work reported here is complemented by a companion article (Abbassi and Aldige: J. Pediatr. 90:298, 1977) with an almost identical quantitative conclusion regarding replacement doses. – T.B.S.] ◀

Case of Myxedema Coma Successfully Treated by Low-Dose Oral Triiodothyronine. J. J. Graham and P. E. Harding[8] (Adelaide) report a case of primary myxedema coma successfully treated with use of no more than 20–40 μg triiodothyronine (T$_3$) daily.

Man, 77, was admitted comatose after having deteriorated in health and activity for 2 years, markedly in the past 6 months. He had felt cold and had a deeper voice for 6 months and in the week before admission had become disoriented and had hallucinations. A below-knee amputation had been done 10 years before for arterial disease. A brother was diabetic. The obese, comatose patient was

---

(8) Aust. N. Z. J. Med. 7:163–168, April, 1977.

grossly myxedematous and had a rectal temperature of 30.4 C and a pulse of 45 per minute. Chest films showed cardiomegaly and early pulmonary edema. The ECG showed sinus bradycardia, small-voltage complexes, flat T waves and a P-R interval of 0.28 second. The effective thyroxine ratio was 0.84 and the circulating T_3 was 0.12 μg/L with a serum thyrotropin of 120 mμ/L. Thyroid microsomal antibodies were positive at 1:51,200.

The patient was ventilated and placed on restricted fluids. He was given 10 μg T_3 every 12 hours by nasogastric tube and also intravenous frusemide for pulmonary edema. Body temperature rose 6 hours after the first dose of T_3 and was normal by day 7. Consciousness began to improve on day 5. The serum sodium rose to normal by day 7, after a cumulative loss of 6.7 L total body water. The creatinine clearance rose from 28 to 98 ml per minute on day

Fig 20.—The changes in serum CPK and cholesterol with respect to therapy are shown. The upper and lower limits of the normal range of serum T_3 is shown with changes in serum T_3 levels. (Courtesy of Graham, J. J., and Harding, P. E.: Aust. N. Z. J. Med. 7:163–168, April, 1977.)

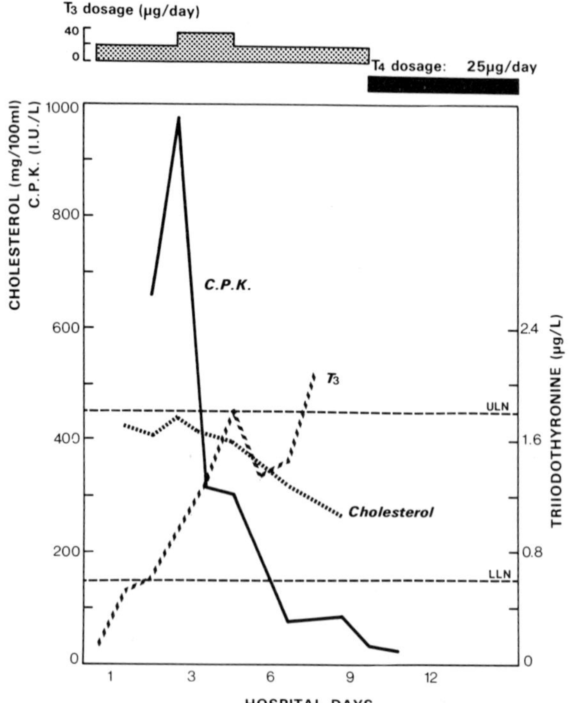

6 and the serum sodium rose despite a net loss of 87 mM sodium. The serum T_3 levels rose steadily to the euthryoid range by day 5. The plasma creatine phosphokinase and cholesterol fell rapidly during treatment (Fig 20). On day 10 the patient was changed from T_3 to thyroxine and increased to 50 μg daily after 1 month. He is presently fully mobile and alert but mildly hypothyroid, with a thyrotropin of 17 mμ/L.

The cause of coma in hypothyroidism remains unclear; hypothermia itself and CO_2 retention may be important factors and hypoglycemia should also be considered. Either low-dose T_3 therapy or high-dose thyroxine therapy appears to be the safest and most productive approach to treatment. Attention to pulmonary function with mechanical ventilation is essential. A dose of 20–40 μg T_3 daily appears to be adequate. Survival depends on adequate supportive therapy until the effects of thyroid hormone become established.

► [Low-dose T_3 versus high-dose T_4. It reminds me of the present views of the treatment of diabetic ketoacidosis. Nonetheless, as Figure 20 shows, low-dose T_3 works and is worth further consideration. However, I am more concerned about the frequency with which the diagnosis of myxedema coma is missed, particularly in elderly people, than with any particular therapeutic regimen. Impallomeni (Age Ageing, 6:71, 1977) is also concerned, because he describes 7 patients with myxedema coma seen over a 2-year period in whom there were frequently unusual clinical features, including generalized seizures. Four of the 7 "were previously diagnosed as suffering from myxedema, but thyroxine therapy had been discontinued." Ah, there's another rub. — T.B.S.] ◄

► ↓ An unusual complication of replacement therapy is reported in the following article. — T.B.S. ◄

Visual Failure during Replacement Therapy in Primary Hypothyroidism with Pituitary Enlargement. Impaired visual fields have been documented in several reports of primary thyroid or gonadal failure with hypersecretion of tropic hormones. J. R. Stockigt, W. B. Essex, R. H. West, R. M. L. Murray and H. D. Breidahl[9] (Alfred Hosp., Melbourne) report data on a patient with long-standing hypothyroidism and pituitary fossa enlargement in whom pressure symptoms developed during T_4 therapy.

Woman, 34, with long-standing hypothyroidism, had headaches associated with an expanded pituitary fossa. She had been seen 6 weeks earlier with a history of cold intolerance and episodic depression since childhood, and hypothyroidism had been diagnosed and treated with 0.1 mg T_4 daily. Increasingly severe headaches

(9) J. Clin. Endocrinol. Metab. 43:1094–1100, November, 1976.

TSH, Prolactin, T$_4$ and T$_3$ Values during Replacement Therapy

Day*	Dose T$_4$ mg/day	Plasma T$_4$ μg/100 ml	Dose T$_3$† μg/day	Plasma T$_3$ ng/100ml	TSH μU/ml	Prolactin ng/ml
0	Nil	1.3	Nil	—	—	—
41	0.1	4.5	Nil	—	250	—
111	0.2	5.5	Nil	—	—	—
115†	0.2	6.4	60	90	46	—
116	0.3	7.4	60	205	30	—
118	0.3	4.6	60	263	28	—
121	0.3	6.9	60	280	18	—
308	0.3	6.1	Nil	68	80	22.5
310†	0.3	7.8	60	200	35	18.9
313	0.3	8.6	60	210	11	12.9
315	0.3	9.0	60	190	7	15.0
317	0.4	11.4	Nil	175	5	14.7
319	0.4	13.0	Nil	140	5	11.7
Normal values:		4–11		75–175	<4	2.4–15.0

*Days after beginning continuous T$_4$ treatment.
†T$_3$ 60 μg/day added on days 115–121 and 309–315.

had ensued while the presenting symptoms resolved. Growth had been retarded from about age 3 and the patient had been slow to learn. She had had 2 normal pregnancies before menses ceased at age 28. Prednisolone had been given intermittently for asthma from age 29. She was about 4½ ft tall and had a hypothyroid facies. The pituitary fossa was markedly enlarged but the anterior clinoids were intact. The estimated bone age was 17. Treatment was continued with 0.2 mg T$_4$ daily and defective peripheral vision was reported after 6 months of treatment. The fields were severely constricted concentrically. An air study showed anterior suprasellar extension. Transfrontal surgery showed suprasellar tissue displacing the optic chiasm and both optic nerves upward. The visual fields were normal postoperatively but diabetes insipidus developed. The epiphyses have shown progressive fusion.

Plasma TSH and prolactin levels were elevated during T$_4$ therapy but were suppressed by hyperreplacement with T$_3$ and T$_4$ preoperatively (table). Examination of the pituitary tissue showed a marked increase in vesiculate mucoid cells on trichrome-periodic acid-schiff staining. This patient appeared to have juvenile familial hypothyroidism of thyroprivic type. Pituitary enlargement appears to have been secondary to hypothyroidism. The paradoxical pressure symptoms suggest imbalance between pituitary TSH content and TSH release during thyroid hormone treatment.

The fact that low-dose replacement aggravates pituitary growth in some animal studies emphasizes the need to closely observe the visual fields in patients with known pituitary enlargement secondary to thyroid hypofunction during thyroid hormone treatment.

▶ [In essence, the authors suggest that inadequate treatment may on occasion be worse than no treatment at all. As shown in the table, the plasma TSH level came down painfully slowly in this patient. — T.B.S.] ◀

THYROID NEOPLASMS

Riedel's Thyroiditis is a rare chronic inflammatory disease of unknown etiology; it may be a manifestation of multifocal fibrosis. The condition was recognized by Riedel (Fig 21) in 1883. D. Katsikas, A. J. Shorthouse and Selwyn Taylor[1] (Royal Postgrad. Med. School, London) encountered 4 patients during a 12-year period, 3 of whom had unusual presentations that caused difficulty in diagnosis. One pa-

Fig 21.—Bernhard Riedel (1846–1916). (Courtesy of Katsikas, D., et al.: Br. J. Surg. 63:929–931, December, 1976.)

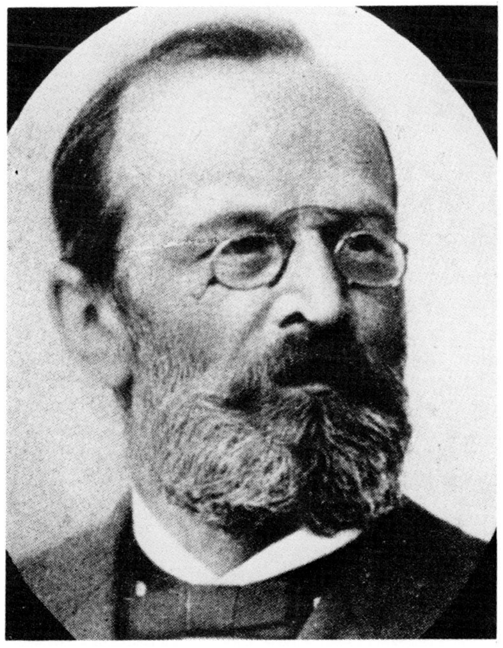

---

(1) Br. J. Surg. 63:929–931, December, 1976.

tient had a sudden painless enlargement of a thyroid swelling present since childhood and another had a gradually enlarging neck swelling present for at least 10 years and associated pain. The third had a 4-week history of a painful, tender goiter, preceded by sore throat and the fourth had progressive, painless enlargement of a neck swelling over 1 year.

Riedel's thyroiditis appears to be a manifestation of a diffuse process when it occurs in association with retroperitoneal fibrosis, mediastinal fibrosis, sclerosing cholangitis and pseudotumor of the orbit. This raises the possibility of autoimmunity. Several associations between Riedel's thyroiditis and autoimmune disease have been described. Eosinophilia suggests that there may be a hypersensitivity response to an unknown antigen. If the etiology is related to an abnormal immune response, cell-mediated immunity may be involved because thyroid antibodies are usually absent or if present are found in titers lower than in Hashimoto's disease.

Histologic confirmation of the disease is mandatory. Needle biopsy is indicated with unilateral involvement of the thyroid. When there is bilateral involvement, a generous wedge of the isthmus is excised. The value of steroids in multifocal fibrosis has been evident in recent years. Two of the present patients improved dramatically on steroid therapy and in 1 of them it was lifesaving. Many patients appear to derive lasting benefit, even after steroids are withdrawn. Possibly the disease is self-limiting; Riedel emphasized its good prognosis.

► [First comes nosologic embarrassment. This first article included in the subchapter Thyroid Neoplasms is a report about patients who don't have a thyroid neoplasm. The problem is that there were not enough selectable papers to warrent a separate section on thyroiditis. The lone representative is placed here because there is plenty of evidence that this inflammatory disease can be destructively invasive, and painfully so, so that clinically it may behave like a neoplasm (see 1977 YEAR BOOK, p. 153).

Second, it is nostalgia time. Look at the photograph (Fig 21). Doctor Riedel was certainly a distinguished-looking man in whom intelligence and accomplishment are wordlessly obvious. Things were done differently in those days. Doctor Riedel recognized the condition in 1883, but he published a description of 2 cases in 1896, 13 years later. I suspect it was not because he was leisurely in his approach to publication that he waited. He was waiting for a broader experience and he didn't feel terribly pressed to get his name into print. Two of my mentors, Drs. Louis Hamman and Arnold Rice Rich, saw, within the space of a couple of years, 4 patients with what has come to be known as Hamman-Rich disease. The publication occurred a decade after the patients were seen, because they thought that they would continue to find more cases at the same rate and that a larger, better-defined description of the syndrome would emerge after the passage of time.

When I was a medical student, my feelings toward these 2 men was best described as *veneration.* Veneration, I had thought, exists for no one these days, but it is still to be found, albeit rarely. My latest encounter occurred several years ago on the last occasion that the "Atlantic City Meetings" were held in Atlantic City. On the short flight from Philadelphia, I sat next to a young investigator from the west coast. We talked amicably. He told me of his abiding interest in hematology and his exhilaration and anxieties about the opportunity to present his work for the first time at a national meeting. I mentioned that, eons ago, I had studied with Dr. Maxwell Wintrobe and had gotten to know his wife. My companion looked at me with new respect and I asked him if he would like to meet the distinguished couple. He agreed. I then suggested that he turn around and I proceeded to introduce him to Doctor and Mrs. Wintrobe, who were seated behind us. What I saw in the young man's eyes and in his respectful smile was veneration.

"Once in the dear dead days beyond recall. . . ." —T.B.S.] ◄

► ↓ Now, back to the subject of an ugly disease. Look below. —T.B.S. ◄

Plasma Thyroglobulin in Detecting Thyroid Carcinoma after Childhood Head and Neck Irradiation. The importance of detecting thyroid nodules has been emphasized recently by the need to evaluate potentially malignant nodular disease in large numbers of patients given head and neck irradiation during childhood. Arthur B. Schneider, Murray J. Favus, Max E. Stachura, John E. Arnold, U. Yun Ryo, Steven Pinsky, Martin Colman, Margaret J. Arnold and Lawrence A. Frohman[2] (Michael Reese Hosp. and Med. Center, Chicago) measured plasma thyroglobulin levels in 904 patients who had histories of head and neck irradiation during childhood, whose records were available and who were examined consecutively during a 9-month period starting in January 1974. Thyroglobulin was determined by radioimmunoassay. Fifty-five control subjects had similar age and sex distributions.

The mean thyroglobulin in control subjects was 15 ng/ml, and the upper limit at 2 SD above the mean was 28 ng/ml. There was a very large overlap of thyroglobulin levels in normal and abnormal subjects. High levels were found in 13% of 608 clinically normal subjects, but the mean level

---

(2) Ann. Intern. Med. 86:29–34, January, 1977.

was significantly elevated in patients with nodular thyroid disease (49.8 vs. 27.0 ng/ml). The mean levels in subjects with benign and malignant thyroid nodules were 48.8 and 53.9 ng/ml, respectively. No significant differences in mean thyroglobulin levels were found when the 52 subjects with thyroid carcinoma were classed by lesion size, histology, vessel invasion, capsule invasion, number of lobes involved, number of malignant foci or nodal involvement. No significant group differences in thyroxine, triiodothyronine or thyrotropin levels were found.

The most complete evaluation of these irradiated subjects includes a detailed history, physical examination and thyroid scintigram. Thyroglobulin assay cannot substitute for the current screening procedures, but scintigraphy conceivably could be reserved for subjects with palpable nodules or elevated thyroglobulin levels to reduce overall costs. A normal circulating thyroglobulin level does not exclude thyroid nodules, but an elevated value indicates a need for thorough thyroid evaluation. Follow-up examination of irradiated subjects with elevated thyroglobulin levels who appear normal will help resolve questions concerning the natural history of clinically undetectable thyroid tumors. Such information is central to the development of a rational approach to the management of radiation-exposed patients.

► [A few years ago (1976 YEAR BOOK, p. 149) I said that a preoperative and postoperative survey in patients exposed to radiation "might be informative." This idea also occurred to the authors of this article and the results are presented. It was no great help. My comment was made in discussing an article in which elevated serum thyroglobulin served as a marker for thyroid cancer metastasis. Similar results have been obtained by LoGerfo (Lancet 1:881, 1977). How else to improve diagnostic accuracy? Look ahead. — T.B.S.] ◄

Fine-Needle Aspiration Cytology in Preoperative Diagnosis of Thyroid Nodules. Fine-needle aspiration biopsy has been used to diagnose abnormalities in a number of organs preoperatively. Marvin C. Gershengorn, Michael R. McClung, Elizabeth W. Chu, Thomas A. S. Hanson, Bruce D. Weintraub and Jacob Robbins[3] (Natl. Inst. of Health) assessed the utility of aspiration cytology in the preoperative diagnosis of thyroid nodules in 50 consecutive adults referred with this diagnosis in 2½ years. The cytolog-

---

(3) Ann. Intern. Med. 87:265–269, September, 1977.

DIAGNOSTIC ACCURACY OF ASPIRATION CYTOLOGY

Cytology		Histology				
Classification	Number	Carcinoma			Occult Carcinoma	Benign
		Papillary	Follicular	Medullary		
Malignant	9	5	1	1	1	1
Suspicious	5	0	1	1	1	2
Benign	18	0	1	0	0	17
Total	32	5	3	2	2	20

ic diagnosis was made without knowledge of clinical or laboratory data and did not influence the decision for operation. The patients had discrete, usually single, thyroid nodules. Aspiration was done in the outpatient clinic with sterile technique and intradermal anesthesia. Two patients bled into evacuated large, hemorrhagic nodules. The major morbidity was mild pain, tenderness or both.

Two patients had cyst evacuation with no recurrence for over a year of follow-up. Thirty-three others had excision biopsy. Five of these patients had two nodules. All but 1 of the 33 had "cold" nodules on technetium scanning; the exception had a "warm" nodule. In 5 of 25 patients given L-thyroxine the nodule became smaller. A satisfactory aspiration specimen was obtained in all but 1 of the 33 patients. Nine malignancies were diagnosed (table); 7 were confirmed histologically. There was 1 false positive finding and 1 occult carcinoma. Histologic studies showed malignancy in 3 of 5 cases with suspicious aspiration findings. One of 18 aspiration diagnoses of benignity was a false negative diagnosis.

Fine-needle aspiration cytologic examination is of definite value in the preoperative evaluation of thyroid nodules. A definite cytologic diagnosis of malignancy warrants excision biopsy, but a negative diagnosis should not at present preclude a decision for excision biopsy. The procedure can help evaluate the need for excision biopsy in aged patients and those with medical complications and can be of value in selection of patients for long-term thyroid suppression therapy.

▶ [Needle biopsy goes back a long way (see 1964–1965 YEAR BOOK, pp. 58–60). It is important to distinguish between the older biopsy, in which a core of tissue was removed, from that presented here, in which there is aspiration of cells. This works better. Walfish et al., in a companion article (Ann. Intern. Med. 87:270, 1977), think so too. These latter workers also thought so when they published essentially the same material in another journal (Walfish et al.: Surgery 82:474, 1977). Naughty!

Are you impressed with the number of patients studied? You are about to be considerably more impressed when you look ahead. — T.B.S.]

Thin-Needle Biopsy of Cold Goiter Nodules in 4,555 Patients: Results and Clinical Significance are reviewed by G. Galvan, G. B. Pohl and I. Skerbisch[4] (Inst. of Radiotherapy and Nuclear Medicine, Salzburg). Although thyroid carcinoma is only occasionally associated with normal or increased iodine or ^{99m}Tc-pertechnetate uptake, each instance of decreased accumulation may be caused by a malignancy. If such a cold nodule is only observed, there is the risk of failure of early diagnosis; if resection is done, this generally prophylactic procedure must be weighed against the rate of complications. Since 1967, fine-needle biopsy and cytologic evaluation have helped solve this problem.

Within a period of 8 years, 4,555 patients were examined in this manner; 1,076 underwent surgery and cytologic diagnoses were histologically confirmed. In 715 patients with normal or degenerative cytologic findings the diagnosis was correct in 95%. Eight malignancies, 13 Hürthle cell adenomas and 26 cases of Hashimoto's thyroiditis were not correctly diagnosed. The diagnostic errors in the case of malignancies were due to puncturing of the wrong nodule in 3 instances and the presence of highly differentiated, partially degenerated, follicular carcinomas in the others. In 322 cases with suspect or malignant cytology, 129 malignancies (40%) were confirmed. False positive diagnoses were mostly determined by histologically atypical adenomas; Hashimoto's thyroiditis was recognized readily in the advanced stage only.

TECHNIQUE. — The biopsy is taken with patient in the sitting position; the nodule is fixated with one hand and the point of entry is disinfected. Care must be taken not to puncture an epidermal vein, which may cause a cosmetically undesirable hematoma. The patient should not swallow during the procedure. Puncture is achieved by a disposable no. 12 needle attached to a disposable 10-ml syringe. After the nodule is punctured, aspiration is carried out. Eventually the cyst is voided by compression; otherwise the needle

---

(4)   Schweiz. Med. Wochenschr. 106:1247–1251, Sept. 11, 1976.

is advanced under suction in two or three directions. The piston is retracted and the needle is pulled out. The puncture site is compressed by moderate pressure.

This technique fills the diagnostic void in cases of so-called cold thyroid nodules. It is quickly accomplished on an outpatient basis, with minimal inconvenience to the patient and practically free of complications, other than occasional hemorrhage into the nodule or transient pain in the cervical region. Reliability is high, although the cytologic findings should be evaluated in relation to the clinical picture. Negative cytologic results should not rule out nodule resection in patients with suspect clinical findings.

▶ [This group took their time and really waited until they had a lot to say. Doctor Riedel would have been proud (see article by Katsikas et al. in this chapter). And, if thyroid aspiration biopsy needs final approval, it receives it from Dr. George Crile, Jr. (Postgrad. Med. 60:105, 1976), an admirable clinical investigator who has been blessed with the happy facility to be mostly correct in his often controversial views.

What prognostic value do histologic findings have? Look ahead.— T.B.S.] ◀

Surgical Significance of Capsule Invasion of Adenoma of the Thyroid. Vascular and capsule invasion of thyroid adenomas have been emphasized as being histologic evidence of malignancy, even if cytologic atypism has not been noted. Futoshi Iida[5] (Shinshu Univ.) established a histologic definition of invasion in a series of 611 adenomas of the thyroid diagnosed as benign based on cytologic atypism, on the basis of the correlation between tumor parenchyma and stromal features, and related it to the postoperative results.

Only marked destructive phenomena in the capsule were considered as invasion. Tissue invasion that cut off and turned out collagen fibers was considered as histologic evidence of capsule destruction (Fig 22) but a localized push-out without cutoff of the fibers was not. Thyroid follicles within the capsule did not indicate invasion if no destruction of surrounding collagen fibers was evident. Capsule invasion so defined was seen in only 8 adenomas (1.3%), 4 tubular and 4 simple adenomas. No colloid adenoma was found to be invasive. None of the 8 patients with invasive adenoma had clinical signs of recurrence on follow-up for

---

(5) Surg. Gynecol. Obstet. 144:710–712, May, 1977.

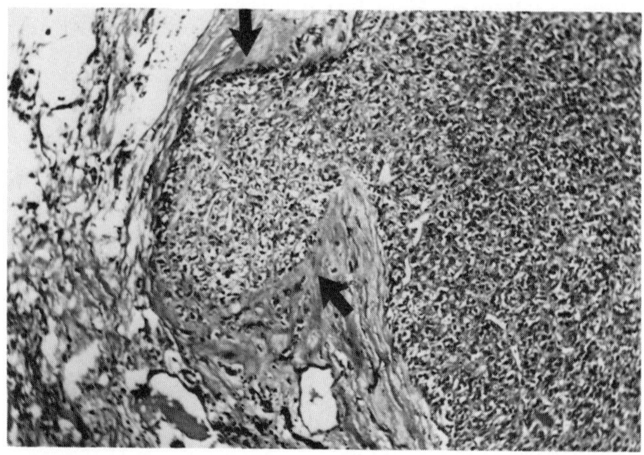

Fig 22. — Tumor tissue invades into the capsule cutting off and turning out the collagen fibers. Hematoxylin-eosin; reduced from ×40. (Courtesy of Iida, F.: Surg. Gynecol. Obstet. 114:710–712, May, 1977.)

2–10 years. Five other patients, none with any evidence of capsule invasion, had repeat operations for recurrence of a thyroid nodule; 3 had colloid adenomas.

This study showed no relationship of invasive thyroid adenoma with recurrence. The capsule invasion noted in adenomas may not be histologic evidence of a malignant condition, but merely an incidental phenomenon in the progress of growth of an adenoma. The malignant potential of a thyroid tumor should be based on the cytologic atypism of the tumor cells, not on the presence of capsule invasion. Recurrences may be due to leaving microadenoma in the thyroid at the initial operation.

► [Invasive, yes; malignant, no! Figure 22 looks frightening enough, but patients harboring such adenomas do well.

Other things you should know follow. (1) A patient with undifferentiated thyroid carcinoma metastatic to the lung also had a leukomoid reaction with a striking increase of blood eosinophils (Miller et al.: Chest 71:6, 1977). (2) Metastasis of thyroid carcinoma to the skin is rare, but does occur (Auty: Arch. Dermatol. 113:675, 1977; and Runne and Mooder: Dtsch. Med. Wochenschr. 101:1831, 1976). (3) There are unusual thyroid cancers such as an apparently primary mucoepidermoid carcinoma (Rhatigan: Cancer 39:210, 1977) and a microfollicular, amyloid-producing carcinoma resembling a medullary carcinoma (ibid., p. 1573).

Are you beginning to feel that I am providing you with more information than you deserve, need or want? Relax! It is difficult, indeed, for anyone to try to recall all that is presented in a volume like this YEAR BOOK; the best one can hope for is not *recall,* but merely recognition. Sometime someone may tell you of a primary mucoepidermoid carcinoma of the thyroid. Ping, you vaguely remember seeing it here. You look it up. You are brilliant. Or, take another tack. An old friend told me that he was one among many who read the YEAR BOOK as a pleasant, guilt-abating technique for falling asleep at night. Slumber on ahead. — T.B.S.] ◄

Papillary Thyroid Carcinoma: Impact of Therapy in 576 Patients. Although a trend toward a more conservative surgical approach to papillary thyroid carcinoma has developed, no uniform opinion exists on how to treat this neoplasm. The wide range of biologic behavior of the tumor makes evaluation of its therapy difficult. Ernest L. Mazzaferri, Robert L. Young, James E. Oertel, William T. Kemmerer and Carey P. Page[6] report a retrospective analysis of the clinical and pathologic findings in 576 patients with papillary thyroid carcinoma. Follow-up averaged 6.9 years (table). Women constituted about 62% of the series. The mean patient age was about 32. A thyroid mass was initially noted by the patient in 40% of cases. Most patients had a single palpable nodule. Nineteen patients were thyrotoxic at some time. A history of head and neck irradiation was obtained in 24 patients (4%). Twenty patients had at least

STATUS OF PATIENTS AS OF SEPTEMBER 1972

Papillary Thyroid Carcinoma (n = 576)

Status	All	Without cancer	With cancer
Alive	532	523	9
(%)*	(92.4)	(90.8)	(1.6)
Dead	19	12	7†
(%)	(3.3)	(2.1)	(1.2)
Lost	25	25	0
(%)	(4.3)	(4.3)	0
Total	576	560	16
(%)	(100)	(97.2)	(2.8)

*Percent of all patients with papillary carcinoma in this study.
†Five patients died of thyroid cancer.

(6) Medicine (Baltimore) 56:171–196, May, 1977.

one other malignancy. Four patients had coexisting hyper-parathyroidism.

The average interval between the discovery of a thyroid nodule and surgery was 13 months. Multiple lesions were found in 29% of thyroid specimens. Nearly all patients received adjunctive medical therapy with thyroid hormone, radioiodine or external irradiation. No deaths resulted from surgery, but 46 patients (44%) had major complications after total thyroidectomy and extensive neck dissection and 27 patients (13%) after total thyroidectomy with regional node excision. Papillary thyroid cancer recurred in 70 patients (12.2%) who were free of disease after treatment; 8 patients had recurrences at distant sites. The mortality was 3.3%; 5

Fig 23.—Cumulative recurrence rates for those in whom follow-up was 1 year or longer divided according to the type of medical therapy used postoperatively. (Courtesy of Mazzaferri, E. L., et al.: Medicine (Baltimore) 56:171–196, May, 1977.)

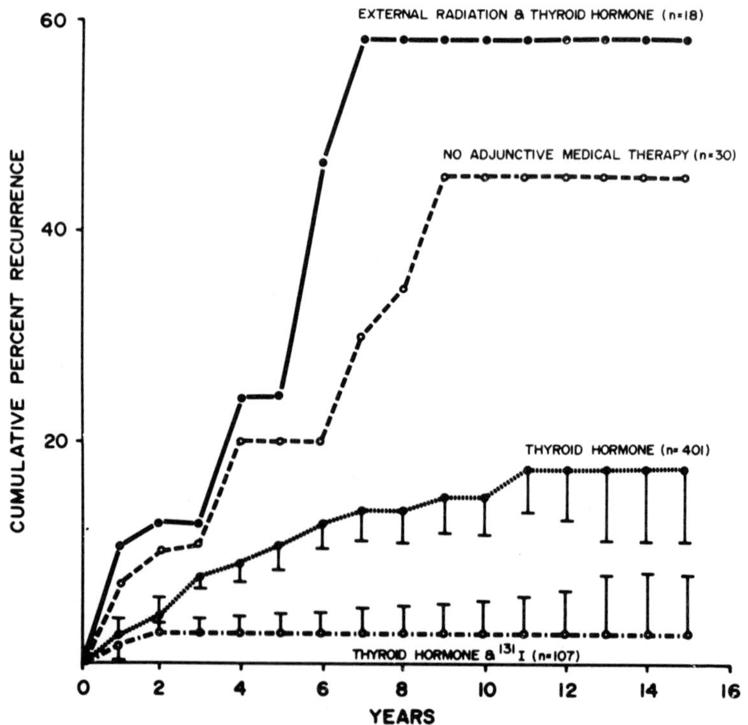

deaths were a direct result of thyroid cancer. Patients under age 30 at diagnosis had a higher rate of recurrence than older patients. Recurrences were most frequent in patients with symptomatic thyroid lesions and in those with lesions 5 cm or larger in diameter. Cervical node metastasis did not influence recurrence or survival. Recurrences were more than twice as frequent in patients having subtotal thyroidectomy initially, but the extent of lymph node surgery did not influence the recurrence or survival rates. Recurrence rates are shown in Figure 23 in relation to adjunctive therapy.

Thyroid hormone therapy is indicated in all patients with papillary thyroid carcinoma. Total or near-total thyroidectomy is preferable to a more limited excision. Local excision of obviously metastatic cervical nodes is appropriate. Ablative doses of ^{131}I are indicated postoperatively, especially in patients with multiple or locally invasive lesions or lesions larger than 2.5 cm and those with metastases.

► [This is an important article and it represents, however imperfect, a rare real contribution in a controversial and emotion-laden area. It should be read in full by anyone with a serious interest in the subject. Several things are noteworthy. First, in this large group of patients treated (or perhaps in some instances, mistreated) by a variety of techniques, only a total of 5 patients died of thyroid cancer in a follow-up averaging nearly 7 years. Second, Figure 23 shows striking differences and makes a strong argument for the use of total thyroidectomy, with postoperative ^{131}I treatment followed by maintenance on TSH-suppressive doses of thyroid hormone. However, one should be aware that Figure 23 speaks to *recurrence*, not mortality or even rates of recurrent symptoms of carcinoma. Whereas recurrences are significantly more likely to occur in patients who initially had symptoms, there's no quantitative information presented as to what percentage of those who had recurrences were symptomatic. I emphasize this point because there are many patients with local lymph node metastases who remain asymptomatic for years. Finally, of the 5 patients who died of cancer of the thyroid, only 1 patient, an elderly man who already had had extension into neck muscles at the time of initial operation, had received suppressive therapy with thyroid.

From Figure 23 it is clear that recurrences are minimized by total thyroidectomy followed by ^{131}I therapy. However, surgical complications are significant and whether this form of therapy serves patients best in terms of longevity and good health remains, in my mind, in question.

There are, as usual, multiple articles on this subject, most of which are not worth mentioning. I will single out only one for comment. Clark and Demling (Am. J. Surg. 132:615, 1976) make the point that in elderly patients with thyroid nodules, those who are multinodular rarely require surgical intervention. — T.B.S.] ◄

Radical Thyroidectomy for Malignant Thyroid Tumor: Prognosis and Complications were investigated by R. Wahl, J. Nievergelt, H. D. Röher and B. Oellers[7] (Univ. of Heidelberg). Based on the frequent reports of microscopically disseminated intraglandular tumoral expansion and because of the effective adjunctive ^{131}I therapy for extrathyroidally accumulating tumor tissue, the necessity of radical thyroidectomy has been increasingly recognized for all cases of thyroid carcinoma.

During 1955–74, 270 patients underwent surgery for thyroid malignancy. Before 1967 less radical surgical methods were preferred in the 117 patients; since 1968, total thyroidectomy has been the choice, if necessary supplemented by selective or radical neck dissection, whenever curative surgery was still feasible. Analysis of histologic types showed an increase of differentiated tumors in the second period of observation (70.6% and 48.7%). There was a clear shift to less advanced tumor stages during this same time.

Between 1955 and 1967 subtotal thyroidectomy or unilateral lobectomy was usually done (48%). Only in 5% of the patients was the entire gland removed and in 25% only a

Fig 24.—Postoperative complications (recurrent nerve paralysis and tetany) during two periods of observation. (Courtesy of Wahl, R., et al.: Dtsch. Med. Wochenschr. 102:13–20, Jan. 7, 1977.)

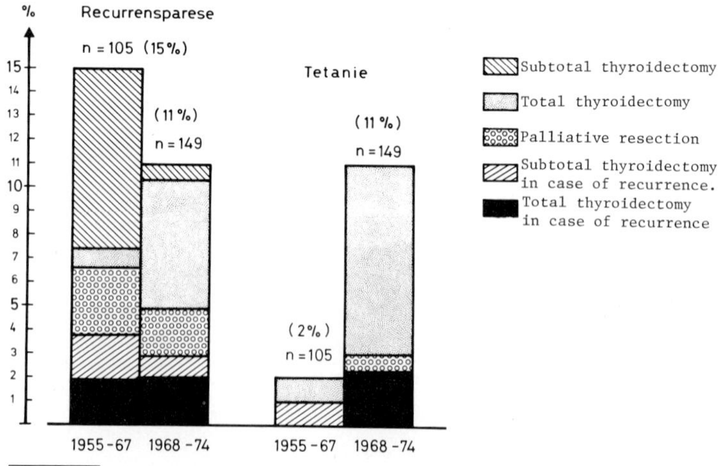

(7) Dtsch. Med. Wochenschr. 102:13–20, Jan. 7, 1977.

palliative operation was possible. During the second time period, most patients underwent radical thyroidectomy; only 7% were treated by lobectomy or subtotal resection and the number of palliative operations was considerably reduced. The most significant complications are shown in Figure 24. Despite the radical nature of surgery no increase in recurrent nerve paralysis occurred during the second time period; a reduction from 15% to 11% was observed. However, a considerable increase in the incidence of tetany, from 2% to 11%, was noted after radical thyroidectomy. Postoperative mortality was reduced by slightly above 4%; it remained high in local palliative procedures, 20% in the second time period, 31% in the first. Even more impressive was the fewer number of recurrences, from 54% in those operated on during 1955–67 to 10.6% in those treated during 1968–74. The larger number of patients in the second time period, the relative increase of histologically differentiated tumor forms and early stage at the start of therapy are functions of improved early diagnostic techniques.

For treatment of a thyroid malignancy, particularly of differentiated types, several mutually supplementary treatments may be considered, including operation, irradiation and hormonal suppression therapy. Even more than the diminished incidence of recurrence, it is the improved survival of patients with differentiated carcinoma which clearly supports radical thyroidectomy. Its advantages outweigh the increased incidence of postoperative hypoparathyroidism.

► [Look at Figure 24. In view of the previous comment, the reader can guess that I do not agree with the judgments reached here.

Since I am taken with thyroid suppression as a form of therapy, it is important for me to be certain that suppression is real. A technique to do this using thyrotropin-releasing hormone is proposed by Hoffman et al. (J. Clin. Endocrinol. Metab. 44:892, 1977). — T.B.S.] ◄

Malignant Lymphomas of the Thyroid: Clinical Pathologic Study of 35 Patients Including Ultrastructural Observations. Jerome S. Burke, James J. Butler and Lillian M. Fuller[8] (Univ. of Texas, Houston) reviewed the findings in 35 patients seen in 1951–75 with malignant lymphoma presenting in the thyroid. The 26 women and 9 men had a mean age at initial diagnosis of 65. All presented

---

(8) Cancer 39:1587–1602, April, 1977.

1977) found that the most common type of carcinoma associated with Hashimoto's thyroiditis is lymphoma. — T.B.S.] ◄

The following review articles are recommended to the reader:

Bernal, J., and Refetoff, S.: The action of thyroid hormone, Clin. Endocrinol. (Oxf.) 6:227, 1977.

DeGroot, L. J., and Niepomniszcze, H.: Biosynthesis of thyroid hormone: Basic and clinical aspects, Metabolism 26:665, 1977.

Irvine, W. J., and Toft, A. D.: The diagnosis and treatment of thyrotoxicosis, Clin. Endocrinol. (Oxf.) 5:687, 1976.

Roche, J., and Michel, R.: Les deux triiodothyronines, T_3 et rT_3, Ann. Endocrinol. (Paris) 38:243, 1977.

Sterling, K.: The mitochondrial route of thyroid hormone action, Bull. N.Y. Acad. Med. 53:260, 1977.

Zachrisson, B. F.: Thyroid angiography, Acta Radiol. [Suppl. 350] (Stockh.), 1976.

The Adrenal Gland

Large Product of Cell-Free Translation of Messenger RNA Coding for Corticotropin. Various endocrine peptides appear to be initially synthesized from larger precursors, which are then converted to their respective peptides by posttranslational cleavage. Multiple molecular forms of ACTH exist in pituitary extracts of many different animals, suggesting that ACTH initially is synthesized as a large precursor molecule. Shigetada Nakanishi, Shunzo Taii, Yukio Hirata, Shigeru Matsukura, Hiroo Imura and Shosaku Numa[9] studied the translation of mRNA coding for ACTH in a heterologous cell-free system in an attempt to demonstrate the initial, direct product of this process. Studies were done with RNA isolated from bovine pituitaries and rabbit antiserums against porcine or synthetic (1–18) ACTH. Cell-free products were immunoprecipitated and solubilized by sodium dodecyl sulfate-polyacrylamide gel electrophoresis.

Polyadenylate-containing RNA prepared from the membrane fraction of anterior pituitaries directed the synthesis of a large translation product related to corticotropin in a cell-free system derived from wheat germ. Further evidence for the identity of the translation product was provided by the presence of a common peptide in the chymotryptic digest of ^{35}S-methionine-labeled cell-free product and in that of authentic corticotropin. The estimated molecular weight of the translation product was about 35,000.

Corticotropin mRNA directs the cell-free synthesis of a product that contains the amino acid sequence of corticotropin but is much larger than this hormone. The large precursor molecules may function to facilitate the transport of secretory proteins through the membrane. The large cell-free product of ACTH may represent the initial precursor that is

---

(9)   Proc. Natl. Acad. Sci. U.S.A. 73:4319–4323, December, 1976.

rapidly converted to the large or intermediate form of ACTH and is finally cleaved to natural ACTH in pituitary tissues.

▶ [Now I know why there is all the fuss about recombinant experiments. Beware of wheat germ extract gone beserk!

A return to reality is hardly less astonishing. Is this large product of cell-free translation of messenger RNA the same large, parent molecule that contains ACTH, lipotropin and endorphin referred to earlier?

Of course, we've heard of large products in relation to ACTH before. "Last week's" designations were "large ACTH" and "big ACTH." In addition, the ACTH produced by a primary pituitary tumor has recently been characterized fully by Krieger et al. (Clin. Endocrinol. (Oxf.) 5:455, 1976). — T.B.S.] ◀

Acute Unilateral Adrenal Hemorrhage Following ACTH Administration in a Patient with Cushing's Syndrome. Adrenal hemorrhage has been reported to be associated with adrenal venography and to follow ACTH administration. Also, remission of Cushing's syndrome after adrenal venography or ACTH administration has been reported.

John F. Redman and Fred H. Faas[1] (Univ. of Arkansas) describe a patient with Cushing's syndrome in whom a clinically significant, pathologically verified adrenal hemorrhage followed ACTH administration.

Woman, 61, had a history of tentative diagnosis of Cushing's syndrome 8 months earlier, weakness for 2–3 years and blackouts and staggering for 1 year. She reported bruising easily. She had been treated for hypertension and diabetes for 5 years.

Centripetal obesity, a florid face, a cervical hump, abdominal striae and large ecchymoses were present. Blood pressure was 170/100 mm Hg. Steroid data confirmed the diagnosis of Cushing's disease (table). Severe pain in the left flank and upper abdomen developed on the 3d day of an ACTH stimulation test and lasted 5 days. A 10% fall in hematocrit was observed. An excretory urogram showed lateral displacement of the superior pole of the left kidney, more marked than was present 3 months before. Ultrasonography showed a sonolucent area, 6×6 cm, above the left kidney.

Surgical exploration 2 weeks after onset of flank pain revealed a large left suprarenal mass and dense fibrosis from the diaphragm to the renal pedicle and to the lower pole of the kidney. The mass was removed with the adrenal gland and kidney. The hyperplastic right adrenal was also excised. A thin rim of left adrenal gland surrounded a 6×4-cm mass of thrombus; no tumor was identified.

---

(1) Am. J. Med. 61:533–536, October, 1976.

STEROID DATA CONFIRMING DIAGNOSIS OF
CUSHING'S DISEASE*

Medication	Date (mo/yr)	24 Hour Urine 17-OHCS (mg/g creatinine)	Plasma Cortisol (µg/dl)
None	2/75	23.9	8 A.M.—21
			Noon—19
			4 P.M.—23
			8 P.M.—16
None		17.9	
Dexamethasone (20 µg/kg/day—day 2)		4.9	13
None	3/75	19.3	
None		17.6	
2nd day of dexamethasone (20 µg/kg/day)		12.9	
2nd day of dexamethasone (8 mg/day)		4.1	
3rd day of ACTH gel (40 U twice a day IM)		222	
4th day of ACTH gel (40 U twice a day IM)		182	
None		20.9	
Day after metyrapone (3 g/day)		166	

*Urine 17-hydroxycorticosteroids (17-OHCS) were determined by the Porter-Silber method. Plasma cortisol was determined fluorimetrically. Normal urine 17-OHCS are 2–7 mg/gm creatinine, with normal suppression of urine 17-OHCS being to less than 1 mg/gm creatinine and plasma cortisol to less than 5 µg/dl on administration of dexameth-asone, 20 µg/kg/24 hours in 4 divided doses.

Patients with Cushing's syndrome and enlarged hypervascular adrenal glands secondary to overstimulation by endogenous ACTH seem to be candidates for adrenal hemorrhage. Adrenal hemorrhage is usually diagnosed post mortem. If it is suspected, steroids should be given to protect against possible adrenal insufficiency, along with supportive measures with volume expansion if necessary. Surgical exploration may or may not be necessary, depending on the amount of adrenal bleeding.

► [In ancient days when I was young and ACTH first became available for clinical use, the question was raised as to whether permanent damage to adrenal glands could result from constant stimulation with ACTH. The only evidence that I could uncover (the reference has been lost but I recall that it was in *Proceedings of the Society for Experimental Biology and Medicine*) was that in unilaterally adrenalectomized mice given constant infusions of ACTH, the hypertrophied remaining adrenal gland could become apoplectic and be destroyed. This is not too far a cry from what we find here. I agree with the authors' retrospective view that 3 days of ACTH administration in such patients is too much and unnecessary.

Hemorrhage is not the only threat to patients with Cushing's syndrome. More often, they are threatened by thrombosis, which has been reported a number of times, most recently by Sjoberg et al. (Acta Med. Scand. 199: 95, 1976). I mentioned about 8 years ago that one of my patients, after successful bilateral adrenalectomy for Cushing's syndrome, suddenly died of a massive pulmonary embolus on the 4th postoperative day.— T.B.S.] ◄

Nelson's Syndrome: Frequency, Prognosis and Effect of Prior Pituitary Irradiation. It is generally estimated that pituitary tumors will develop in 10% of patients after adrenalectomy. The natural history of these tumors is not clear. Thomas J. Moore, Robert G. Dluhy, Gordon H. Williams and John P. Cain[2] (Boston) reviewed 120 cases of Cushing's disease in patients who were followed for 2–20 years after adrenalectomy for bilateral adrenal hyperplasia. In 9 patients (8%), there was radiographic evidence of a pituitary tumor associated with progressive cutaneous melanosis after adrenalectomy (Nelson's syndrome) during the mean follow-up of 8 years. Three other patients had radiographic evidence of pituitary tumors before adrenalectomy.

The patients with and without pituitary tumors are compared in the table. Two tumor patients presented with headache and 2 with visual field disorders, whereas the others were discovered on follow-up sellar x-ray studies. The time from adrenalectomy to discovery of the pituitary tumor ranged from 6 months to 16 years; four tumors were discovered more than 9 years after adrenalectomy. All study patients had some cutaneous hyperpigmentation. All 3 patients with evidence of pituitary tumor before adrenalectomy had cutaneous melanosis. Two of them were over age 50, whereas the study patients tended to be younger when Cushing's disease was diagnosed. Tumors causing compressive symptoms generally were treated surgically first and then irradiated. Four of 5 patients operated on had chromophobe adenomas. Seven patients are living an average of 9.7 years after the pituitary tumors were found. Two of the patients with preadrenalectomy pituitary tumors are living and well. Three study patients required thyroid supple-

---

(2)   Ann. Intern. Med. 85:731–734, December, 1976.

COMPARISON OF PATIENTS AT THE TIME OF DIAGNOSIS
OF CUSHING'S DISEASE*

	BAH without Nelson's Syndrome	BAH with Nelson's Syndrome
Number	111	9
Mean age at diagnosis of Cushing's disease (range)		
Male	35 yrs (19 to 55)	21 yrs
Female	35 yrs (15 to 67)	31 yrs (14 to 52)
Male:female ratio	1:4	1:8
Mean 17-hydroxycorticoid excretion, $mg/24\,h$	19	20
Mean 17-ketosteroid excretion, $mg/24\,h$	24	22
Mean duration of symptoms before diagnosis of BAH (range)	2.8 yrs (1 month to 11 yrs)	2.9 yrs (4 months to 10 yrs)

*BAH = bilateral adrenal hyperplasia.

ments for secondary hypothyroidism. Two have stable visual field defects. One manifested a 3d nerve palsy after irradiation of the pituitary.

Most patients in this series with Nelson's syndrome are clinically stable several years after pituitary tumors were discovered. One of the 2 deaths was due to breast cancer, and the other was directly related to a malignant pituitary neoplasm. The pathogenesis appears to differ from that of tumors present at the time Cushing's disease is diagnosed. All patients should be followed indefinitely by sellar x-ray studies after adrenalectomy for bilateral adrenal hyperplasia, regardless of previous pituitary irradiation.

► [The last sentence of this article should be modified to read, "All patients *who develop some degree of hyperpigmentation* should be followed . . ." Postadrenalectomy pituitary tumors developing without increasing pigmentation is unheard of in the literature and unspoken of in my experience.

The prevalence of sella enlargement in patients with Cushing's disease varies. The present authors quote a figure of about 10% but MacErlean et al. (Br. J. Radiol. 49:820, 1976) found sella enlargement in 20 of 80 patients (23%) with Cushing's disease.

Are the pituitaries of patients with Nelson's syndrome stimulable? Studies by Krieger and Luria (J. Clin. Endocrinol. Metab. 44:361, 1977) indicate that they are, suggesting again, that Cushing's syndrome is primarily a hypothalamic disease with the corticotrophs being driven by an abnormal hypothalamic stimulus. Indeed, Liberman et al. (ibid. 43:913, 1976) followed for nearly a year before operation a patient with Cushing's disease due to a chromaphobe adenoma and demonstrated periodic hormonogenesis at 86-day intervals and with paradoxical dexamethasone responses, further evidence suggesting aberrant hypothalamic modulation.

How sexy are patients with Cushing's syndrome (not sexy looking, sexy feeling)? I ask this question to (1) regain your wandering attention and (2) glide to the following article. — Ed.] ◄

Plasma Testosterone Profiles in Cushing's Syndrome. Gonadal and sexual disturbances are frequent in both women and men with Cushing's syndrome. A. G. H. Smals, P. W. C. Kloppenborg and Th. J. Benraad[3] (Univ. of Nijmegen) obtained testosterone profiles during adrenocortical suppression and stimulation in 8 women and 2 men with Cushing's disease and 2 men with Cushing's syndrome due to adrenal adenoma. Six women had serious hirsutism and all premenopausal women reported menstrual abnormalities. Loss of libido and impotence were mentioned by 3 of the 4 men with Cushing's syndrome. ACTH was given intravenously over 8 hours and dexamethasone was given for 6 days. Plasma testosterone was radioimmunoassayed.

The mean plasma testosterone concentration in women with Cushing's disease, 43 ng/100 ml, was significantly above that in 23 control women. Five of the 6 women with severe hirsutism had supranormal values. The men with Cushing's syndrome had a mean plasma testosterone concentration of 320 ng/100 ml, significantly lower than that in control men; 2 had subnormal mean values. Serum LH levels were normal in the 4 men with Cushing's syndrome. The mean ACTH-induced plasma testosterone rise was significantly increased in the women with Cushing's disease, but the declines in men with Cushing's syndrome were comparable to those in control men. Dexamethasone reduced plasma testosterone levels significantly more in women with Cushing's disease than in control women. Testosterone levels were essentially unchanged by 8 mg dexamethasone in both men with Cushing's syndrome and control men. The plasma testosterone concentration fell sharply after 16 mg dexamethasone in the men with Cushing's syndrome, whether or not cortisol levels were suppressed. Serum LH levels did not change significantly during dexamethasone

(3)   J. Clin. Endocrinol. Metab. 45:240–245, August, 1977.

administration. Adrenalectomy reduced the elevated plasma testosterone levels in women with Cushing's disease to values significantly below those in control women. In the men with Cushing's syndrome testosterone levels rose sharply after adrenalectomy or adenotomy to values twice the preoperative value, whereas serum LH levels were essentially unchanged. Menses became regular and hirsutism decreased after adrenalectomy in all the premenopausal women. In the men with Cushing's syndrome, libido and potency returned to normal.

The findings suggest that the gonadal and sexual disturbances that often occur in men and women with Cushing's syndrome may have different causes: adrenal hyperandrogenism in women and glucocorticoid-induced Leydig cell suppression in men. A direct effect on hypercortisolism at the hypothalamic, pituitary or ovarian level cannot be excluded in women as a cause of gonadal and sexual dysfunction.

► [First, the authors stand accused of sexist attitudes. They examined the libido of men with Cushing's disease but only discussed the menstrual cycle and hirsutism of the women.

The findings are interesting and the interpretations plausible but both must be accepted with some caution, because the only androgen measured was testosterone. Other androgens like dehydroepiandrosterone and dehydroepiandrosterone sulfate might undergo fluctuations that would lead to some rethinking of what has transpired. The decreased testosterone levels are confirmed by the studies of Luton et al. (J. Clin. Endocrinol. Metab. 45:488, 1977), and Anderson and Walters (Aust. N.Z. J. Obstet. Gynecol. 16:225, 1976) describe the course of a pregnant patient with Cushing's syndrome. She was treated by external radiation and a normal female infant was born.

Lest you forget, relative testosterone deficiency in male patients with Cushing's syndrome has been reported before (1975 YEAR BOOK, p. 294). — T.B.S.] ◄

Spontaneous Hypercortisolism without Cushing's Syndrome. Hyposensitivity of target tissues to hormone action has been described in many clinical states but peripheral hyposensitivity to cortisol has not been reported. A. C. M. Vingerhoeds, J. H. H. Thijssen and F. Schwartz[4] (Univ. of Utrecht) report data on a hypertensive, hypokalemic patient with hypercortisolism apparently of the pituitary dependent type, in whom no changes in outward appearance

---

(4)   J. Clin. Endocrinol. Metab. 43:1128–1133, November, 1976.

BASELINE VALUES*

	Father	Son Age 20 yrs.	Daughters Age 14 yrs.	Age 10 yrs.
Cortisol production rate (mg/24 h) (6–25)	135 and 126	42	—	—
Urinary 17 KGS-excretion (mg/24 h) (8–25)	108.4, 97.3, and 86.9	45.5	17.5 (14.2)	11.8 (10.9)
Urinary 17 KS-excretion (mg/24 h) (8–30)	41.0, and 42.0	30.2	15.1 (8.5)	7.6 (5)
Urinary pregnanetriol-excretion (mg/24 h) (<1.5)	0.98	—	—	—
Aldosterone secretion rate on 1 g salt (μg/24 h) (200–500)	330	—	—	—
Aldosterone secretion rate on 9 g salt (μg/24 h) (50–200)	18	—	—	—
Plasma renin activity on 1 g salt (angiotension I/100 ml/h)(200–500)	315	—	—	—
Plasma renin activity on 9 g salt (angiotension I/100 ml/h) (50–200)	75	—	—	—
Plasma transcortin at 0930 (μg/dl) (20–30)	23.9	28	—	—
Total plasma cortisol at 0930 (μg/dl) (9–25)	77.0, 63.2, and 61.1	37.8	—	—
Free plasma cortisol at 0930 (μg/dl) (5–10% of total plasma cortisol)	24	5.8	—	—

*Normal values in parentheses.
Total plasma cortisol levels and plasma ACTH levels throughout day.

occurred during a 3-year follow-up period despite persistent hypercortisolism.

Man, 51, who had always felt healthy, was found to be hypertensive and hypokalemic, with low urinary aldosterone excretion. Excretion of urinary corticoids was grossly elevated. Sexual function was normal. The patient was slightly obese but had normal body hair, well-developed muscles and no buffalo hump or striae. The results of endocrine studies are given in the table. Chlorthalidone, α-methyldopa and potassium supplements were given. The patient's appearance was unchanged after 33 months and there were no changes in the laboratory data, which still indicated severe hypercortisolism. The cortisol production rate on follow-up was 110–143 mg per 24 hours.

One of 3 children of this patient also showed hypertension and hypercortisolism. More recently the patient had been treated with dexamethasone to eliminate the mineralocorticoid action of endogenous cortisol. Potassium supplementation could be withdrawn with this treatment. The hypertension persists but all other features of Cushing's syndrome are still lacking.

A possibly genetically determined hyposensitivity to the glucocorticoid action of cortisol is postulated. Study of glucocorticoid receptors in the patient's tissues has not yet been possible but the patient's 2 daughters have slightly elevated urinary steroid excretion.

▶ [The title of this article looked mighty familiar to me. Almost, but not quite! Some years back (1971 YEAR BOOK, p. 268) we included an article entitled "Cushing's Syndrome without Cortisolism." Whoever said, "You can't have it both ways," is obviously wrong. Dr. Grant Liddle's previously described patient had ACTH secretion characteristic of Cushing's disease, but Cushing's disease could not develop because of previously existing Addison's disease.

Here, we are one step beyond, with, presumptively, a hereditary receptor deficiency for cortisol. If so, tissues perceive this as they should, as cortisol deficiency, and signals are sent to activate the hypothalamic-pituitary-adrenocorticol axis with the result that is described here. We have, in effect, still another example of receptor loss, the equivalent, say, of testicular feminization. Could there be another variant called "Cushing's syndrome without Cushing's syndrome"? Look ahead. — T.B.S.] ◀

Alcohol-Induced Pseudo-Cushing's Syndrome. Abnormalities of adrenocortical function have been described after excessive alcohol ingestion, and clinical evidence of corticosteroid excess may be observed in patients with some chronic liver diseases, notably chronic active hepatitis. Recently, Smals et al. described 3 alcoholics with findings strongly suggestive of Cushing's syndrome. L. H. Rees, G. M. Besser, W. J. Jeffcoate, D. J. Goldie and V. Marks[5] describe 4 patients in whom Cushing's syndrome was strongly suspected but subsequently disproved, and in whom the initial biochemical abnormalities appear to have been caused by alcohol abuse.

Man, 30, a known alcoholic for 13 years, had some features suggestive of Cushing's syndrome on admission, including plethoric facies, easy bruising and truncal obesity. The 9-A.M. plasma fluorogenic corticosteroid levels were elevated on consecutive days. In several further admissions in the next 3 years the plasma corticosteroid levels were 840–1,260 nM/L. Urinary 17-oxosteroids and 17-oxogenic steroids were high on a number of occasions, and the midnight plasma corticosteroid level on one occasion was 364 nM/L. After an admission the 9-A.M. plasma corticosteroid level fell over 5 days from 1,260 to 364 nM/L. An overnight dexamethasone suppression test with 2 mg reduced the morning plasma cortisol value to 84 nM/L, excluding true Cushing's syndrome. There was no clinical evidence of liver disease, and liver function values were normal or only slightly abnormal.

Cushing's syndrome was suspected mainly from the biochemical findings in 2 cases and on both clinical and biochemical grounds in 2. The mechanism of severe alcohol-

---

(5) Lancet 1:726–728, Apr. 2, 1977.

induced hypercortisolemia is unknown. Corticotropin secretion was deranged in 1 of the 3 patients in whom it was evaluated. Impaired hepatic function might be expected to result in a lower metabolic clearance rate for cortisol, but it is unlikely to be the cause of the clinical and biochemical abnormalities in these patients. In some patients alcohol ingestion may result in severe hyperlipemia, which may cause interference in the fluorogenic corticosteroid assay.

▶ [The authors mention a potential fly in the ointment in the last sentence of this article; the fluorogenic corticosteroid assay is less specific than receptor assays or radioimmunoassays. Other authors who describe a similar patient made no mention of the procedure used to measure plasma cortisol (Smals et al.: Br. Med. J. 2:1298, 1976).

In the 1977 YEAR BOOK (p. 258), the work of Krieger et al. with the use of cyproheptadine in the treatment of Cushing's disease generated enthusiasm and excitement. For what's happened since, look ahead. — T.B.S.]

Suppression by Cyproheptadine of Human Growth Hormone and Cortisol Secretion during Sleep. Accumulating evidence suggests that serotonergic mechanisms are implicated in the regulation of both growth hormone (GH) and ACTH in animals. Release of GH and cortisol induced by hypoglycemia and the plasma GH response to exercise are significantly blunted in man by pretreatment with the serotonin antagonist cyproheptadine. Kazuo Chihara, Yuzuru Kato, Kiyoshi Maeda, Shigeru Matsukura and Hiroo Imura[6](Kobe Univ.) studied the effect of cyproheptadine on the nocturnal rise in plasma GH and cortisol levels in 7 healthy men aged 19–23 years, all of whom were nonobese and had apparently normal endocrine and autonomic nerve function. Infusions of saline and 5 mg cyproheptadine were given over 3 hours after the onset of sleep. Some subjects received infusions of cyproheptadine starting a 7 P.M. also.

Plasma GH rose significantly in early sleep periods on baseline nights (Fig 26); the first increase occurred 25–35 minutes after the onset of sleep. Release of GH was sometimes suppressed when cyproheptadine was infused after onset of sleep. In the subjects in whom it was not, cyproheptadine infusion at 7 P.M. delayed or abolished the plasma GH increase. Plasma cortisol showed a progressive rise in the early morning on baseline nights, and this was inhibited by infusion of cyproheptadine from 4 A.M. to 7 A.M. Sleep

____

(6) J. Clin. Invest. 57:1393–1402, June, 1976.

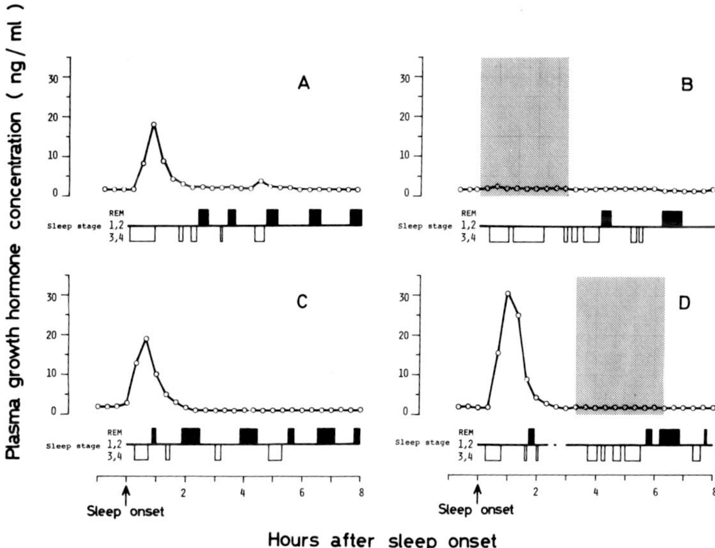

Fig 26. – Plasma GH concentrations after onset of sleep (entry into stage 2) during baseline nights and nights of cyproheptadine infusion in 1 subject. Sleep histogram is shown beneath each panel. Open histograms show slow wave stages 3 and 4, solid histograms indicate REM stage and solid lines denote stages 1 and 2. Brakes in lines represent waking periods. Stippled areas indicate periods of cyproheptadine infusion. **A,** 1st baseline night; **B,** night with cyproheptadine infused after sleep onset; **C,** 2d baseline night; **D,** night with cyproheptadine infused from 4 A.M. (Courtesy of Chihara, K., et al.: J. Clin. Invest. 57:1393–1402, June, 1976.)

stages 3 and 4 were increased by cyproheptadine infusion after onset of sleep, whereas rapid eye movement (REM) sleep was significantly reduced, compared with baseline nights. Total REM sleep time was also significantly reduced when cyproheptadine was infused at 4 A.M.

Intravenous cyproheptadine suppresses GH release during early sleep periods in man. The agent appears to inhibit GH and ACTH release by antagonizing brain serotonergic mechanisms controlling secretion of these hormones. The apparent dissociation between the GH rise and slow-wave step after cyproheptadine administration suggests that subcortical mechanisms in the brain stem may act independently on cortical and hypothalamic areas under certain circumstances.

► [Are you surprised that Figure 26, which shows suppression of the rise in *growth hormone,* is included in this chapter, The Adrenal Cortex? So am I. I had forgotten that I had selected this particular figure, but changes in cortisol are similar. Figure 26 nicely shows both the experimental design and the dramatic suppressive effect of cyproheptadine. While there are reports (1977 YEAR BOOK, p. 258) cyproheptadine blocks ACTH secretion after L-dopa or metyrapone administration, this apparently is not true for vasopressin-stimulated cortisol release in a patient with Cushing's syndrome (George et al.: Horm. Res. 7:308, 1976). This last patient, however, had a pituitary tumor that could well have become autonomous, and unresponsive to serotonin antagonism.

Wouldn't it be interesting to treat patients with Nelson's syndrome with cyproheptadine? Well, yes, as shown below. — T.B.S.] ◄

Effectiveness of Cyproheptadine in Decreasing Plasma ACTH Concentrations in Nelson's Syndrome. Cyproheptadine reverses the clinical and laboratory abnormalities of Cushing's disease, possibly via its antiserotonergic effects. There is evidence that pituitary function in patients with Nelson's syndrome is not autonomous and that these patients might therefore respond to this drug. Dorothy T. Krieger and Martin Luria[7] (Mt. Sinai School of Medicine, New York) evaluated cyproheptadine in 4 patients with Nelson's syndrome, treated for periods of 3–5 months.

Three patients had highly significant reductions in mean plasma ACTH concentrations. Two had visible lightening of skin pigmentation with treatment. The plasma ACTH rose significantly above treatment levels in 1 patient 1 month after cyproheptadine was stopped. No change in sellar size was observed during treatment. Plasma prolactin levels decreased significantly in 3 patients and increased in 1. The plasma growth hormone decreased significantly during cyproheptadine therapy in all cases.

Cyproheptadine reduces the plasma ACTH in some cases of Nelson's syndrome, providing additional evidence of the nonautonomous nature of pituitary function in such patients and its dependence on central nervous system "drive." It remains to be seen whether cyproheptadine therapy after bilateral adrenalectomy for Cushing's disease will prevent the occurrence of Nelson's syndrome or whether it will permanently reduce ACTH secretion and reverse abnormal pigmentation in established cases of Nelson's syndrome.

► [This is encouraging, particularly regarding the emergence of the question of whether cyproheptadine, given prophylactically, would pre-

---

(7)   J. Clin. Endocrinol. Metab. 43:1179–1182, November, 1976.

vent Nelson's syndrome. It would be a great help to have a marker to indicate which patients are at risk to acquire Nelson's syndrome.

Sadly, not all experiences are favorable. We must record that Vetter et al. (Schweiz. Med. Wochenschr. 106:1320, 1976) treated a patient with Cushing's disease and found that after 2 months there was an escape from the cyproheptadine effect, with a biochemical relapse. Cyproheptadine failures in 2 children were also recorded by D'Ercole et al. (J. Pediatr. 90:834, 1977), although the therapeutic trial may have been too short.

Metyrapone continues to have adherents for adjunctive treatment of Cushing's syndrome (Jeffcoate: Br. Med. J. 2:215, 1977). — T.B.S.] ◄

ADRENAL INSUFFICIENCY

Ossification of the Helix of the Ear in Addison's Disease is described by R. E. Siebenmann[8] (Pathological Inst., Zurich) in order to clarify the pathology and clinical aspects of the effect of adrenocortical deficiency on the entire organism.

Man, 65, had had tuberculous Addison's disease for 20 years and had been treated only with desoxycorticosterone, except for a few days of glucocorticoid administration. An acute infection triggered a crisis and the patient committed suicide several days later due to the effect of an endocrine organic psychosis. A terminally demonstrated massive calcific opacity of the helix of the ear bilaterally proved to be a subtotal ossification of the elastic cartilage of the ear

Fig 27.—**A,** x-ray film of traumatically severed helix of the ear with massive opacity of cartilaginous structure, particularly along helix and antihelix, as well as within area of meatus and tragus. Between these areas are thinner sections of helix with fine trabecular structure. **B,** x-ray film of prepared epiglottis, with homogeneous dense opacity in upper segment. **C,** x-ray film of prepared lower trachea with increased ossification of cartilage rings and incipient tracheopathia osteoplastica. (Courtesy of Siebenmann, R. E.: Schweiz. Med. Wochenschr. 107:468–474, Apr. 9, 1977.)

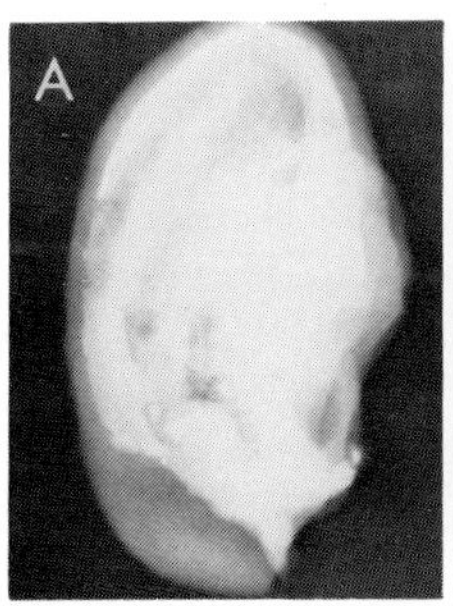

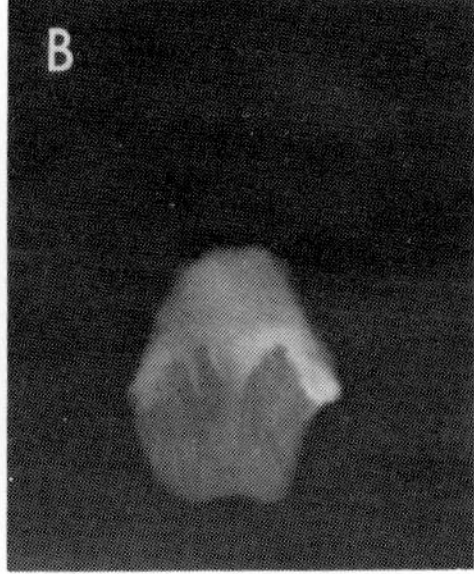

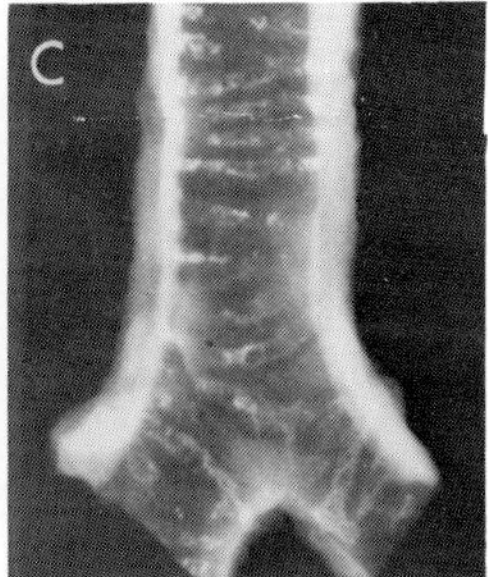

(8)   Schweiz. Med. Wochenschr. 107:468–474, Apr. 9, 1977.

(Fig 27). The elastic cartilage of the epiglottis was also ossified; the hyaline cartilage showed increased ossification only in the trachea, partly in the form of tracheopathia osteoplastica. There were no signs of metastatic ossifications.

Systematic anatomical and histologic investigations of the helix of the ear are not readily possible on an external level and thus little is known about physiologic age-determined changes or other pathologic findings of this cartilage. Radiologic demonstration of opacity does not differentiate between calcification and ossification. Current reported data indicate that these alterations have been observed only in male patients treated exclusively with mineral corticoids and experiencing long-term glucocorticoid deficiency. In the present patient it could be demonstrated that these lesions constituted a pathologic ossification and not a metastatic calcification of the ear cartilage.

Several pathogenic possibilities must be considered. Hypercalcemia can be ruled out in the absence of the typical metastatic calcifications. Long-term desoxycorticosterone substitution carried out in all these patients has been considered, although no relationship has been demonstrated between the extent of ossification and duration and dosage of this treatment. An endocrine regulatory disturbance must be considered. In the untreated, uncomplicated, congenital adrenogenital syndrome the congenital adrenocortical enzyme defect leads to long-term glucocorticoid deficit. Chronically increased ACTH and MSH secretion must be assumed and these patients at times show striking, unusually extensive cartilage ossification. This parallel should stimulate the search for a possible mutual pathogenic factor. Perhaps it is not the long-term glucocorticoid deficit itself, but an abnormally increased hypophyseal secretion, which is of importance, and in case of ossification of the helix of the ear in acromegaly, an increased GH secretion might be considered, paralleling the increased ACTH secretion.

▶ [Striking roentgenograms, yes? Calcification of the epiglottis and trachea is new to me, but I was aware of calcification of the ear. In truth, I could not resist including this article because it provides an opportunity for me to tell a flattering story. Several years ago, while a visiting professor, I was presented with a young man who was early in his workup for possible Addison's disease. I palpated his ears in front of a large group and asserted that I could feel calcification and, therefore, diagnosis of

Fig 28.—Calcification of the ear. (Courtesy of T. B. Schwartz.)

Addison's disease was established. Seeing expressions varying from admiration through incredulity to contempt, I invited members of the audience to come forward and palpate the patient's ears. Some were convinced, but in others the disapproving expressions were intensified. Several weeks later I received the roentgenogram shown in Figure 28, along with a letter admitting to a grudging respect for my clinical prowess.

This story of self-aggrandizement reminds me of another one, and, because there aren't very many, I'm going to tell it, too. Several years ago I was asked to serve as a consultant to evaluate the department of medicine of one of our medical schools. It happened that this was among the medical schools to which I had applied for admission in ancient days. It was the first medical school to respond and it responded with a resounding rejection. I was saved from suicide by an acceptance elsewhere shortly thereafter. I performed my consultant's duties studiously and conscientiously, but could not forebear saying at the summing up, "Your first mistake goes back quite a few years . . . ." What I felt is best described as delicious.

Among the other weird things noted with Addison's disease is "salty sweat and ichthyosis" (Chan and Gwee: Br. Med. J. 1:81, 1977) and polyradiculoneuropathy (Abbas: Neurology (Minneap.) 27:494, 1977).—T.B.S.] ◄

► ↓ For another irresistible article, look ahead.—T.B.S. ◄

Treatment of Hereditary Angioedema with Danazol: Reversal of Clinical and Biochemical Abnormalities.

Hereditary angioedema is thought to be due to deficient activity of the inhibitor of the activated 1st component of complement, C1 esterase. The effective prophylactics, antifibrinolytic agents and androgens, may cause side effects, the former, thrombophlebitis and myositis, and the latter, virilization and hepatotoxicity. Jeffrey A. Gelfand, Richard J. Sherins, David W. Alling and Michael M. Frank[9] (Natl. Inst. of Health) performed a double-blind study of the efficacy of a synthetic androgen, danazol, that is mildly anabolic.

The subjects were 5 women and 4 men, aged 25–63 years, with hereditary angioedema. All had had at least one attack a month and had low serum levels of C4 and C1 esterase inhibitor (C1EI) activity. Eight patients had low serum levels of C1EI protein, and 1 patient had normal levels of a functionally deficient inhibitor protein. Danazol was given orally, 200 mg 3 times daily for 28 days or until an attack occurred.

The 9 patients completed a total of 93 courses, 47 with placebo and 46 with danazol (table). The rate of attacks was significantly lower with the active drug than with placebo. Only minor side effects were noted. The mean C1EI serum level increased threefold on drug therapy, reaching normal or near-normal levels in 4 patients. Serum C4 levels showed

RESULTS WITH DANAZOL AND PLACEBO IN PATIENTS WITH HEREDITARY ANGIOEDEMA

Patient No.	Sex	Age (Yr)	Courses with Danazol		Courses with Placebo		Totals
			Attacks	Attack-Free	Attacks	Attack-Free	
1	F	25	0	5	5	0	10
2	M	34	0	5	5	0	10
3	F	38	0	4	5	0	9
4	F	28	1	6	7	1	15
5	F	36	0	6	5	2	13
6	F	33	0	4	5	0	9
7	M*	28	0	5	5	0	10
8	M	29	0	5	3	0	8†
9	M	63	0	5	4	0	9†
Totals			1	45	44	3	93
% Courses with attacks‡			1/46 = 2.2%		44/47 = 93.6%		

*Patient with abnormal C1EI protein.
†Study terminated.
‡Chi-square = 77.8; $P < 0.001$.

(9) N. Engl. J. Med. 295:1444–1448, Dec. 23, 1976.

a 15-fold rise on danazol therapy, often increasing to the normal range. The only patient who had an attack on drug therapy had the smallest increments in C1EI and C4 levels. Attacks occurred later in the course of placebo administration if the preceding course was danazol than if it was placebo.

Danazol was highly effective in preventing attacks of hereditary angioedema in patients of both sexes. Side effects were minimal. Danazol appears to act by increasing serum levels of C1EI.

▶ [You ask, "The selection of this article is apropos of what?" My feeble defenses are that I have taken a monitory interest in anabolic steroids (1976 YEAR BOOK, pp. 237–239) and, also, that I was seduced by the results obtained. Look at the table. A clinical investigator's dream come true!

It is possible that the abusers of anabolic steroids may be impressed by horror stories. Prat et al. (J.A.M.A. 237:2322, 1977) report the appearance of Wilms' tumor in a man who used large amounts of anabolic steroids as part of a body-building program. – T.B.S.] ◀

ALDOSTERONE

Possible Role of Renin in Hypertension as Suggested by Renin-Sodium Profiling and Inhibition of Converting Enzyme. David B. Case, John M. Wallace, Hans J. Keim, Michael A. Weber, Jean E. Sealey and John H. Laragh[1] (New York Hosp.-Cornell Med. Center) evaluated seated hypertensive patients on a normal or low-sodium regimen with the nonapeptide inhibitor of angiotension I-converting enzyme, SQ20881, an agent that competitively blocks the conversion of angiotensin I to angiotensin II by pulmonary and plasma enzymes. Sixty-five hypertensive patients had SQ20881 injected in a dose of 1 mg/kg at least 3 weeks after the withdrawal of antihypertensive medications. Sodium depletion was induced by giving a 10-mEq sodium diet for 5 days.

Blood pressure responses to SQ20881 are shown in Figure 28A. High-renin patients had greater falls in blood pressure at all intervals and greater maximum decreases than did normal-renin patients; smaller changes were seen in low-renin patients than in either. High-renin patients had simi-

(1) N. Engl. J. Med. 296:641–646, Mar. 24, 1977.

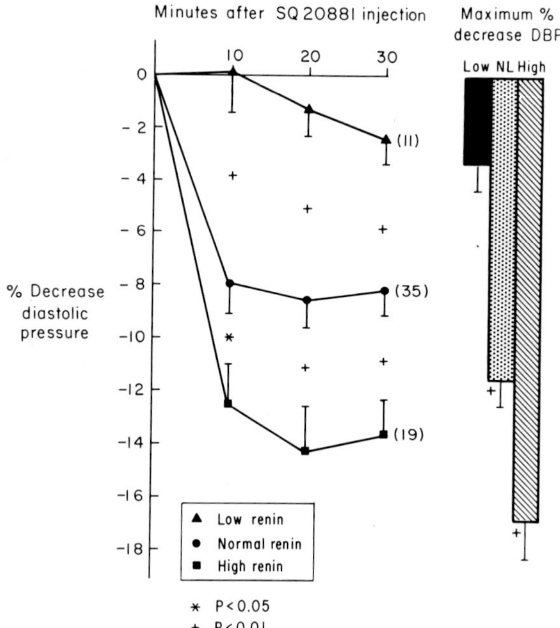

Fig 28A.—Diastolic blood pressure responses to converting-enzyme inhibitor SQ20881, 1 mg/kg, in 65 hypertensive patients profiled as high, normal *(NL)* and low renin (values are mean ±SEM). The left panel represents the time course of the depressor responses, comparing the values of the low-renin *(triangle)*, normal-renin *(circle)* and high-renin *(square)* patients. The right panel compares the maximal percent decreases in diastolic blood pressure *(DBP)* of the three subgroups. Figures in parentheses denote number of patients. (Courtesy of Case, D. B., et al.: N. Engl. J. Med. 296:641–646, Mar. 24, 1977.)

lar maximum responses with or without sodium depletion, but the effect occurred more rapidly after sodium depletion. Sodium-depleted normal-renin patients had greater falls in blood pressure than did the group on a normal sodium intake. No pressor responses to SQ20881 were observed. A direct relationship was found between pretreatment plasma renin activity and the maximum percentage fall in diastolic blood pressure. Plasma renin activity increased after SQ20881 in all normal-renin and high-renin patients on either a normal or low-sodium intake but not in the low-renin patients. The maximum fall in diastolic pressure was closely related to the induced increment in renin levels.

The induced depressor responses observed were apparently largely if not completely related to blockade of angiotensin II formation. If this is so, the findings validate by functional testing the degrees of participation of renin activity in hypertension, as also indicated by renin-sodium profiling. Testing for the presence and magnitude of this factor could become more clinically relevant for baseline definition as well as for selecting either acute or long-term therapy directed at reducing angiotensin II levels. More work is needed to determine whether the suggested renin participation is primary or secondary and to what extent it may differ from renin participation in normal homeostasis.

▶ [Figure 28 clearly tells the story. Blocking the genesis of angiotensin II reduces diastolic pressure, and the higher the pretesting renin level, the greater the fall. So, for the nth time, there is telling evidence that renovascular effects are operative in patients with essential hypertension. Similar conclusions have been drawn using saralasin, an angiotensin II antagonist (1976, YEAR BOOK, p. 255).

This is a very active field and I do not pretend to have covered it thoroughly nor digested all that I have read. There exists now not only angiotensins I and II, but also angiotensin III and angiotensin III A (J. Clin. Endocrinol. Metab. 43:940, 1976), as well as naturally occurring and synthetic analogues of each. Furthermore, they vary considerably in relative ability to induce hypertension or to stimulate aldosterone production. They even behave differently on renal vasculature and in general systemic effects (Taub: J. Clin. Invest. 59:528, 1977).

Ferguson et al. (Lancet 1:775, 1977) are enthusiastic about a new inhibitor of converting enzyme that appears to be effective by mouth. Williams and Hollandberg (N. Engl. J. Med. 297:184, 1977) add another dimension by showing changes not only in the renin-angiotensin system, but also in the kallikrein-bradykinin systems after the administration of a converting enzyme inhibitor to salt-depleted normal and hypertensive persons. Furthermore, don't go away thinking that renovascular hypertension is not affected by prostaglandins. Romero and Strong (Circ. Res. 40:35, 1977) found that indomethacin blockade of prostaglandin synthesis in rabbits led to an inhibition of the expected increase in plasma renin and a salutary effect on the blood pressure in some rabbits.

For those readers who would become anxious were I to become less compulsive, three additional articles on saralasin were published this year (Baer et al.: Ann. Intern. Med. 86:257, 1977; Marks et al.: ibid. 87:176, 1977; and Anderson et al.: ibid., p. 183).

Having read all this, now go back and reread the first sentence of this article. Can't you visualize a very nervous patient sitting on an ornate regimen (a regimen looks something like a hassock) with the nonapeptide inhibitor (which looks something like a shillelagh) by his side. I'm reminded of a picture hung on the wall of the basic science building of my medical school. It showed a group of ancient and honorable histologists. One of them, with a faraway look in his eyes, was seated, with a little wooden box on his lap. I was told that the seated figure was Doctor Golgi and the little box was, of course, his apparatus.

Enough nonsense! Let's look more at patients with low-renin hypertension. — T.B.S.] ◄

Evidence for an Unidentified ACTH-Induced Steroid Hormone Causing Hypertension. Dexamethasone-suppressible hyperaldosteronism is a form of low-renin hypertension in which dexamethasone rapidly suppresses aldosterone to very low levels. Maria I. New, Ralph E. Peterson, Paul Saenger and Lenore S. Levine[2] (New York Hosp.-Cornell Med. Center, New York) studied a male patient, aged 18, to determine if hyperaldosteronism alone accounts for the hypertension in this syndrome. Little or no treatment had been given for 6 years. The patient was kept on a constant diet containing 100 mEq daily of sodium and potassium during the studies.

Hypertension and mild hyperaldosteronism were promptly reduced by a small dose of dexamethasone. When the patient was normotensive and aldosterone secretion was below normal, treatment with 1 mg aldosterone or 18-hydroxydesoxycorticosterone (18-OH-DOC) daily or 30 mg desoxycorticosterone (DOC) daily did not cause hypertension, but sodium retention and potassium loss were noted during aldosterone and DOC infusion. Hypertension appeared within 5 days during infusion of ACTH or oral metyrapone administration. The hypertensive effect of metyrapone was abolished by adding aminoglutethimide treatment.

A steroid other than aldosterone, 18-OH-DOC or DOC may have been the cause of the ACTH-induced hypertension in this patient. The steroid may have been an 11-desoxysteroid. Further studies with the use of blood and urine samples collected under ACTH and metyrapone stimulation may provide a source from which this steroid may be characterized.

► [First, it should be noted that the constancy of this patient is equaled only by the devotion of his physician. The report of the patient's first studies occurred 10 years ago.

Read the article. The evidence is certainly strong that ACTH stimulates the secretion of a hypertension-producing mineralocorticoid other than aldosterone. Candidates for this elusive steroid abound. Tan et al. (Clin. Sci. Mol. Med. 51:311s, 1976) found 11-deoxycorticosterone plasma levels to be elevated in some patients with primary aldosteronism,

---

(2)   J. Clin. Endocrinol. Metab. 43:1283–1293, December, 1976.

Cushing's syndrome and low-renin hypertension and in adults with elevated urinary 17-ketosteroid excretion. Another candidate (Melby and Dale: Mayo Clin. Proc. 52:317, 1977) is dihydroxy-11-deoxycorticosterone, while Dr. Grant Liddle's group (Sennett. et al.: Circ. Res. (Suppl.) 36:1, 1977) prefer 16-β-hydroxydehydroepiandrosterone. Finally, Doctor New, with a different set of collaborators (J. Clin. Endocrinol. Metab. 44:924, 1977), describe a 3-year-old child with hypertension, hypokalemia and suppressed plasma renin activity. All of the mineralocorticoids measured were very low and showed a blunted response to ACTH administration. Nonetheless, ACTH infusion aggravated the hypertension and hypokalemia.

After looking ahead, one might wonder whether these patients have overproduced endogenous licorice. — T.B.S.] ◄

Licorice Toxicity and the Renin-Angiotensin-Aldosterone Axis in Man.

M. T. Epstein, E. A. Espiner, R. A. Donald and H. Hughes[3] (Christchurch, New Zealand) evaluated the renin-angiotensin-aldosterone axis and electrolyte status in 4 ill women, aged 38–55 years, admitted with chronic licorice intoxication, after the withdrawal of licorice. They had consumed 25–200 gm licorice daily for 6 months to 5 years. Urinary potassium excretion exceeded 40 mM/24 hours in all patients in the face of plasma potassium values of 1.6–2 mM/L. Sodium balance was negative on a fixed 10-mM low-salt diet, but potassium balance was positive, and the plasma potassium became normal by the 6th day of the low-salt diet. In 3 patients, potassium supplements had to be stopped. Plasma electrolytes remained normal thereafter on follow-up examination for up to 4 months. Subnormal urinary aldosterone and plasma renin levels persisted on the low-salt challenge (table). Plasma aldosterone and angiotensin II levels were relatively normal under basal conditions but abnormally low during low-salt challenge.

Signs of mineralocorticoid excess in these cases are presumably due to the continued action of the glycyrrhizinic acid component of licorice on renal tubular potassium secretion. A phase of sodium loss and potassium retention follows, contrasting with the findings in Conn's syndrome. These effects are presumably related to the effects of extracellular volume expansion and paralysis of the renin-angiotensin-aldosterone system. The electrolyte response to intravenous salt loading is normal. The renin-angiotensin-

---

(3) Br. Med. J. 1:209–210, Jan. 22, 1977.

ASSESSMENT OF RENIN-ANGIOTENSIN-ALDOSTERONE AXIS ON FOUR DAYS
IN FOUR PATIENTS WITHDRAWN FROM LICORICE*

	Case No: 1	2	3	4	Normal range (10-am standing)
On admission (normal diet)					
Urinary aldosterone (nmol/24 h)	2·8	8·3	2·8	4·0	8·3–50
Plasma aldosterone (pmol/l): 8 am	111	139	83	306	
10 am		278	111		139–556
PRA (nmol/l/h): 8 am	0·26	0	0·11	0·09	0·15–1·54
10 am		0·17	0·43		0·38–2·69
Plasma angiotensin (pmol/l): 8 am		28·5	28·5	38	
10 am		35·2	28·5		19–66·5
5th day of low-salt diet					
Urinary aldosterone (nmol/24 h)	5·5	22·2	2·8	6·0	41·6–221·6
Plasma aldosterone (pmol/l): 8 am	167	139	195		
10 am	195	445	167	390	445–2224
PRA (nmol/l/h): 8 am	0·04	0·45	0·25		
10 am	0·23	2·07	0·26	0·25	3·85–30·8
Plasma angiotensin (pmol/l): 8 am	26·6	38	23·8		
10 am	28·5	47·5	26·6	46·6	76–200
Last day of salt depletion					
	(Day 12)	(Day 7)	(Day 11)	(Day 11)	
Urinary aldosterone (nmol/24 h)	11·1	12·5	11·1	8·0	
Plasma aldosterone (pmol/l): 8 am	167	222	167	445	
PRA (nmol/l/h): 10 am	1·94			3·2	
Follow-up					
Urinary aldosterone (nmol/24 h)	24·9	36	30·5	8·3	
Plasma aldosterone (pmol/l): 10 am	361	334	189	360	
PRA (nmol/l/h): 10 am	2·45	0·77	0·75	0·67	
Plasma angiotensin (pmol/l): 10 am	52·3	29·0	35	35	

*Patients were supine when 8 A.M. values were measured and standing when 10 A.M. values were measured.

Conversion: SI to traditional units – Urinary aldosterone: 1nM/24 hours≈361 ng/24 hours. Plasma aldosterone: 1 pM/L≈0.036 ng/100 ml. PRA: 1 nM/L/hour≈1.3 ng/ml/hour. Plasma angiotensin II: 1 pM/L≈1.05 pg/ml.

aldosterone axis was suppressed in all patients, and in 1 case it remained suppressed for at least 2 weeks after the withdrawal of licorice. Paralysis of the axis led to mineralocorticoid deficiency. Long-term suppression of the renin-angiotensin-aldosterone axis is uncommon despite several years of licorice ingestion, in contrast to the prolonged suppression observed after the removal of some aldosterone-secreting tumors.

▶ [This study is a model of brevity, taking up less than one full page of the *British Medical Journal.* In commenting on a previous report of licorice-induced pseudoaldosteronism, I confessed to an addiction to licorice. It may not be so funny though, as evidenced by another report of these same authors (Br. Med. J. 1:488, 1977), who fed licorice to volunteers and found that eating moderate amounts of licorice daily for less than a week could provoke serious hypokalemia. Damn it! I've already abandoned my pipe, and now this! — T.B.S.] ◄

Dexamethasone-Modified Adrenal Scintiscan in Hyporeninemic Aldosteronism (Tumor versus Hyperplasia): Comparison with Adrenal Venography and Adrenal Venous Aldosterone. Until recently it has remained necessary for patients who harbor an aldosterone-producing adenoma to undergo invasive localizing procedures preoperatively. J. W. Conn, E. L. Cohen and Karl R. Herwig[4] (Univ. of Michigan) report experience with the dexamethasone-modified adrenal scintiscan (DS) in 26 hyporeninemic patients with adrenal hyperplasia or tumors

Fig 29. — A, standard scintiscan. B, dexamethasone-modified scintiscan at 4 days; C, at 6 days; and D, at 7 days. The left adrenal is seen on the left side of each photograph. In B it is clear the tumor appears to be on the right side, but by the 7th day the advantage of the dexamethasone scan over the standard scintiscan has been lost. (Courtesy of Conn, J. W., et al.: J. Lab. Clin. Med. 88:841–856, November, 1976.)

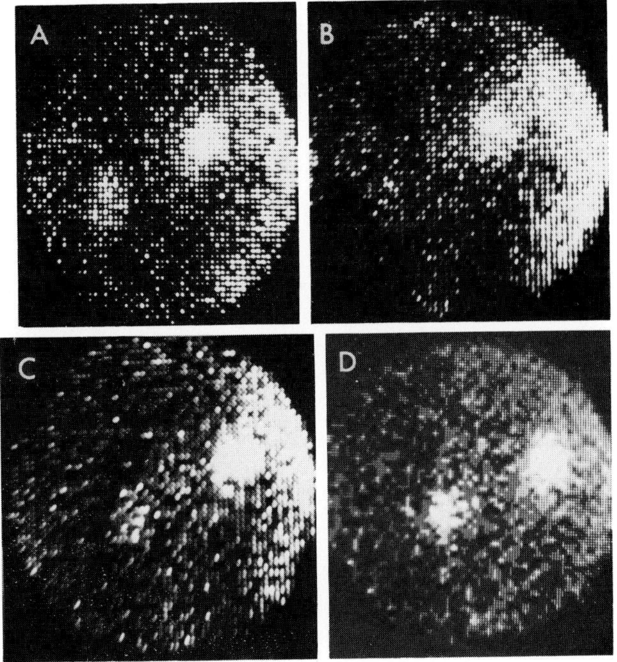

---

(4)   J. Lab. Clin. Med. 88:841–856, November, 1976.

producing excessive aldosterone. Twenty-two patients were surgically explored. Patients received a basic diet containing 10 mEq sodium and 70 mEq potassium, and 110 mEq sodium was added for 3 days. Dexamethasone was given in a dose of 0.5 mg every 6 hours for 48 hours before the administration of [131]I-19-iodocholesterol. Scanning was begun as early as 3 days after radiocholesterol administration and continued for up to 2 weeks. Patients received Lugol's solution for 2–3 weeks starting 48 hours before radiocholesterol injection to minimize thyroidal uptake of [131]I.

Seventeen patients had aldosterone-producing tumors. Presumed bilateral hyperplasia was confirmed at exploration in 5 of 9 patients; 4 of the 5 had extreme macronodular hyperplasia. The other 4 patients were diagnosed on the basis of negative venograms and nonlateralizing standard scintiscans. All but one of the tumors were solitary. The standard adrenal scintiscan (SS) lateralized tumors correctly in 88% of 17 cases. The effect of the DS is illustrated in Figure 29. The DS is most important in cases of bilateral hyperplasia, when there is unequal uptake of activity in the SS study, since it prohibits uptake in both glands and provides the potential for distinguishing between adenoma and hyperplasia. The findings in patients with aldosterone-producing tumors are summarized in the table.

The dexamethasone-modified adrenal scintiscan is at least as effective in lateralizing aldosterone-producing tumors as are invasive procedures, and it is less costly and eliminates the frequent difficulties of catheterization and

---

Aldosterone-Producing Tumor: 17 Cases*

	No. performed	*Positive lateralization*	*No lateralization*	*Effectiveness*
DS	17	15	2†	88%
SS	14	10	4†	71%
Adrenal venography	15	12	3‡	80%
Adrenal venous aldosterone levels	10	8	2‡	80%

*Comparative effectiveness for tumor localization of the DS, the SS, adrenal venography and adrenal venous levels of aldosterone.

†One case was a carcinoma. These usually do not show uptake of radioactivity. One case showed no uptake in either adrenal both in the SS and in the DS.

‡In 2 cases the right side (side of tumor) could not be catheterized. Negative left side, however, gave useful information.

adrenal venous injections. The DS is also at least as effective in distinguishing between tumor and bilateral adrenal hyperplasia. The DS is simple enough to be used as an outpatient procedure.

► [Doctor Conn and his associates continue the saga of adrenal scinti-scanning. The addition of dexamethasone administration, as I and my associates have also found in a recent patient, helps considerably. In our case, it established the diagnosis of unilateral adrenal adenoma. It was much less obvious before dexamethasone suppression was invoked.

Mantero et al. (Clin. Sci. Mol. Med. 51:329S, 1976) attempt to differentiate between adenoma and hyperplasia by examining steroids and plasma renin activity in patients in the supine and upright positions. Danforth et al. (J. Urol. 117:140, 1977) point out that treatment of primary aldosteronism should be prompt if one is to avoid irreversible parenchymatous renal damage, and Kramer et al. (Clin. Endocrinol. (Oxf.) 7:151, 1977) recommend amiloride, a potassium-conserving diuretic, for the treatment of primary hyperaldosteronism. They found it effective even for patients with adenoma.

These patients are notorious for not becoming edematous. What's new about those who do? Look below. — T.B.S.] ◄

Catecholamine Excretion in "Idiopathic" Edema: Decreased Dopamine Excretion, a Pathogenic Factor?

Idiopathic edema affects almost exclusively women of reproductive age. Swelling is associated with neurogenic, particularly emotional, stimuli. There is some evidence that affected patients behave as though hyperreactive to catecholamines acting on β-adrenergic receptor sites. O. Kuchel, J. L. Cuche, N. T. Buu, G. P. Guthrie, Jr., T. Unger, W. Nowaczynski, R. Boucher and J. Genest[5] (Univ. of Montreal) examined the role of catecholamines in sodium retention in 16 women with idiopathic edema who had typical histories of edema and diurnal oliguria and nocturia unrelated to apparent cardiorenal, hepatic or other systemic disease. Body weights fluctuated greatly, and 13 patients had a weight increase usually exceeding the morning-evening difference in the premenstrual period. The cases are summarized in the table. Ten healthy subjects were also evaluated. Eight recumbent patients and 10 controls received 40 mg furosemide intravenously.

Urinary norepinephrine and epinephrine excretions were similar in the patients and controls and increased with upright posture in both groups, but urinary dopamine excretion was lower in the patients in the recumbent position.

---

(5)   J. Clin. Endocrinol. Metab. 44:639–646, April, 1977.

CLINICAL PRESENTATION OF PATIENTS WITH IDIOPATHIC EDEMA

Patients	Age	Weight (kg)	Morning–evening weight differences (normal: <0.6 kg)	Associated conditions	History of oral contraceptives or estrogen treatment	Premenstrual accentuation of edema
B.L.	23	57	0.7–1.1	increased salt appetite and consumption	−	−
B.D.	23	53	0.6–2.2	paroxysmal supraventricular tachycardia, mucous colitis, dysmenorrhea, family history of "swelling"	+	−
C.P.	41	79	0.7–2.6	labile hypertension, obesity, asthmatic bronchitis	−	+
G.D.	25	53	0.8–1.5	labile hypertension, history of pre-eclampsia, depression	+	+
G.H.	32	57	0.7–1.6	labile hypertension, gastric ulcers, hysterectomy, depression	−	formerly +
L.L.	31	62	0.5–1.2	family history of "swelling", anxiety, mild diabetes, hysteriform behaviour	+	+
P.S.	21	54	0.8–2.2	"swelling" up to hydrothorax, orthostatic proteinuria	+	+
St.A.G.	35	53	0.7–0.9	orthostatic hypotension, excessive salt appetite, dysmenorrhea	+	+
St.P.L.	50	61	0.9–3.4	history of kidney ptosis, treated by nephropexy and decapsulation, oligohypermenorrhea	−	+
St.P.M.	25	58	1.2–1.8	kidney ptosis, ovarian cyst	−	−
T.G.	35	85	0.6–1.2	obesity, labile hypertension, increased salt appetite	+	+
T.J.	23	45	0.8–3.2	oligohypomenorrhea, thirst, orthostatic hypotension, hypokalemia	−	+
M.L.	34	59	1.3–1.8	dysmenorrhea, pregnancy with edema and proteinuria, frigidity, dyspareunia, anxiety	−	+
B.D.	49	56	0.7–1.4	migraine headaches, orthostatic hypotension, hyperlipidemia type IV, prediabetes	−	+
C.J.	38	63	0.8–2.1	hyperlipidemia type IIa, orthostatic hypotension	+	+
B.Y.	35	58	0.6–5.9	hysterectomy and bilateral oophorectomy, extreme anxiety, polydipsia, palpitations, peptic ulcers, depression	+	formerly +

Tubular rejection fraction of sodium was reduced in upright patients. Plasma renin activity and plasma aldosterone were higher in patients than in controls in both the upright and the recumbent positions. Patients with idiopathic edema excreted significantly less dopamine and sodium after furosemide injection than did controls.

The findings suggest that a decrease in urinary dopamine, a catecholamine with natriuretic action, may reflect suppression of the renal dopaminergic system and may contribute to excessive sodium retention in idiopathic edema, either directly or indirectly through the renin-aldosterone system. The favorable results obtained with bromocriptine in women with premenstrual tension, often associated with unexplained edema, suggest that a more general defect of the dopaminergic autonomic nervous system may be present in this syndrome.

▶ [Another promising approach is discussed here. The mention of treatment with bromocriptine refers to an article in the 1977 YEAR BOOK (p. 290). In a subtractive sort of way, these findings are supported by those of Katz (J. Clin. Endocrinol. Metab. 45:419, 1977) who found that circadian rhythms of plasma aldosterone in these patients were similar to those of normal subjects, and he concluded, "Excessive renin and aldosterone are not usually found in recumbent patients with idiopathic edema." – T.B.S.]

Amelioration of Metabolic Acidosis with Fludrocortisone Therapy in Hyporeninemic Hypoaldosteronism. In contrast to the renal potassium-wasting characteristic of patients with distal (type 1) and proximal (type 2) renal tubular acidosis, some patients with renal hyperchloremic acidosis have persisting hyperkalemia. Nearly all such patients have impaired renal renin secretion and a resultant reduction in adrenal aldosterone secretion but otherwise normal adrenocortical function. The urine is acidic and bicarbonate free during spontaneous acidosis, but reabsorption of filtered bicarbonate is subnormal at normal plasma bicarbonate levels. Anthony Sebastian, Morris Schambelan, Stanley Lindenfeld and R. Curtis Morris, Jr.[6] (Univ. of California, San Francisco) believe that this is a pathophysiologically distinct form of renal tubular dysfunction, termed type 4 renal tubular acidosis. Four patients with stable chronic renal insufficiency, persisting hyperkalemia and hyperchloremic metabolic acidosis (Table 1) were studied. The renal disease was clinically characteristic of interstitial nephritis. Five balance studies were done with mineralocorticoid administration during spontaneously occurring acidosis. In two added studies the effects of discontinuation of fludrocortisone were examined.

Net acid excretion increased in all studies and systemic acidosis was corrected or nearly corrected (Table 2). Increased urinary ammonium excretion contributed to the

---

(6) N. Engl. J. Med. 297:576–583, Sept. 15, 1977.

TABLE 1.—Clinical and Biochemical Features in Patients with Hyporeninemic Hypoaldosteronism

Case No.	Age & Sex	Blood Pressure	Creatinine Clearance	Serum Electrolytes				Plasma Renin Activity*		Urine Aldosterone*
				NA^+	K^+	CL^-	HCO_3^-	SUPINE	UPRIGHT	
		mm Hg	ml/min/ 1.73 m²		meq/liter			ng/ml/3 hr		µg/24 hr
1	76M	131/70	13	141	6.0	114	16	0.8	2.4	2.0
2	61M	122/66	35	141	6.7	116	21	0.7	0.9	6.2
3	68M	74/45	31	138	5.8	111	17	3.3 (0.6)†	11.0 (1.2)†	3.8
4	32M	118/80	44	138	6.0	113	17	3.0	4.4	6.8

*Range of values in normal subjects: plasma renin activity (supine-upright), 2 – 10/5 – 32 ng/ml/3 hours; urinary aldosterone excretion, 4 – 17 µg/24 hours.
†After partial correction of hypovolemia during sodium bicarbonate therapy.

TABLE 2. – EFFECT OF FLUDROCORTISONE ON ACID-BASE BALANCE IN PATIENTS WITH HYPORENINEMIC HYPOALDOSTERONISM[*]

CASE No.	TIME OF MEASUREMENT	ARTERIAL BLOOD PLASMA			Δ PLASMA HCO_3^-	$\Sigma\Delta$ NAE	$\%\Delta$ PLASMA $[HCO_3^-]$[†] EXPLAINED BY $\Sigma\Delta$ NAE
		pH	Pco$_2$	HCO_3^-			
			mm Hg	meq/ liter	meq/ liter	meq	
1	C	7.34	24	12.7			
	F	7.39	35	20.5	7.8	96	45
2A	C	7.27	33	14.5			
	F	7.42	37	23.5	9.0	213	59
2B	C			20.6[‡]			
	F			24.1[‡]	3.5[‡]	180	78
3	C	7.25	39	16.7			
	F	7.33	44	22.5	5.8	220	146
4	C	7.27	44	19.6			
	F	7.39	41	24.1	4.5	40	36

[*]C and F denote respectively values before and at the completion of treatment; Δ plasma HCO_3^-, the change in plasma bicarbonate; $\Sigma\Delta NAE$, the cumulative increase in net acid excretion during the period of treatment.

[†]Calculated on basis of an assumed bicarbonate space equal to 50% of body weight.

[‡]Serum carbon dioxide content.

increase in net acid excretion in each study. Urinary potassium excretion increased with fludrocortisone therapy and normokalemia was restored. Discontinuance of therapy in two studies led to a prompt rise in urinary pH and a reduction in net acid excretion, with recurrence of acidosis.

In hypertensive patients, fludrocortisone therapy might exacerbate the hypertension and lead to other deleterious effects of extracellular-fluid volume expansion. Such patients might be treated by dietary potassium restriction, potassium-binding resins, sodium bicarbonate and loop diuretics.

▶ [First, some of you who are still awake are wondering what happened to type 3 renal tubular acidosis. Well, it was preempted by a variant of type 1 (Sebastian et al.: in Brenner, B. M., and Rector, F. C. (eds.): *The Kidney* [Philadelphia: W. B. Saunders Company, 1976] pp. 615).

We've been following the evolution of our knowledge of this disease for some years (see 1972 YEAR BOOK, p. 274; 1973 YEAR BOOK, pp. 306–308; 1976 YEAR BOOK, p. 264; and 1977 YEAR BOOK, p. 269).

The present findings suggest that the renal resistance to steroid action (pseudohypoaldosteronism) is relative and can be overcome by larger doses than would be necessary to repair the mineralocorticoid defect in the absence of renal insufficiency.

Having come this far, let's complete the review. Petersen et al. (Acta Endocrinol. (Kbh.) 84:605, 1977) describe a patient with typical familial hypoaldosteronism. These persons make glucocorticoids, but they have no zona glomerulosa. Sometimes, though, the lesion is due to an enzyme defect as was found in 2 infants by Milla et al. (Arch. Dis. Child. 52:580, 1977), who adduced evidence for an inability to dehydrogenate 18-hydroxycorticosterone to aldosterone. Another form of acquired hypoaldosteronism was reported by Perez and Oster (South. Med. J. 70:363, 1977), who recognized the disorder in a patient after renal transplantation, who had an allograft rejection. And, interestingly, Lebel and Grose (Clin. Sci. Mol. Med. 51:335S, 1976) infused, in a 63-year-old woman with hyporeninemic hypoaldosteronism, both ACTH and angiotensin II. They found a blunting of the plasma aldosterone response and suggested that the renal deficiency could contribute to impaired functioning of the zona glomerulosa. This form of pseudohypoaldosteronism must be differentiated from the genetic kind. Look ahead. — T.B.S.] ◄

The Nature of Defect in a Salt-Wasting Disorder in Jews of Iran was investigated by Ariel Rösler, David Rabinowitz, Rachel Theodor, Leyla C. Ramirez and Stanley Ulick.[7] A salt-wasting syndrome has been discovered in Jewish children of Iranian origin. Their response to sodium-retaining steroids suggested hypoaldosteronism, but their normal or elevated plasma aldosterone levels seemed to indicate decreased renal tubular responsiveness to the hormone. The plasma aldosterone levels were noted to be achieved at the expense of markedly elevated plasma renin activity. Aldosterone biosynthesis was examined in 12 patients from 8 families. All patients were Iranian Jews. There was parental consanguinity in all except 2 siblings.

All patients had sodium depletion and hypovolemia, but the spectrum of severity was wide. Some patients were discovered by screening apparently asymptomatic relatives of patients by the urinary C-18 oxygenated steroid ratio. The electrolyte abnormalities generally included hyponatremia, hyperkalemia, acidosis and prerenal axotemia. Plasma renin activity was markedly elevated, but this was corrected by sodium repletion therapy. All patients showed marked overproduction of the 18-hydroxy metabolite relative to that of

---

(7)   J. Clin. Endocrinol. Metab. 44:279–290, February, 1977.

aldosterone, the excretory ratio decreasing strikingly on sodium repletion. Aldosterone secretory responses were nearly maximal on a normal-salt diet. Acute dehydration was treated with parenteral fluids and DOCA; a glucocorticoid was not necessary.

Aldosterone deficiency in this condition is due to an inborn error involving the terminal biosynthetic pathway and characterized by marked overproduction of zona glomerulosa 18-hydroxycorticosterone relative to aldosterone. Plasma aldosterone is a less reliable index of the disorder than the excretory ratio of the major urinary metabolites. The disorder can readily go undetected and be underdiagnosed because of the subtlety of manifestations of hypoaldosteronism, especially in adults. It is important to detect even asymptomatic adults, since they are at risk for the development of lethal hyperkalemia, particularly when salt depleted.

▶ [This disorder has been found to occur as an autosomal recessive trait (Cohen et al.: Clin. Genet. 11:25, 1977).

The authors' study suggests that despite the normal or elevated levels of aldosterone, the primary defect is one of impairment of the conversion of 18-hydroxycorticosterone, to aldosterone, as mentioned in a prior comment on other patients, and they feel that they have been successful in differentiating this disease from true pseudohypoaldosteronism (Rosler et al.: J. Clin. Endocrinol. Metab. 44:292, 1977). True pseudohypoaldosteronism! Sorry about that! — T.B.S.] ◀

Postural Changes in Plasma Renin Activity and Responses to Vasoactive Drugs in a Case of Shy-Drager Syndrome. C. J. Mathias, W. B. Matthews and J. M. K. Spalding[8] studied the records of a patient with the Shy-Drager syndrome and gross autonomic insufficiency to determine cardiovascular and hormonal responses to head-tilt and cardiovascular responses to vasoactive drugs. The patient was a man aged 47 who for 8 years had had impotence, for 5 years had had urinary symptoms and for 3 years had had shortness of breath and fainting on exertion and on standing. He had had progressive worsening of symptoms for a few months before admission. Increasing "lack of balance" and slurring of speech had also been noted in the past year, and he had had attacks of "sighs." Emergency gastrectomy had been done for a duodenal ulcer and cardiac arrest had occurred 5 weeks postoperatively. The supine and stand-

---

(8) J. Neurol. Neurosurg. Psychiatry 40:138–143, February, 1977.

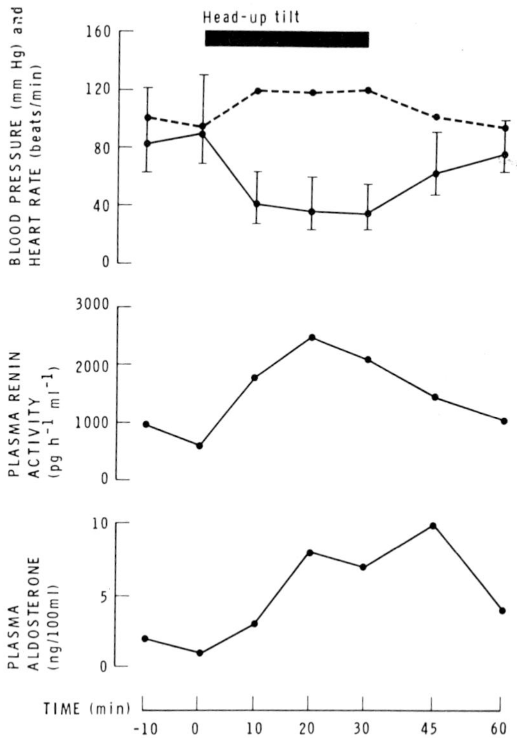

Fig 30. — Blood pressure (systolic, mean, diastolic), heart rate, plasma renin activity and plasma aldosterone in patient with Shy-Drager syndrome before (−10 and 0 minutes), during (10, 20 and 30 minutes) and after (45 and 60 minutes) head-up tilt. *Solid line,* mean blood pressure; *broken line,* heart rate. (Courtesy of Mathias, C. J., et al.: J. Neurol. Neurosurg. Psychiatry 40:138–143, February, 1977.)

ing blood pressures were 150/100 and 90/70 mm Hg, respectively. Mild cerebellar ataxia of all limbs was noted.

Heavy sweating on the palms, face and axillae but no sweating on the lower arms or trunk below the waist or the lower limbs were noted. The Valsalva maneuver resulted in abnormal cardiovascular responses of the "blocked" type. Responses to tilt testing are shown in Figure 30. Noradrenaline infusion caused a marked rise in blood pressure and a concomitant fall in heart rate. Angiotensin infusion increased the blood pressure more than in control subjects and lowered the heart rate. Isoprenaline injection resulted in a marked fall in pressure and rise in heart rate. The responses were greater than those in 3 paraplegics who were studied as controls.

The profound orthostatic hypotension in this patient was indicative of his inability reflexly to increase sympathetic nervous activity. The patient had exaggerated responses to vasoactive drugs of differing pharmacologic properties. Increased receptor sensitivity may play a part in these responses, but it is more likely that they were due to the absence of those baroreflexes that involve sympathetic efferent pathways.

▶ [This patient had quite classic symptoms of the Shy-Drager syndrome and the changes in blood pressure and pulse rate shown in Figure 30 are quite typical. The responses in plasma renin activity and plasma aldosterone are exaggerated and the authors make the point, "plasma renin activity is not dependent on sympathetic nervous activity . . . ." This is not to say that nervous sympathetic activity has no effect on renin secretion; anyone coming to such a conclusion would be guilty of what I have come to call the "Collip fallacy." Just about everyone, now, is too young to recall that Fuller Albright contended that parathyroid hormone acted primarily on the kidney while Collip insisted that its primary action was on bone. Professor Collip then did a "crucial" experiment. He injected a parathyroid hormone extract into nephrectomized rats and found a rise in serum calcium. He then insisted that the kidney had nothing to do with the action of parathyroid hormone and Doctor Albright agreed with him. Clearly, Doctor Collip's experiment could lead to *no* conclusions about the effect of parathyroid hormone on the kidney; there were no kidneys in the experiment!

Speaking of oldtimers, I must remind you that two senior citizens, Drs. Eugene Stead and Richard Ebert, published one of the important articles related to what we now call the Shy-Drager syndrome (Arch. Intern Med. 67:546, 1941).—T.B.S.] ◀

The following review articles are recommended to the reader:

Brunner, H. R., and Gavras, H.: Les inhibiteurs de l'angiotensine II pour le diagnostic et le traitement de l'hypertension, Schweiz. Med. Wochenschr. 106:1791, 1976.

De Wardener, H. E.: Natriuretic hormone, Clin. Sci. Mol. Med. 53: 1, 1977.

Frohlich, E. D., et al.: Second Pan American symposium on hypertension (continued), Mayo Clin. Proc. 52:361, June, 1977.

Kaplan, N. M.: Renin profiles: The unfulfilled promises, J.A.M.A. 238:611, 1977.

Laragh, J. H., et al.: Symposium on hypertension, Am. J. Med. 61: 721, November, 1976.

McGiff, J. C.: Bortter's syndrome results from an imbalance of vasoactive hormones, Ann. Intern. Med. 87:369, 1977.
Stockigt, J. R.: Potassium homeostasis, Aust. N.Z. J. Med. 7:66, 1977.
Weidmann, P., and Reubi, F.: Renale hypertonie, Schweiz. Med. Wochenschr. 106:1778, 1976.

The Ovary

Relaxin: Product of Human Corpus Luteum of Pregnancy. Gerson Weiss, E. M. O'Byrne and B. G. Steinetz[9] describe relaxin as a peptide hormone identified in several mammalian species during pregnancy. Its reported actions include cervical dilation and softening, inhibition of uterine contractions, and relaxation of pelvic joints. The major source of the hormone is the corpus luteum of the pregnant sow. Relaxin has been reported to be present in human pregnancy. A specific radioimmunoassay for porcine relaxin has been developed with ^{125}I-labeled polytyrosylrelaxin.

The source of human relaxin in late pregnancy was sought in 7 women at term undergoing cesarean section. Plasma was sampled from the ovarian veins 20–30 minutes after the placenta was delivered. Plasma progesterone concentrations were higher in the ovarian vein of the corpus luteum-bearing ovary than in peripheral plasma or on the contralateral side. Relaxin concentrations were also significantly higher in the ovarian vein on the corpus luteum-bearing side than in the peripheral plasma or the plasma of the contralateral ovary. Increased luteal progesterone secretion was accompanied by increased relaxin secretion. An increase of 1 ng/ml in relaxin was associated with an increase of about 30–50 ng/ml in progesterone. Such concentrations of relaxin are too low to be detected by current bioassays.

A peptide is present in the serum of pregnant women at term, which competes with porcine relaxin in a specific radioimmunoassay. The substance is secreted by the pregnancy corpus luteum, and its secretion correlates with luteal progesterone secretion.

► [That evidence should be found that the ovary of a pregnant woman is a major source of relaxin should not come as a surprise, because preparations are routinely obtained from the pregnant sow. (I've just reread this awkward and misinterpretable sentence. No offense intended!) The differ-

(9) Science 194:948–949, Nov. 26, 1976.

ence is that we used to *think* that relaxin came from the human corpus luteum of pregnancy; now we know. Furthermore, if there is a relaxin, there must also be a prorelaxin, right? Right, and this is shown by Frieden and Yeh (Proc. Soc. Exp. Biol. Med. 154:407, 1977). What else is new among ovarian products? Look ahead. — T.B.S.] ◄

Catechol Estrogens Inhibit Estrogen-Elicited Accumulation of Hypothalamic Cyclic AMP Suggesting Role as Endogenous Antiestrogens. The catechol estrogens, including 2-hydroxyestradiol and 2-hydroxyestrone, are major metabolic products of estrogen. They are present in the pituitary and hypothalamus in concentrations at least 10-fold higher than those of the parent estrogens, and they compete with estradiol-17β (E_2) for soluble estrogen receptors of the pituitary and hypothalamus, suggesting a role for these compounds in the control of gonadotropin secretion. Steven M. Paul and Phil Skolnick[1] (Natl. Inst. of Health) studied the effects of 2-hydroxyestradiol on the estrogen-elicited accumulation of cyclic adenosine monophosphate (AMP) in intact hypothalami in vitro. Cyclic AMP accumulation was elicited by diethylstilbestrol (DES) and E_2 in hypothalami of immature female rats.

Both DES and E_2 significantly stimulated the accumulation of cyclic AMP in incubated rat hypothalami. Preincubation of hypothalami with equimolar concentrations of 2-hydroxyestradiol significantly inhibited the effects of DES and E_2 on cyclic AMP accumulation, by 57% and 68%, respectively. This agent alone did not significantly stimulate cyclic AMP accumulation. The O-methylated metabolite 2-methoxyestradiol was inactive in high concentrations. Equimolar concentrations of estrone and estriol inhibited DES-elicited accumulation of cyclic AMP only marginally. Clomiphene antagonized the effects of DES.

The ability of estrogenic compounds to stimulate the formation of cyclic AMP in the hypothalamus in vitro seems to parallel their estrogenic potency in vivo. The catechol estrogen 2-hydroxyestradiol, like clomiphene, antagonizes the effects of both DES and E_2 on generation of cyclic AMP in the hypothalamus, whereas weakly estrogenic compounds are ineffective as either agonists or antagonists. The catechol estrogens could function as endogenous antiestrogens and thus regulate the actions of estrogens in situ. Reports

(1)   Nature 266:559–561, Apr. 7, 1977.

that 2-hydroxyestrone produces elevations of plasma LH in ovariectomized, estrogen-primed female rats and immature male rats are consistent with an antiestrogen action for the catechol estrogens.

▶ [A new category is heard from. I remind you that a catechol is an organic compound consisting of a six-carbon aromatic ring with two hydroxyl groups attached. These are naturally occurring antiestrogens, and they antagonize the actions of estrogen in the hypothalamus. In effect, catechol estrogens are to clomiphene as endorphins are to heroin. The analogy is not entirely frivolous, because the impact of catechol estrogens in terms of animal behavior and diseases like depression and migraine may be very real. — T.B.S.] ◀

Mefenamic Acid in Dysmenorrhea. Several gynecologists have stressed a functional etiology for dysmenorrhea, especially since the prostaglandins were found to contract the uterus. Martti O. Pulkkinen and H.-L. Kaihola[2] (Univ. of Turku) evaluated treatment with mefenamic acid (Ponstan), which interferes with the binding of prostaglandins to the cell, in dysmenorrheic patients. Eleven patients with severe dysmenorrhea, who had used other drugs without significant benefit, received 750 mg mefenamic acid on the 1st day of the menses. Intrauterine pressures were measured with the microballoon technique during 30 minutes before and 3 hours after medication. Plasma prostaglandins were determined by radioimmunoassay before and 3 hours after medication.

Uterine pressure and the frequency of contractions declined about 2 hours after mefenamic acid and active pressure decreased slightly (Fig 31). Dysmenorrheic pain was relieved as the uterine activity declined. One patient taking oral contraceptives had no further fall in intrauterine pressure and obtained no pain relief. Plasma prostaglandin E fell from 39 to 32 pg/ml 3 hours after mefenamic acid administration. The prostaglandin F level fell from 9 to 5 pg/ml. No significant changes in the ratio of prostaglandin to progesterone were observed. In 26 patients given 500 mg mefenamic acid every 6–8 hours, 67 of 75 treated cycles became painless, whereas in 4 cycles no pain relief was obtained. Two gynecologists used this regimen in about 200 cycles of 50 dysmenorrheic subjects and found that about 90% of the cycles became painless.

---

(2)   Acta Obstet. Gynecol. Scand. 56:75–76, 1977.

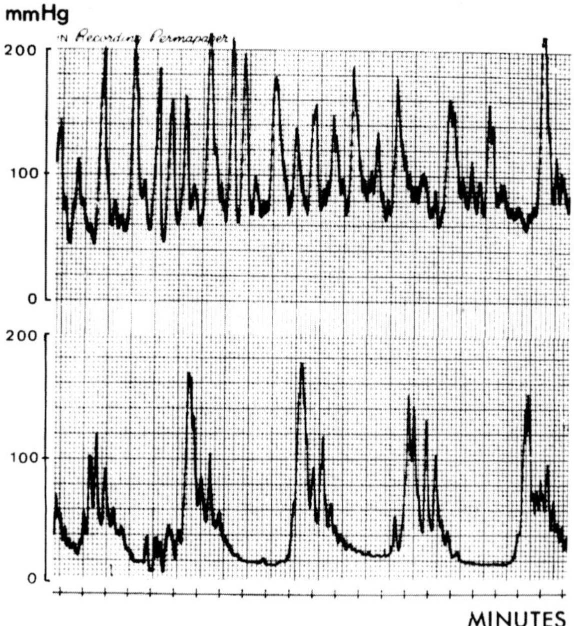

Fig 31.—Uterine activity before *(upper panel)* and after *(lower panel)* a single dose of mefenamic acid during the 1st day of menstruation. Original recording. Note the decrease in uterine resting pressure and frequency of contractions and nearly unchanged active pressure (decreasing later on), coincident with the disappearance of dysmenorrheic pain. (Courtesy of Pulkkinen, M. O., and Kaihola, H.-L.: Acta Obstet. Gynecol. Scand. 56:75–76, 1977.)

Mefenamic acid reduces uterine activity in dysmenorrheic patients and relieves pain so frequently that it can be used clinically in the management of true dysmenorrhea. Double-blind observations with placebo are needed for final conclusions to be drawn as to the clinical efficacy of this drug.

► [This is a nicely documented confirmation of a study reported in the 1977 YEAR BOOK (p. 291).

The authors are also to be congratulated for their cautionary last sentence. Despite the "experience" in use of these agents, disorders like dysmenorrhea may be strikingly susceptible to placebo effect. For instance, in the 1977 YEAR BOOK (p. 290) there also appeared an article proclaiming the efficacy of bromocriptine in the treatment of the premenstrual syndrome. Since then, two other double-blind studies were carried out. Andersen et al. (Br. J. Obstet. Gynecol. 84:370, 1977) discovered "medication considerably improved all the menstrual symptoms, but mastodynia was the only one where bromocriptine was significantly better than the placebo," whereas Ghose and Coppen (Br. Med. J. 1:147, 1977) found no effect at all for bromocriptine. Finally, we should mention an adolescent girl who became psychotic with each menstrual period (Kramer: Am. J. Dis. Child 31:316, 1977). Your first guess is that she was cured with mefenamic acid or indomethacin, right? No, the attacks have been virtually eliminated by phenytoin.—T.B.S.] ◄

Serum Cortisol and 11-Desoxycortisol Levels in Hirsute Premenopausal Women. It has been postulated that hirsute patients may have a relative deficiency in 11β-hydroxylase activity in the adrenal cortex. George B. Maroulis, Fredesminda S. Manlimos, Romula Garza and Guy E. Abraham[3] tested this postulate by measuring serum levels of cortisol (Cp F) and 11-desoxycortisol (Cp S) in 34 hirsute premenopausal women. Nine nonhirsute premenopausal women were also evaluated. Serums Cp F and Cp S were measured by radioimmunoassay. As a group, the hirsute patients had significantly elevated mean Cp F and Cp S levels, but the mean Cp S/Cp F ratio was not significantly different from normal. Only 3 hirsute patients had a ratio more than 2 SD above the normal mean. A patient with documented 11β-hydroxylase deficiency had a Cp S of 218 ng/ml and a Cp S/Cp F ratio of 0.7.

These findings suggest that 11β-hydroxylase deficiency is not a common cause of hirsutism. Only 3 of 34 patients in the present study had a significantly elevated Cp S/Cp F ratio, and the elevations were not marked. Other factors that are not well understood at present appear to be involved in hyperandrogenism in women. Further studies should be directed toward gaining an understanding of the mechanisms controlling androgen secretion by the adrenal cortex under normal and pathologic conditions.

► [This is a disappointing study. I had always thought that because these hirsute women often responded so well to adrenocortical suppression, that they, like the children with hereditary pseudohermaphroditism, have an enzyme defect. Indeed, we've often spoken of this disorder as "adult adrenogenital syndrome." But wait! If you look ahead, you'll see that all is not yet lost.—T.B.S.] ◄

Partial 11- and 21-Hydroxylase Deficiencies in Hirsute Women. Some hirsute patients in most series respond favorably to suppressive therapy with glucocorticoids or estrogens, but pretreatment steroid studies often fail to predict the source of androgen or the response to therapy. Ste-

---

(3)   Obstet. Gynecol. 48:388–391, October, 1976.

phen Newmark, Robert G. Dluhy, Gordon H. Williams, Peter Pochi and Leslie I. Rose[4] (Harvard Med. School) sought
to devise a means of screening women for partial adrenocortical enzyme deficiencies to identify those who might
benefit from glucocorticoid suppression. Thirty-one hirsute
female patients, aged 16–46 years, were studied. Cushing's
syndrome had been excluded by dexamethasone suppression
testing in each. Nine of 15 patients with menstrual abnormalities had ovarian pathologic changes, but none had enlarged polycystic ovaries. Eight nonobese, normal women
aged 21–29 years were also evaluated.

Fig 32.—Mean ± SEM steroid excretion values in control, nonhirsute female subjects *(clear bars)* and in group I *(hatched bars)* and group II *(solid bars)* hirsute female
patients, basally and after 50 units (0.5 mg) of α-1–24 ACTH cosyntropin continuously infused over 24 hours. (Courtesy of Newmark, S., et al.: Am. J. Obstet. Gynecol.
127:594–598, Mar. 15, 1977.)

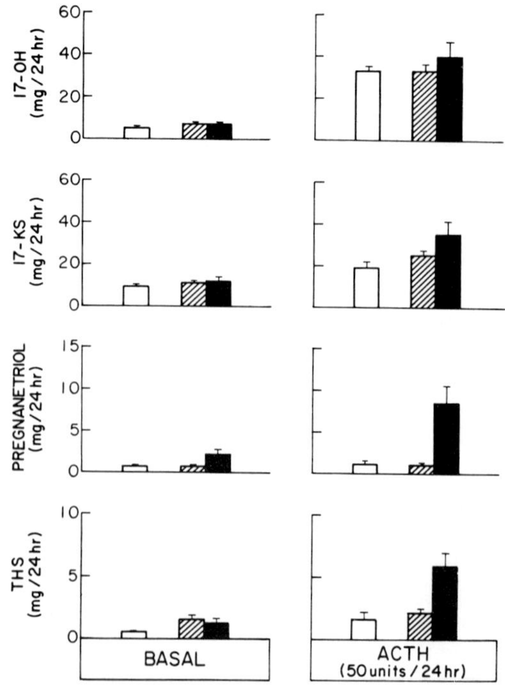

(4)   Am. J. Obstet. Gynecol. 127:594–598, Mar. 15, 1977.

The results of steroid studies are shown in Figure 32. Eighteen hirsute patients (group I) had normal basal and cosyntropin-stimulated tetrahydro compound S (THS) and pregnanetriol responses, whereas the other 13 (group II) had values more than 2 SD from the control mean. Group II patients also showed increments in 17-ketosteroid excretion on cosyntropin stimulation that were significantly greater than those in the control group. Group II patients had sebum production rates significantly above those of normal females, whereas group I patients had rates similar to those of normal females. Basal morning plasma testosterone values were in the high-normal range or were slightly elevated in groups I and II.

Some hirsute women have partial adrenocortical 21- and 11-hydroxylase deficiencies that can be detected after a 24-hour infusion of ACTH. Such testing may identify patients who will respond favorably to glucocorticoid suppressive therapy. Further study is needed of the results of long-term glucocorticoid suppression in these patients.

▶ [Here it is apparent that what we have come to call "the syndrome of functional androgen excess" is a mixed bag. (Honest, ladies, no pun is intended.) The technique used here has appeal because ACTH stimulation would exaggerate the shortcomings of partially deficient androgen-producing enzymes.

What else is new? Well, Meikle et al. (Trans. Assoc. Am. Physicians 89: 133, 1976) offer plasma 5-α-androstanediol as a good androgen marker of hirsutism, but I am more attracted to the views of Paulson et al. (Am. J. Obstet. Gynecol. 128:851, 1977), who have successfully used serum free testosterone concentrations to monitor the treatment of patients with hirsutism. They found that in half of their hirsute patients suppression of free testosterone to normal occurred with dexamethasone treatment alone. In the others, suppression was accomplished with the addition of Enovid-E.

Finally, I should mention what interests many patients most. Dewhurst et al. (Br. J. Obstet. Gynecol. 84:119, 1977) successfully treated severely hirsute patients with cyproterone, although relapses with discontinuance of the therapy were frequent. For the first time, in this article I saw convincing photographs showing that therapy for hirsutism was effective.

It's worry time. Look ahead. — T.B.S.] ◀

Upper Genital Tract Changes Associated with Exposure In Utero to Diethylstilbestrol. Besides adenocarcinoma of the upper vagina and cervix, various vaginal and cervical abnormalities have been described in association with female exposure in utero to diethylstilbestrol (DES).

Raymond H. Kaufman, Gary L. Binder, Paul Milton Gray, Jr., and Ervin Adam[5] (Baylor Univ.) studied by hysterosalpingography a group of young women, exposed in utero to DES. The exposure was documented in 46 of the 60 young women studied; in 14 instances the mothers were certain they had received DES. Hysterosalpingograms of 23 women being studied for infertility in the same period also were reviewed. In 28 of the women with documented drug exposure, medication was begun before 13 weeks' gestation. Dosages ranged from 5 to 300 mg daily. Mean age of the exposed group was 22.3 years and that of the controls was 27.6.

Upper genital tract changes were detected in 40 exposed subjects. In 21 instances the changes included a T-shaped appearance of the uterus, with widening of the interstitial and isthmic parts of the oviducts and narrowing of the lower uterine cavity. Constriction bands were present in the dilated lateral parts of the T in several cases (Fig 33). In 5 instances the uterus appeared to be generally small. Defects were seen within the uterine cavity in 4 patients. In 36 of these 40 subjects the cervix showed gross anatomical changes, and

Fig 33. – Note T-shaped appearance with well-demarcated annular constriction of proximal horns. Lower segment appears wide. (Courtesy of Kaufman, R. H., et al.: Am. J. Obstet. Gynecol. 128:51–59, May 1, 1977.)

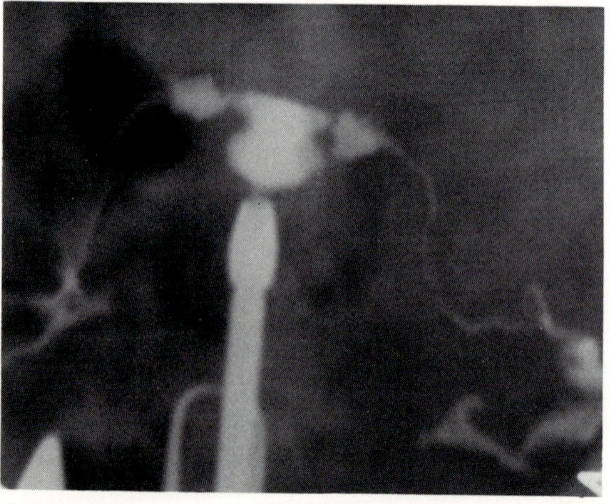

(5)   Am. J. Obstet. Gynecol. 128:51–59, May 1, 1977.

this was also true of 4 patients with normal uteri on x-rays. Adenosis was diagnosed in 28 patients with abnormal x-rays and in 10 with normal x-rays. Twenty of 28 women whose mothers began using DES in the first 12 weeks of pregnancy had abnormal x-rays, as did 2 of 5 women exposed at 19 weeks or later during gestation. No comparable changes were found in controls.

The clinical significance of these findings is unclear. Three of 4 live births were premature and 2 of these women had abnormal uteri. One of 2 women who had spontaneous abortions had an abnormal uterus.

▶ [The deformed uterus, shown in Figure 33, is obviously not the only worry of these patients. They are relatively infertile and they very often, as everyone now knows, have adenosis, if not adenocarcinoma of the vagina and cervix. Fortunately, Herbst et al. (Am. J. Obstet. Gynecol. 128:43, 1977) found that the highest incidence of carcinoma occurs at the young age of 19, and then the incidence declines dramatically. Furthermore, the risk of exposed female subjects is only about 1/1,000. On the one hand, this is outrageously high because there should be no risk but, on the other, for those unwittingly at risk, 999 of the 1,000 get by harmlessly. As indicated in this article, however, abnormalities of one sort or another, including vaginal adenosis, are very common, the latter occurring in 35% of one series (Poskanzer and Herbst: Cancer 39:1892, 1977).

Those of you who have assumed that male offspring of DES-treated mothers get off scot-free are wrong. Cosgrove et al. (J. Urol. 117:220, 1977) and Gill and associates (ibid., p. 477) both found genitourinary abnormalities and pathologic semen in such offspring. — T.B.S.] ◀

Plasma Estrogen in Patients with Endometrial Hyperplasia and Carcinoma. Fatma A. Aleem, Mamdouh A. Moukhtar, Hin Cheung Hung and Seymour L. Romney[6] (Albert Einstein College of Medicine) determined plasma estrogens by gas-liquid chromatography in 53 women, most of them over age 40, who presented with vaginal bleeding, and examined the clinical correlates. Twenty-eight patients had proved endometrial carcinoma, 8 had endometrial hyperplasia of various types and 7 had abnormal uterine bleeding with no apparent histologic endometrial lesion. Ten normal postmenopausal women were used as controls.

The controls had a mean total plasma estrogen content of 47 ng/100 ml, with a SE of 4.7. Only 2 of the patients with endometrial carcinoma were nulliparous. Over half the patients were obese, half were hypertensive and 12 of the 28 were diabetic. Mean total estrogen concentration was 76.65

---

(6) Cancer 38:2101–2104, November, 1976.

ng/100 ml plasma, significantly above the control mean. Obese patients with endometrial carcinoma had significantly higher estrogen values than nonobese patients, whose values did not differ significantly from control values. Five of the 8 patients with endometrial hyperplasia were obese, 6 were hypertensive and 5 had diabetes. Mean plasma estrogen concentration was 117.1 ng/100 ml, significantly above the control value. The other patients with abnormal uterine bleeding had a mean plasma estrogen concentration of 64.2 ng/100 ml, not significantly different from the control mean.

Clinical correlates, as well as significantly higher plasma estrogen values, occur in patients with endometrial cancer and in those with endometrial hyperplasia. A positive correlation between hyperestrogenism and obesity is evident. Increased plasma estrogen values and obesity are significant, but not the only, etiologic factors in the development of endometrial carcinoma.

► [The constellation of symptoms noted in these patients was first discussed in the 1969 YEAR BOOK (p. 290), and the evidence seems to be sustained that in its naturally occurring form, "carcinoma of the endometrium is a complication of a chronic hypothalamic disorder" and the relative hyperestrogenism of these patients fits nicely. The iatrogenic variety was first reported in the 1977 YEAR BOOK (p. 310). The subject has become controversial. There are some supportive articles (Gordon et al.: N. Engl. J. Med. 297:570, 1977; Gambrel: J. Reprod. Med. 18:301, 1977; and Schumaker et al.: J.A.M.A. 238:1524, 1977), as well as some suggestion that perhaps low-dose estrogens, along with some progesterone, may prevent endometrial carcinoma. An interesting study was done by Byrd et al. (Ann. Surg. 185:574, 1977), who found that *hysterectomized* women treated with estrogen showed a striking decrease in mortality from heart attack and cancer, as compared to nonhysterectomized, non-estrogen-treated women. Could the beneficial effects be attributable to hysterectomy rather than the estrogens?

Onward and upward (literally) to consider estrogens and breast cancer. — T.B.S.] ◄

Menopausal Estrogens and Breast Cancer. Since reproductive factors and ovarian hormones have long been implicated in the origin of breast cancer, administration of estrogens to healthy women is controversial. Much laboratory evidence supports the idea that estrogens are harmful, but observations on women suggest protection against breast cancer.

Robert Hoover, Laman A. Gray, Sr., Philip Cole and Brian

MacMahon[7] did a follow-up study of 1,891 women in Louisville, Kentucky, given conjugated estrogens for the menopause since 1939 in order to determine the incidence of breast cancer. All women were white and in the upper-middle or upper socioeconomic class. The average age at start of therapy was 49 years. Mean follow-up was 12 years. A total of 22,717 person-years of follow-up was accumulated, and 620 women were followed for over 15 years.

Breast cancer developed in 49 women, with 39.1 cases expected from rates in the general population, for a relative risk of 1.3. The relative risk increased with duration of follow-up, reaching 2.0 after 15 years. The excess risk after 10 years was not due simply to prolonged estrogen use, since there was no clear dose-response relationship to accumulated years of use. The risk was higher in women using higher-dose tablets and those taking the medication on an other than daily basis (table). After 10 years of follow-up, both

OBSERVED AND EXPECTED CASES OF BREAST CANCER ACCORDING TO FOLLOW-UP DURATION AND STRENGTH AND FREQUENCY OF ESTROGEN USED*

FOLLOW-UP DURATION (YR)	STRENGTH			FREQUENCY	
	0.3 MG (873)[†]	0.625 MG (1262)	>0.625 MG (246)	DAILY (1830)	OTHER (278)
<10:					
Observed	13.0	17.0	4.0	25.0	5.0
Expected	13.8	16.5	3.2	25.4	4.1
Relative risk	0.9	1.0	1.3	1.0	1.2
95% confidence interval	0.5 - 1.5	0.6 - 1.6	0.4 - 3.3	0.7 - 1.5	0.4 - 2.8
10+:					
Observed	14.0	11.0	8.0	20.0	9.0
Expected	8.5	9.8	3.0	14.8	3.9
Relative risk	1.6	1.1	2.7	1.4	2.3
95% confidence interval	0.9 - 2.7	0.5 - 2.0	1.2 - 5.3	0.9 - 2.2	1.1 - 4.4

*Tabulated according to whether the woman ever used a particular type of therapy. Number of women more than total in study since a woman could be in more than one category.

†Figures in parentheses denote number of women.

(7) N. Engl. J. Med. 295:401–405, Aug. 19, 1976.

multiparity and oophorectomy were no longer related to a low risk of breast cancer. Estrogen use was associated with a particularly high risk in women who developed benign breast disease after they started using the drug.

These findings clearly indicate the menopausal estrogen use does not protect against breast cancer. The data do not in themselves indict exogenous estrogens as a cause of breast cancer. However, they suggest this as a definite possibility and indicate that a thorough evaluation is needed. Factors such as latent period, risk indicators for breast cancer, type of treatment and total accumulated dosage will have to be incorporated into a full evaluation of estrogens.

► [I've seen a number of women desperately drinking from the estrogenic fountain of youth develop remarkably lumpy breasts. Certainly, one might conclude from this study that they ought to stop taking estrogens. It is good to know that Cole (Cancer 39:1906, 1977) agrees. — T.B.S.] ◄

Changed Levels of Endogenous Sex Steroids in Women on Oral Contraceptives. The mechanism of action of oral contraceptives is not yet clear, but they are thought to inhibit gonadotropin release or to affect the ovaries and genital tract directly. J. M. Kjeld, C. M. Puah and G. F. Joplin[8] (Royal Postgrad. Med. School, London) studied the effects of oral contraceptives on serum levels of sex hormones in 19 healthy women aged 18–34 years. Ten not on medication were studied in the first 10 days of the menstrual cycle. Nine had taken oral contraceptives for at least 2 months. Five women were taking Ovran (50 μg ethinyl estradiol and 250 μg D-norgestrel); 2, Eugynon 50 (50 μg ethinyl estradiol and 500 μg DL-norgestrel); and 2, Gynovlar 21 (50 μg ethinyl estradiol and 3 mg norethisterone acetate).

The contraceptive group had higher mean values of serum testosterone and dihydrotestosterone than did controls and significantly lower serum estradiol values, similar to those of postmenopausal women. Mean serum values of dihydrotestosterone and estradiol correlated well in the control group but poorly in the contraceptive group. The women using contraceptives excreted less unconjugated estradiol than did controls; the difference between the means of the

---

(8) Br. Med. J. 2:1354–1356, Dec. 4, 1976.

MEAN (± SD) SERUM AND URINARY LEVELS OF UNCONJUGATED TESTOSTERONE, DIHYDROTESTOSTERONE AND ESTRADIOL IN 10 HEALTHY WOMEN IN EARLY FOLLICULAR PHASE OF MENSTRUAL CYCLE AND 9 WOMEN ON ORAL CONTRACEPTIVES. RANGES GIVEN IN PARENTHESES

	Testosterone	Dihydrotestosterone	Oestradiol
Serum levels (nmol/l)			
Control group	0·722 ± 0·184 (0·451–1·041)	0·313 ± 0·145 (0·082–0·616)	0·126 ± 0·054 (0·044–0·217)
Contraceptive group	0·972 ± 0·382 (0·382–1·596)	0·623 ± 0·243 (0·372–1·118)	0·038 ± 0·012 (0·022–0·051)
t Test	NS*	P <0·01	P <0·001
Urinary excretion (nmol/24 h)			
Control group	320 ± 264 (115–902)	134 ± 81·2 (36·5–282)	88·1 ± 91·8 (20·9–274·52)
Contraceptive group	694 ± 579 (108–1947)	259 ± 146 (68·1–488·5)	25 ± 21·3 (5·5–73·8)
t Test	NS*	P <0·05	P <0·05

*NS, not significant at 5% level.

Conversion of SI to traditional units: serum testosterone, 1 nM/L≈288 pg/ml; urinary testosterone, 1 nM/24 hours≈0.288 pg/24 hours; serum dihydrotestosterone, 1 nM/L≈290 pg/ml; urinary dihydrotestosterone, 1 nM/24 hours≈0.29 pg/24 hours; serum estradiol, 1 nM/L≈272 pg/ml; urinary estradiol, 1 nM/24 hours≈0.27 pg/24 hours.

two groups was just significant. Serum and urine values for both groups are given in the table.

This study showed profound changes in endogenous sex hormone concentrations in women using oral contraceptives, compared with normal early follicular phase values. The contraceptive users had about twice the urinary excretion of unconjugated testosterone and dihydrotestosterone as did the controls, but their excretion of unconjugated estradiol was almost threefold lower. The great increase in serum and urinary androgens and the suppression of estradiol may be related to the antiovulatory effect of oral contraceptives. The dihydrotestosterone-estradiol ratio in contraceptive users was over 6 times higher than that in the control group. Further study might show whether this ratio could be used as an index of the antiovulatory efficiency of contraceptive preparations.

► [Interesting! First, one might suspect that the rise in serum androgens was simply the result of increased sex steroid-binding globulin concentrations induced by the estrogens present in the oral contraceptives. This idea is weakened substantially by the fact that androgen excretion in the urine is increased. The reason androgen levels are increased in these patients in whom gonadotropins are suppressed escapes me. Do estrogens directly stimulate Leydig's cells to produce androgens? At a tissue level the androgen-estrogen ratios would tend to be maintained (the low estradiol levels plus the estrogen contained in the oral contraceptives); certainly androgenic effects are not a prominent consequence of pill taking. — T.B.S.] ◄

► ↓ I have been so critical of the unthinking, large-scale dissemination of contraceptive steroids to women that I have tended to blind myself to possible ameliorating aspects. I try to make amends in the following two articles. — T.B.S. ◄

Amenorrhea Following Use of Oral Contraceptives. Postoral contraceptive amenorrhea is rare. Jacques Van Campenhout, Pierre Blanchet, Hugues Beauregard and Said Papas[9] (Univ. of Montreal) retrospectively studied 86 patients with postoral contraceptive amenorrhea of over 6 months' duration. Serum and plasma levels of hormones were determined by radioimmunoassay. There were 55 amenorrheic patients without detectable galactorrhea (group I) and 31 with amenorrhea associated with galactorrhea (group II). The groups were comparable in age and gravidity. The prevalence of previous oligomenorrhea was 60% in group I and 48.4% in group II. Late menarche had occurred in 10.9% of group I patients and 6.4% of group II. Mean durations of contraceptive pill use were 29 months in group I and 34.5 months in group II. The respective mean durations of amenorrhea were 17.5 and 27.7 months.

Hypothalamic-pituitary dysfunction was diagnosed in 70.9% of group I patients (table). A psychologic factor was identified at the onset of amenorrhea in 12.7% of this group. Primary ovarian failure was confirmed in 3 patients. One patient had a prolactin-secreting tumor. Causes of amenorrhea probably unrelated to the pill were identified in 5 patients. Eighteen group II patients had intermittent spontaneous galactorrhea, 3 of them before oral contraceptive use and 4 concomitantly with the amenorrhea. Ten group II patients (32.3%) were found to have a pituitary tumor, and 9 were proved to have pure prolactin-secreting tumors; 1 is awaiting surgery. The other 21 group II patients had diagnoses of hypothalamic-pituitary dysfunction. One had primary hypothyroidism. Fourteen others had high serum prolactin concentrations.

---

(9)　Fertil. Steril. 28:728–732, July, 1977.

ETIOLOGIC FACTORS FOUND IN PATIENTS WITH POSTPILL
AMENORRHEA WITHOUT GALACTORRHEA (GROUP I) AND WITH
GALACTORRHEA (GROUP II)

Etiologic factor	No. of cases	
	Group I: 55 patients	Group II: 31 patients
Pituitary tumor	1	10
Hypothalamic-pituitary dysfunction	39	20
Psychogenic	7	
Premature ovarian failure	3	
Primary hypothyroidism		1
Other	5	

Galactorrhea should be carefully sought in all patients
with postpill amenorrhea. When galactorrhea is present,
study of the hypothalamic-pituitary axis is mandatory, including repeated prolactin assays and tomographic study of
the sella. When galactorrhea is not elicited, the chance of
finding a pituitary prolactin-secreting tumor is low. It seems
to be acceptable in the absence of galactorrhea to reassure
the patient and to wait 1 year before requesting an expen-
sive and not readily available endocrine work-up.

▶ [It is reasonable to conclude from this study of postpill amenorrhea
that, in part, oral contraceptives have suffered "a bum rap." It may be that
they serve as precipitating rather than causal agents of amenorrhea, like
the diuretic-induced severe hypokalemia in patients who have primary
aldosteronism, or the hypercalcemia similarly induced in patients harboring a parathyroid adenoma. Perhaps patients harboring the nidus of a
prolactin-secreting tumor rock along until exposed to oral contraceptives.
The supraphysiologic levels of estrogens then attained stimulate prolactin-secreting cells so that when the pill is stopped, the prolactinoma has
achieved autonomy. This explanation will serve until the true one comes
along.

The "bum rap" in this instance does not exonerate oral contraceptives
from their well-known deleterious side effects, and I am incapable of
completing YEAR BOOK chores without listing some. The hyperlipemic
effect of oral contraceptives is probably due to a decrease in hepatic triglyceride lipase (Applebaum et al.: J. Clin. Invest. 59:601, 1977), and the
megaloblastic anemia occasionally encountered is due to pyridoxine deficiency (Tant: Br. Med. J. 2:979, 1976). Estrogen-associated skin eruptions
are described by Wilkin (Arch. Dermatol. 113:486, 1977) and Cosky (ibid.
p. 333). Did you know that in patients using oral contraceptives postoperative localized osteitis is more frequent after tooth extraction? To find
details, see Sweet and Butler (Am. J. Obstet. Gynecol. 127:518, 1977). And
the association of pill taking with ulcers of the colon is reported by Berna-
dino and Lawson (Am. J. Dig. Dis. 21:503, 1976).

Finally, I have before me thirteen articles from twelve journals on the subject of oral contraceptives and hepatic disease, particularly focal nodular hyperplasia. They were all published in 1977, and the interested reader is referred, as always, to *Index Medicus*. While the message may be muddled to some gynecologists, to me it is clear. The incidence of these previously rarest of liver neoplasms has greatly increased with increased use of oral contraceptives. Only a very small minority of pill users are presently afflicted. — T.B.S.] ◄

Oral Contraceptives for Prophylaxis of Acute Exacerbations of Intermittent Porphyria. G. Schley, M. Anlauf and K. D. Bock[1] (Univ. of Essen). Because acute intermittent porphyria occurs in a temporal relationship to menstruation, various authors have reported trials with ovulation inhibitors for prevention of exacerbations. In the present study the illness was observed in 14 women with acute intermittent porphyria, 7 of whom were treated with ovulation inhibitors an average of 5 years. In 2 others bilateral oophorectomy and irradiation castration were performed, respectively; 5 untreated women served as controls.

In contrast to the control group, there were no further acute exacerbations in the group treated with oral contraceptives. The 2 patients treated by oophorectomy and irradiation died after repeated acute bouts. Persistent, at times severe, arterial hypertension developed in 4 women taking oral contraceptives; its pathogenesis is unexplained.

Statistical analysis of all observations confirms the favorable influence of ovulation inhibitors on the number of exacerbations in acute porphyria, although the action mechanism is unclear. It is known that δ-aminolevulinic acid synthetase activity is increased by estrogens, whereas estrogen secretion is diminished by ovulation inhibitors. This might mean that the oral contraceptives also inhibit the increased δ-aminolevulinic acid synthetase characteristic in acute porphyria by diminished endogenous estrogen formation. The effect of oral contraceptives on ovulation is mainly caused by inhibition of FSH and LH and thus the effect of ovulation inhibitors in intermittent porphyria may be explained on the basis of inhibited gonadotropin secretion. However, the initially promising prophylactic action of oral contraceptives in acute intermittent porphyria becomes somewhat questionable due to the seemingly frequent de-

---

(1)   Dtsch. Med. Wochenschr. 101:1901–1907, Dec. 24, 1976.

velopment of arterial hypertension, which was not observed in the untreated patients. These observations need further confirmation in more patients.

▶ [But, even my best efforts at optimism about the pill are suspect. Four of the 5 successfully treated patients developed severe hypertension. What's more, Leonhardi (Dtsch. Med. Wochenschr. 102:160, 1977) found 4 patients who fell ill with cutaneous hepatic porphyria after taking oral contraceptives for from 3 to 8 years.

I insist on finishing this comment on an upbeat note. Did you know that Rothman (N. Engl. J. Med. 297:468, 1977) found that the rates of spontaneous abortion and stillbirth was smaller for former pill users than nonusers, and that the occurrence of twins was higher? This, of course, was good news only for the dwindling segment of the population that remains interested in parenthood. — T.B.S.] ◀

Catamenial Pneumothorax: Bilateral Occurrence while on Suppressive Therapy. Catamenial pneumothorax was first reported in 1958; in 26 of the subsequent 29 cases the right side of the chest has been affected. John L. Wilhelm and Antonio Scommegna[2] (Chicago) report the first occurrence of bilateral catamenial pneumothorax.

Woman, 32, a nulligravid black, reported having had painful menses since the menarche at age 13 and had been effectively treated with cyclic Norinyl. Right shoulder pain had occurred with menses at age 28 and recurred the next year, when endometriosis had been diagnosed and treated with cyclic Ortho-Novum and then cyclic Enovid. Dysmenorrhea had persisted despite treatment and at age 30 the patient presented with sudden substernal chest pain and dyspnea, starting 24 hours after the onset of menses. Bilateral pneumothorax with effusion was diagnosed and water-seal-type drainage was used to reexpand the right lung. Similar symptoms occurred the next month and the pleural surfaces were abraded at exploratory thoracotomy. Pericardial endometriosis was discovered at this time (Fig 34). An asymptomatic left pneumothorax occurred after 9 months of continuous Ovral therapy and was treated with thoracotomy and abrasion of the left pleural surfaces. Endometriosis and decidual change were found in the diaphragm and pericardial tissue and decidual change in a pleural biopsy specimen. Hypertension developed 2 months later and Ovral was discontinued. Cyclic Duphaston then controlled the dysmenorrhea that followed, but shortness of breath was noted and Depo-Provera therapy was instituted. The patient has since been amenorrheic and had no pelvic discomfort or chest symptoms.

Catamenial pneumothorax repeatedly occurred bilateral-

---

(2) Obstet. Gynecol. 50:227–231, August, 1977.

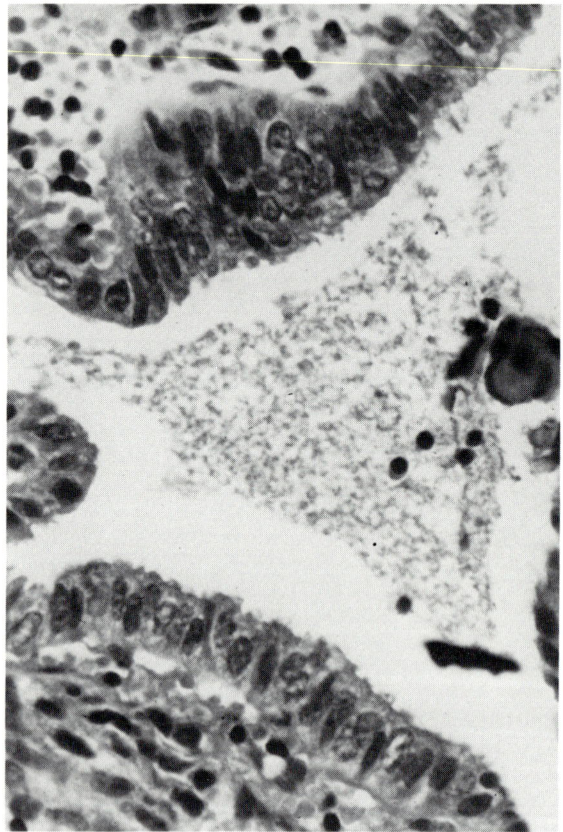

Fig 34.—Portion of endometrial tissue in the pericardium. Note the active glandular epithelium with intraluminal hemorrhage; reduced from ×40. (Courtesy of Wilhelm, J. L., and Scommegna, A.: Obstet. Gynecol. 50:227–231, August 1977.)

ly in this case, in association with anovulatory bleeding. Not all patients with catamenial pneumothorax have diaphragmatic defects. The ideal treatment of a patient with extensive disease is suppression of all growth and bleeding of intrathoracic endometrial implants. This can be achieved by increasing the dose of continuous oral contraceptives until amenorrhea persists. When hypertension develops, the same effect can be achieved with Depo-Provera.

► [As you see in Figure 34, endometrial mucosa is the most itinerant tissue in the body. You may know that it doesn't stop at the pleura or pericardium. It can invade bronchi and produce monthly hemoptysis and may show up in the nasal mucosa (Fliess spots), provoking monthly nose bleeds. Catamenial pneumothorax may be a serious event, and deaths have been reported (1969 YEAR BOOK, p. 308).—T.B.S.] ◄

The following review articles are recommended to the reader:

Channing, C. P., and Tsafriri, A.: Mechanism of action of luteinizing hormone and follicle-stimulating hormone on the ovary in vitro, Metabolism 26:413, 1977.

Fishman, J.: The catechol estrogens, Horm. Res. 8:363, 1977.

Hoffbrand, B. I., and Lawson, J. P.: The menopause and its treatment, Postgrad. Med. J. 52 (Suppl. 6), 1976.

Jewelewicz, R.: The diagnosis and treatment of amenorrheas, Fertil. Steril. 27:1347, 1976.

Klatskin, G.: Hepatic tumors: Possible relationship to use of oral contraceptives, Gastroenterology 73:386, 1977.

McCann, S. M.: Luteinizing hormone-releasing hormone, New Engl. J. Med. 296:797, 1977.

Szego, C. M.: Steroid-protein binding: From circulating blood to target cell nucleus, Gynecol. Invest. 7:251, 1976.

Yen, S. S. C.: The biology of menopause, J. Reprod. Med. 18:287, 1977.

The Testis

Sex Hormones and Vocal Pitch in the Male. W. Meuser and E. Nieschlag[3] (Univ. of Münster) investigated this relationship in 102 male vocalists. The difference in pitch between the male and female voice has been attributed to the difference in androgen production. The high eunuchoid voice as a result of early castration in the man, the coincidence of increased androgen levels and voice change during puberty in boys and the deepening voice of women under androgen treatment support this assumption. However, other than the effect of androgen on the larynx, little is known about the role of sex hormones in the development and maintenance of the bass, baritone and tenor registers of the male voice.

In the present study the plasma concentrations of testosterone, estradiol, LH and FSH were determined (table). As compared to tenors, higher testosterone and lower estradiol concentrations were found in bass and baritone singers, resulting in a higher testosterone-estradiol ratio in the deeper registers due to increased androgen. Deeper voices were also associated with taller and heavier body build. At younger age, sexual activity was (and had been) highest in those with bass voices; middle-aged and older tenors were most active in this regard. There appeared to be no vocal pitch-related differences in terms of sequence and occurrence of various puberal characteristics; the only significant factor was that subsequent bass singers had a higher incidence of acne.

These results suggest that the pitch of the male voice is influenced by the different concentrations of circulating sex hormones as well as the androgen sensitivity of the target organs. Because an increased plasma estrogen value is viewed as a predisposing factor in myocardial infarction, it might be interesting to investigate whether tenors show a

---

(3) Dtsch. Med. Wochenschr. 102:261–264, Feb. 25, 1977.

HORMONE CONCENTRATIONS IN PLASMA OF VOCALISTS, GROUPED BY
VOCAL PITCH AND AGE ($\bar{x}\pm s$).

VOCAL PITCH AND AGE (YEARS)	NO.	TESTOSTERONE [NMOL/L]	ESTRADIOL [PMOL/L]	LH [IU/L]	FSH [IU/L]
Tenor					
20–40	15	10.4±0.7	106±11	9.8±1.0	5.9±0.6
41–50	9	11.3±1.5	145±14	14.7±1.4	7.9±1.5
51–70	16	7.8±0.6	117±10	13.2±1.7	11.1±1.6
Baritone					
20–40	10	13.6±1.8	125±16	11.5±1.4	7.8±0.9
41–50	11	12.5±1.1	114±11	10.1±0.8	7.1±1.1
51–70	6	13.7±1.7	88±10	19.7±3.6	12.0±3.6
Bass					
20–40	12	13.0±1.1	82±56	10.7±1.2	7.2±1.3
41–50	6	13.1±1.8	88±13	10.6±1.3	6.7±0.9
51–70	8	15.0±0.6	116±23	15.9±3.6	9.2±2.2

higher incidence of infarction, which may be of prophylactic and therapeutic significance.

▶ [It is enough to make an endocrinologist's heart sing! Yes, I know that only one androgen and one estrogen were measured, that the differences are not dramatic, that the numbers are not large, that only one casual sample was obtained and that German males might not behave in the same way as do Parisian males (1977 YEAR BOOK, p. 322) and not change testosterone levels with the season of year. Still, the results make endocrinologic sense and no aspersions are cast on anybody. Those who want to make jokes should pick an article like that of Barkey et al. (Fertil. Steril. 28: 175, 1977), entitled "Effect of Caffeine in Increasing the Motility of Frozen Human Sperm." Comment: There's nothing like a good "cuppa coffee" to get a body moving.—T.B.S.] ◀

Mechanism of Feminization in Primary Liver Cancer. Precocious puberty due to ectopic gonadotropin production by primary liver cancer has been reported. Michael C. Kew, Marvin A. Kirschner, Guy E. Abrahams and Maurice Katz[4] studied a case of primary liver cancer in which the associated feminization resolved after removal of the tumor.

Man, 19, had first shown signs of puberty at age 13. Gynecomastia had been noticed at age 17 years and had progressed, and bilateral mastectomies were done at age 18, when hepatomegaly was observed. The patient had not had to shave, but reported normal libido and sexual function. He had rather delicate, feminine features, with smooth skin, and a high-pitched voice. Pubic hair had a feminine pattern. The testes were soft and small. The liver edge was 5 cm below the costal margin. An extended hemihepatectomy

(4) N. Engl. J. Med. 296:1084–1088, May 12, 1977.

SERUM AND URINARY HORMONE VALUES IN PATIENT*

HORMONE	VALUE		NORMAL VALUE
	PREOPERATIVE	POSTOPERATIVE	
Serum:			
E₁ (pg/ml)	1113	14;12.	20–50
E₂ (pg/ml)	140	127	8–25
E₃ (pg/ml)	117	117;3.	<50
Tes (ng/ml)	0.72	2.74	3–14
FSH (mIU/ml)	3	5	1.5–12
LH (mIU/ml)	9.9	17.2	5–25
PR (ng/ml)	10.5	5.4	<15
HPL (μg/ml)	0.52	<0.05	<0.05
HCG_β (mIU/ml)	<5	<5	<5
Urine:			
Est (μg/24 hr)	455;356;217;392.	22	4–25
LH (IU/24 hr)	92;55.	27	25–110
FSH (IU/24 hr)	2	2	2–22
HCG (IU/24 hr)	0	0	
17-K (mg/24 hr)	6	8	6–25
17-H (mg/24 hr)	6	9	5–23

*E₁, estrone; E₂, estradiol; E₃, estriol; Tes, testosterone; FSH, follicle-stimulating hormone; LH, luteinizing hormone; PR, prolactin; HPL, human placental lactogen; HCG_β, β-subunit of human chorionic gonadotropin; Est, estrogens; 17-K, 17-ketosteroids; and 17-H, 17-hydroxycorticosteroids.

was done to remove tumor in the right hepatic lobe and a satellite nodule in the same lobe. The patient has been well for 5 years since operation. He now has normal-sized testes and a deeper voice and shaves daily.

Hormone concentrations are given in the table. Serum and urine estrogens were markedly elevated preoperatively and returned to normal after operation, except for serum estradiol. Serum testosterone was moderately low preoperatively and returned nearly to normal after surgery. Human placental lactogen was measurable in preoperative serum. Tumor extracts contained high levels of β-subunits of chorionic gonadotropin. Both dehydroepiandrosterone and its sulfate were transformed primarily to estrone in primary tumor incubations.

The similarity of the findings in this patient to those obtained in patients with choriocarcinoma and ectopic chorionic gonadotropin syndromes makes it most probable that the tumor tissue was extracting circulating dehydroepiandrosterone sulfate for conversion to estrogen and was the site of excessive estrone production.

► [The authors' thesis is that human placental lactogen (HPL) or its beta subunits, or both, present in the tumor and secreted into the serum led to the feminization noted in this patient. This view is strongly championed by Vaitukaitis (Cancer 37(Suppl.):567, 1976). Indeed, tumors not containing or secreting HPL seem to have become hard to find.

There are less exotic ways for males to become feminized. Alcoholism is one (1977 YEAR BOOK p. 324). Green et al. (Gut 17:426, 1976) found, as have others, that only estrone is significantly elevated in feminized alcoholics, whereas Persky et al. (Am. J. Psychol. 134:6, 1977) were able to follow serum testosterone levels down, as alcoholics previously withdrawn from alcohol were permitted to drink and smoke ad libitum—presumably, very libidum. Other ways to become demasculinized and feminized are shown below. —T.B.S.] ◄

Pathophysiology of Spironolactone-Induced Gynecomastia. Gynecomastia and impotence may develop in patients given moderate to high dosages of spironolactone for prolonged periods. Leslie I. Rose, Richard H. Underwood, Stephen R. Newmark, Eldad S. Kisch and Gordon H. Williams[5] (Harvard Med. School) evaluated the possibility that an effect of spironolactone on the metabolism or peripheral action of testosterone or estrogen, or both, alters the testosterone-to-estrogen ratio and produces gynecomastia. Sixteen men with hypertension, aged 35–61 years, were studied. All had supine diastolic pressures over 90 mm Hg and had been hypertensive for at least 6 months. Six patients were treated with spironolactone; in the others all medications were withheld for at least 2 weeks before hospitalization. The two groups were comparable in age, blood pressure, duration of hypertension and liver function test results.

All spironolactone-treated patients had significant gynecomastia. They had been taking a mean of 300 mg spironolactone daily for a mean of 7 months. No control patient had gynecomastia. Serum FSH levels were similar in the two groups, but LH levels were significantly greater in the spironolactone-treated patients. Blood testosterone levels were significantly less and estradiol levels greater in the spironolactone-treated patients. Blood testosterone levels were normal in all patients, but only 2 spironolactone-treated patients had normal estradiol levels. Testosterone clearance

(5) Ann. Intern. Med. 87:398–403, October, 1977.

was significantly greater in spironolactone-treated patients. Estradiol clearance was also greater, but not significantly so. The production rate of estradiol was significantly greater in these patients. The conversion ratio and transfer constant of testosterone to estradiol were significantly greater in the spironolactone group. All 5 patients studied 3–6 months after spironolactone was stopped showed significant falls in estradiol concentrations, with a mean decrement of 10 pg/ml, whereas testosterone values had increased by 1.3 ng/ml.

Spironolactone may alter liver function to increase the extraction of testosterone and thus its metabolism, or the drug may increase the amount of unbound testosterone available for transformation either by competing with testosterone for binding on its plasma carrier protein or by reducing synthesis of the carrier protein. The latter hypothesis seems more plausible. A unifying hypothesis for most if not all of the antiandrogen effect of spironolactone may be its ability to inhibit testosterone binding to specific receptor sites in the cytosol of target tissue and on plasma proteins, thus reducing its effect on target tissue and increasing its metabolic inactivation, including conversion to estradiol.

▶ [This is a well-conceived, well-executed and well-analyzed study, a clinical investigation as we like to see it. While the fact that spironolactone induces gynecomastia may not be clinically earthshaking, or even important, the study of its effect has led to new sights, extending, possibly, to the cellular level.

Still, the authors aren't perfect. They speak of "supine diastolic pressures." Is this in contrast to prone diastolic pressures, upright diastolic pressures or uptight diastolic pressures? Jargon often leads me to the *Oxford English Dictionary* and this *gaffe* was no exception. What I have to report is that supine used as "morally or mentally inactive, inert or indolent" has been part of the stock in trade of an astonishing array of British writers, including: 1603, Ben Jonson; 1621, Burton; 1630, Donne; 1732, Bishop Berkeley; 1761, David Hume; 1779, Boswell; 1807, Thomas Jefferson; 1819, Shelley; and 1852, Thackeray. So, a nice excursion without an alarum (*Oxford English Dictionary: alarum.* "from the earliest period there was a variant, alarum, due to rolling the *r* and prolonging the final syllable of the call. . ." Which call? The call *à l'arme*. Of course! To arms! And so on. . .).

Hmm! Having waxed ecstatic about this article, I must bring to the reader's attention the work of Caminos-Torres et al. (J. Clin. Endocrinol. Metab. 45:225, 1977). These workers could demonstrate no change in serum concentrations of FSH, LH, testosterone or estradiol after spironolactone administration. They did find that canrenone, a metabolite of spironolactone, displaces testosterone from its binding protein. We'll have to wait to see whether the article selected here was ill conceived, poorly executed and ill analyzed. — T.B.S.] ◄

Partial Androgen Insensitivity: The Reifenstein Syndrome Revisited. Reifenstein described a clinical phenotype of hereditary male pseudohermaphroditism consisting hypospadias, gynecomastia with incomplete virilization at puberty and infertility. James A. Amrhein, Georgeanna Jones Klingensmith, Patrick C. Walsh, Victor A. McKusick and Claude J. Migeon[6] (Johns Hopkins Univ.) reinvestigated 1 member of each of two original families with the Reifenstein syndrome and studied 6 other patients with the syndrome. Plasma hormones were measured by radioimmunoassays. Fibroblast strains were established from explants of genital or pubic skin from 5 patients and 22 normal subjects for assays of dihydrotestosterone receptor and 5 α-reductase. All the patients, aged 16–64 years, had normal karyotypes. All had reduced penile size, small testes and various genital abnormalities. Sex assignment had been incorrect in 2 and delayed in 2 others. Azoospermia was confirmed in all 7 patients evaluated. Three patients had similarly affected maternal relatives. Five patients received 200 mg testosterone intramuscularly per week for 6 weeks, followed by 400 mg weekly for another 6 weeks.

All patients had normal or above-normal plasma testosterone values, and no abnormality in androgen production was evident. All patients had serum LH values more than 2 SD above the mean for normal adult males, whereas concentrations of FSH were normal in 5 and elevated in 3. The metabolic clearance rate of testosterone was definitely low in 2 of the 3 patients in whom it was studied. Fibroblast 5α-reductase activities were normal, as was the whole-cell dihydrotestosterone-binding capacity of fibroblasts in 4. Pubic skin fibroblasts from 1 patient showed extremely low dihydrotestosterone binding. Plasma testosterone values increased and LH levels fell during testosterone therapy, but 2 patients had persistently elevated LH concentrations. All patients showed a slight clinical response to treatment. The 2 patients who continued to have elevated serum LH values on 200 mg testosterone weekly showed no clinical response until given 400 mg weekly.

---

(6)   N. Engl. J. Med. 297:350–356, Aug. 18, 1977.

The Reifenstein syndrome appears to result from defective androgen action rather than reduced androgen synthesis. The designation partial androgen insensitivity syndrome is suggested. The cause of androgen insensitivity in patients with normal cytoplasmic dihydrotestosterone binding is unknown. Routine use of testosterone in these patients is not recommended until more is known of the long-term effects of such therapy.

▶ [So, of the 8 patients, all showed normal serum androgen levels and unresponsiveness to androgen administration. Of the 5 patients studied, only 1 showed a significant reduction in cytosol receptors; the reason for the androgen insensitivity in the other 4 remains unknown. Other investigators, like Kenan et al. (Pediatrics 59:224, 1977) and Barragry et al. (Clin. Endocrinol. (Oxf.) 7:137, 1977), have described similar patients. Another excursion into feminization is discussed below. − T.B.S.] ◀

Leydig Cell Agenesis: Cause of Male Pseudohermaphroditism. Most cases of male pseudohermaphroditism have been due to errors affecting synthesis of either corticosteroid and testosterone or testosterone alone. François Berthezène, Maguelone G. Forest, Jean Alexis Grimaud, Bruno Claustrat and René Mornex[7] (Lyon, France) report a case of male pseudohermaphroditism apparently due to agenesis of Leydig's cells. The plasma FSH level was normal but increased after castration, suggesting that its secretion is regulated, at least in part, by a substance secreted by Sertoli's cells.

Woman, 34, had been considered normal until puberty, when failure of breast development and of menses became apparent. Three brothers and 2 sisters had had normal puberty. Examination showed a high voice, no breast tissue, poor muscle development and a female distribution of pubic hair but no axillary hair. The labia were fused posteriorly. The vagina was 4 cm deep. Bilateral inguinal masses were found. The patient had an X chromatin-negative buccal smear and a blood XY karyotype. Laparotomy revealed 3×1.5-cm testes, which were removed. Estradiol was administered postoperatively but only minimal breast development was present 8 months later.

The plasma testosterone level was 11 ng/100 ml, in the range for prepuberal children, but levels of Δ^4-androstenedione and dehydroepiandrosterone were in the normal range for adult women and the levels doubled after ACTH infusion and after metyrapone administration. Oral dexa-

---

(7) N. Engl. J. Med. 295:969–972, Oct. 28, 1976.

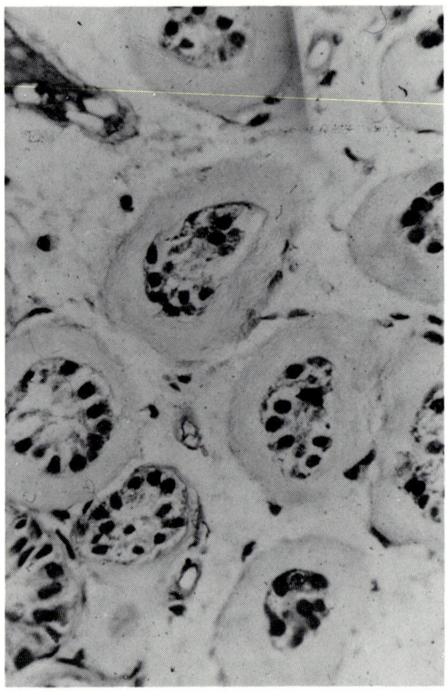

Fig 35.—Hyalinization of seminiferous tubules shown by light microscopy. Hematoxylin-eosin; reduced from ×425. (Courtesy of Berthezène, F., et al.: N. Engl. J. Med. 295:969–972, Oct. 28, 1976.)

methasone reduced all the substances to nearly undetectable levels. No substantial changes occurred on chorionic gonadotropin injection for 3 days. Basal levels of LH were high and levels increased dramatically after injection of luteinizing hormone-releasing hormone (LHRH), whereas the plasma testosterone level remained low. Plasma FSH content was normal and only a small rise was noted after injection of LHRH. Intramuscular estradiol injection reduced the plasma LH level. The level of testosterone in spermatic vein plasma was 152 ng/100 ml. No Leydig's cells were seen in the gonads (Fig 35). The concentration of FSH was much higher after castration and increased after injection of LHRH. After injections of 5 mg estradiol hexahydrobenzoate twice monthly for 8 months, the plasma LH value was 4 and the FSH level was 1.5 mIU/ml.

The mechanism by which the testes exert a feedback inhibitory effect on secretion of FSH is unknown. At least in the present patient, FSH secretion was regulated by a substance that is not testosterone and is not secreted by the Leydig cells, but presumably by Sertoli's cells.

▶ [An interesting, albeit, confusing, patient is described here. If there never were Leydig's cells, whence came the fetal androgens to induce male differentiation? Another point: Look at Figure 35. Agreed, one sees no interstitial cells in the interstitium. But why the hyalinization of the tubules?

Another case reported by Park et al. (Acta Endocrinol. (Kbh.) 83:173, 1976) sounds somewhat similar. Indeed, a photograph of the testes looks much the same, except that scant Leydig's cells can be seen. The authors suggest that perhaps, in their patient, the elevated immunoassayable LH was biologically inactive.

Okay, agenesis of Leydig's cells causes male pseudohermaphroditism. What would a Leydig cell tumor cause? Shimp et al. (Am. J. Med. Path. 67: 562, 1977) found their patient to have gynecomastia and elevated estrogen levels. — T.B.S.] ◀

Feminizing Adrenal Adenoma in a Boy: Case Report and Literature Review. Adrenal tumors may cause gynecomastia, but they are rare in childhood. Campbell P. Howard, Hiroaki Takahashi and Alvin B. Hayles[8] (Mayo Clinic) describe a boy with an adrenocortical tumor, who presented with bilateral gynecomastia, accelerated growth rate and advanced bone age, but no signs of virilization.

Fig 36. — Nephrotomogram, showing large, calcified left adrenal. (Courtesy of Howard, C. P., et al.: Mayo Clin. Proc. 52:354 – 357, June, 1977.)

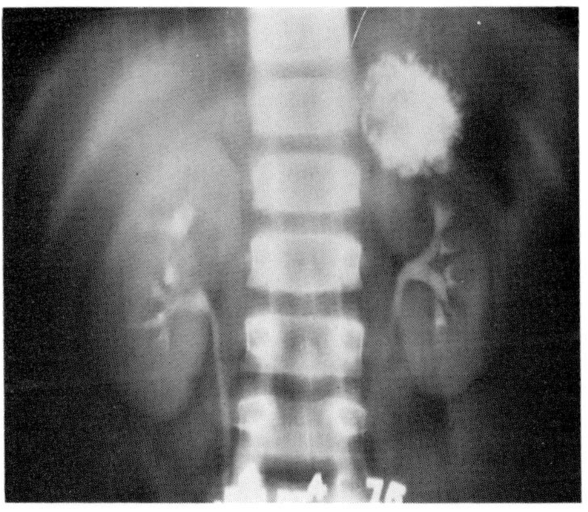

____

(8)   Mayo Clin. Proc. 52:354 – 357, June, 1977.

Boy, aged 5 years 10 months, had had bilaterally symmetric breast enlargement for 2 years. There was no history of exposure to estrogens, and his general health had always been good. At age 4½ years, the boy was 104 cm tall and weighed 16 kg. The breasts were 4 cm in diameter. Urinary 17-ketosteroids were 1.2 mg/24 hours and total urinary estrogens were 17.1 mg/24 hours. A left orchiopexy was done for undescended testis at age 5 years 2 months. At present admission, the boy was 120 cm tall and weighed 20.5 kg. His span was 116.5 cm and his lower segment measurement, 60 cm. The breasts measured 5×6 cm, with normally pigmented, 1-cm areolae. There was no axillary or pubic hair. The penis was 4.5 cm long and 1 cm in diameter. The plasma testosterone concentration was less than 10 ng/dl. A nephrotomogram showed a large, calcified adrenal tumor on the left side (Fig 36). A 3.5×3.5-cm adrenocortical tumor was removed and was found to be a benign, multinodular cortical adenoma with massive central calcification. The patient has been well for over a year, and the breast tissue has regressed.

All 7 patients with reported cases of feminizing adrenal tumor, including this patient, had bilateral gynecomastia and an advanced bone age. Signs of virilization were found in all but 2 of the patients. Four patients had benign adenomas and 3 had carcinomas. The present patient is unique in that urinary steroid excretion was normal for a boy of his age. Bilateral gynecomastia with no other signs of feminization or virilization and with normal 17-ketosteroids and elevated urine estrogens has not previously been described.

▶ [You are right. This article was selected primarily because of the dramatic roentgenogram (Fig 36). A similar patient is described by Wirth et al. (Schweiz. Med. Wochenschr. 107:411, 1977). This patient, however, had an uncalcified adrenal carcinoma.

Lest you begin to feel comfortable, I should point out that males with adrenocortical carcinoma may become virilized as well. Nogeire et al. (Cancer, 40:307, 1977) describe a patient who had much-elevated DHEA and DHEA-sulfate levels in the presence of normal plasma testosterone and elevated plasma estradiol concentrations. – T.B.S.] ◀

The Immotile Cilia Syndrome: Congenital Ciliary Abnormality as an Etiologic Factor in Chronic Airway Infections and Male Sterility. Rune Eliasson, Björn Mossberg, Per Camner and Björn A. Afzelius[9] (Stockholm) investigated 6 men and 1 woman suspected of having congenital immotility of cilia. All had chronic airway infections, and the men had immotile spermatozoa. The woman and 3 men

---

(9)   N. Engl. J. Med. 297:1–6, July 7, 1977.

CLINICAL DATA ON 7 PATIENTS WITH CONGENITALLY NONFUNCTIONING CILIA

Case No.	Sex	Age (Yr)	Smoking	Situs Inversus	Bronchitis, Rhinitis & Sinusitis	Otitis	Sterility
1*	M	37	——	+	+	+	+
2*	M	33	——	−	+	−	+
3	M	32	40–60 cigarettes daily for 15 yr	+	+	−	+
4	M	32	——	−	+	−	+
5	M	31	Ex-smoker for 4 yr	−	+	+	+
6	M	40	20–30 cigarettes daily for 14 yr	+	+	+	+
7	F	28	——	+	+	+	?

*Brothers.

had Kartagener's syndrome. The clinical data are summarized in the table. All patients had histories of chronic or recurrent infections of the upper and lower airways. All, with 1 possible exception, had had chronic expectoration of mucopurulent sputum since early childhood. Obstructive pulmonary changes were present in 3 patients and probably in a fourth. Lung clearance studies were done with ^{99m}Tc-labeled Teflon particles in all cases and biopsies were done in 3.

Patients had significantly higher particle retention values than did healthy controls, and smoking did not influence this finding. The dynein arms of sperm tails were completely absent, and the coarse fibers surrounding the axoneme were irregular in size and arrangement. The fibrous sheath around these structures was also irregular. The dynein arms were nearly absent in cilia from the nasal and bronchial mucosae in some patients. A diffuse matrix material occupied much of the space within the cilium. Neighboring cilia did not have a fixed orientation in the 3 patients in whom they were studied.

The findings in these patients strongly suggest an association between sperm immotility and chronic airway infections and also an association between sperm immotility and the occurrence of Kartagener's syndrome. All patients had extremely slow, probably absent mucociliary transport. The results are in accord with a hypothesis explaining Kartagener's syndrome as a genetic defect in the ultrastructure of cilia, resulting in immotile ciliated epithelia. The observations are compatible with the postulate that immotility of embryonic cilia results in situs inversus in about half the cases.

▶ [First, Kartagener's syndrome, described in 1933, consists of situs inversus, chronic sinusitis and bronchiectasis. Second, here is demonstrated an astonishing relationship, not based on some esoteric functional enzymic defect, but rather on a microscopic *structural* abnormality, shared by distant body parts.

I had a male chauvinist uncle, now deceased, who was a mine of misinformation. At last, one of his dicta makes sense, "One piece of tail is no different from any other."

So much for this rare form of sterility. Before moving on, we should take note of an unexpectedly common form, namely, impaired testosterone production and spermatogenesis, which occurs with chronic renal failure (Holdsworth et al.: N. Engl. J. Med. 296:1245, 1977). About a year ago, I saw one such patient and treated him with testosterone, both of us unaware of the relationship between testicular deficiency and uremia. For more about testicular deficiency, look below. — T.B.S.] ◀

Isolated Follicle-Stimulating Hormone Deficiency in Man. The roles of FSH and LH in human spermatogenesis have not been clearly defined. George B. Maroulis, Albert F. Parlow and John R. Marshall[1] (Univ. of California, Los Angeles) describe 2 men with serum FSH levels persistently below 3 mIU/ml and normal levels of LH, thyrotropin, growth hormone, prolactin, cortisol and testosterone. The patients were found in the course of infertility evaluations.

CASE 1.—Man, 26, with a normal male karyotype and normal appearance, had a serum FSH concentration that was repeatedly below normal. It rose from 2 to 4 mIU/ml after LH releasing factor injection. A value of 5 mIU/ml was observed on treatment with 50 mg clomiphene citrate twice daily for 10 days, and the serum testosterone concentration rose from 3.3 to 7 ng/ml. Testicular biopsy showed arrest at the spermatid level, and semen analysis showed many immature forms.

CASE 2.—Man, 30, who had sired 2 pregnancies ending as spontaneous abortions, the second 5 years previously, had FSH values below the normal range on repeated occasions. Clomiphene therapy increased the serum FSH concentration from 3 to 5 mIU/ml; this was the only normal baseline value obtained.

Apparent FSH deficiency was associated with abnormal spermatogenesis in these patients. Clomiphene administration led to FSH increases to within the normal male range.

---

(1) Fertil. Steril. 28:818–822, August, 1977.

The findings indicate a relatively intact hypothalamic-pituitary axis, and the low baseline values of FSH may be due to a defect above the level of the pituitary. Serum FSH determination is indicated in the evaluation of infertile men with abnormal semen.

▶ [First, we wish to welcome Dr. George Maroulis, one of the authors, to our medical community. Doctor Maroulis is now the head of gynecologic endocrinology at our institution. Second, years ago, in commenting on patients with isolated LH deficiency known as "fertile eunuchs," we speculated that there must also be "sterile studs," and, sure enough, here we have some examples. The authors' thesis that this is a suprahypothalamic lesion is reasonable, but another possibility comes to mind. Could it be that these testes, full of spermatids, make enough inhibin to block FSH secretion? Third, you should know that Bremner et al. (Acta Endocrinol. (Kbh.) 86:1, 1977) found that patients with hypogonadotropic eunuchoidism responded to LH releasing factor infusions with measurable increases in serum LH and FSH, indicating the hypothalamic or suprahypothalamic origin of the lesions. Lipshultz (Clin. Endocrinol. (Oxf.) 7:103, 1977) found that men with severe oligospermia but normal serum levels of FSH and LH hyperresponded to LH releasing factor as compared to normal persons. Is this an inhibin deficiency? — T.B.S.] ◀

Double-Blind Crossover Trial of Gonadotropin-Releasing Hormone (LHRH) in Sexually Impotent Men. Some patients with male hypogonadism who were given LHRH had increased potency before their plasma androgens returned to normal. It has been reported that LHRH induces mating behavior when injected into oophorectomized rats. Terry F. Davies, C. Q. Mountjoy, A. Gomez-Pan, M. J. Watson, J. P. Hanker, G. M. Besser and Reginald Hall[2] report a double-blind crossover trial of 500μg of LHRH and placebo, given subcutaneously every 8 hours for 4 weeks, in 10 men with secondary sexual impotence of unknown cause. Impotence was defined as the inability to achieve or maintain an erection adequate for coitus on more than a quarter of opportunities presented to male patients who previously experienced normal potency. The mean patient age was 40 years, and the average duration of impotence was 2 years. Plasma testosterone and serum gonadotropins were measured by specific radioimmunoassays. Both LHRH and placebo were given for 4-week periods, and libido scores were obtained at weekly intervals.

Two men had elevated prolactin levels, possibly secondary to the stress of venipuncture. Patients found it difficult to

---

(2) Clin. Endocrinol. (Oxf.) 5:601–607, November, 1976.

distinguish between treatment periods, but analysis of questionnaire responses indicated a barely significant improvement during LHRH treatment. The only result that was significant at the 5% level was for spontaneity of erection, but success in ejaculation just fell short of being significant at that level. There was no evidence that LHRH therapy significantly improved the quality of erections or altered mood.

In this trial, LHRH had no obvious clinical effect on the sexual performance or mental well-being of men with secondary impotence. Statistical analysis indicated that LHRH did improve libido, but the treatment effect was rather small and not likely to be clinically significant. The negative results should not, however, be taken to indicate that LHRH normally has no influence on sexual behavior in man, because psychologic factors in the impotent patients may have been powerful enough to suppress any stimulant effects.

► ["A good try but no cigar," as they were wont to say on the carnival midway. Still, the last sentence of this article should be given consideration; there is no question but that LHRH in estrogen-primed, oophorectomized rats leads to dramatic behavioral changes, including the prompt assumption of the lordotic position by which the female invites a sexual advance. Besides, LHRH is good for something. Illig et al. (Lancet 2:518, 1977) found that its administration intranasally provides a quite good stimulus for the descent of cryptorchid testes into the scrotum. — T.B.S.]

The following review articles are recommended to the reader:

Amelar, R. D., and Dubin, L.: The management of idiopathic male infertility, J. Reprod. Med. 18:191, 1977.

Braunstein, G. D., et al.: Germ cell tumors of the testes, West. J. Med. 126:362, 1977.

Bremner, W. J., and de Kretser, D. M.: The prospects for new, reversible male contraceptives, N. Engl. J. Med. 295:1111, 1977.

Sexual Differentiation

Seasonal Rhythm in Plasma Testosterone Levels in the Rhesus Monkey *(Macaca mulatta)*: Three-Year Study. A broad variety of vertebrates engages in reproductive activity only during a discrete, often brief period of each year, and many species exhibit unique behavior or form social aggregates in association with the seasonal mating pattern. Some nonhuman primate species are now known to breed with a distinct annual cycle or rhythm. Observations have linked seasonal sexual behavior to endocrine variables in the rhesus monkey. Thomas P. Gordon, Robert M. Rose and Irwin S. Bernstein[3] monitored behavior patterns and plasma testosterone concentrations of adult males in a rhesus breeding colony for 3 years. The population included 7 sexually mature males, 40 mature females and 14 immature animals at the outset of the study. Testosterone was determined by radioimmunoassay. Blood samples were obtained at least once a month from the sexually mature males.

The breeding group exhibited a seasonal pattern of matings and births. Copulatory activity was restricted to a 5-month period starting in the early fall of each year, with all births recorded in a corresponding span between March and August. Plasma testosterone concentrations showed a distinct seasonal rhythm, peaking in October or November at a mean of about 1,200 ng/100 ml (Fig 37). Plasma testosterone values fell to a low of about 200 ng/100 ml during periods of sexual inactivity.

This study showed a correlation between seasonal breeding activity and increased levels of circulating testosterone in the rhesus monkey. The findings support the postulate that other seasonal behavior patterns, such as increased aggression, may also be mediated by higher testosterone levels. The environmental or social stimuli that control the seasonal patterns have not been identified. Individual vari-

---

(3)   Horm. Behav. 7:229–243, June, 1976.

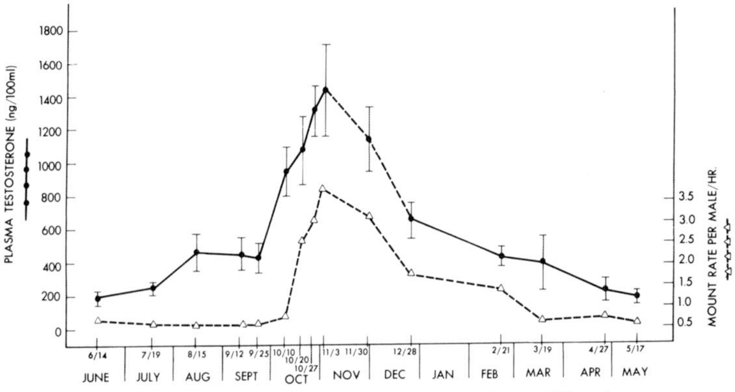

Fig 37.—Mean plasma testosterone value *(solid circles)* ± SE and mean mount rate *(open triangles)* per hour for 7 sexually mature male members of rhesus monkey breeding colony at each of 15 sample points in 12-month span. (Courtesy of Gordon, T. P., et al.: Horm. Behav. 7:229–243, June, 1976.)

ability in sexual behavior or testosterone concentration has not been fully explained.

▶ [Figure 37 is admirable. Note that the rise in mean serum testosterone *precedes* the rise in the mount rate, although both curves fall concurrently. Ah well, this is simple enough to demonstrate in placid, caged monkeys who are incapable of experiencing the emotional spectrum open to man. If man has such seasonal tendencies, they would certainly be dampened to extinction by psychologic factors, right? Hardly! The studies in young Parisian men (1977 YEAR BOOK, p. 322) and in Dutchmen (ibid., p. 324) show almost identical curves, with serum testosterone levels peaking in October!

Incidentally, if serum testosterone levels are suddenly reduced in male rats by castration, the rats can still respond to precopulatory behavior in females. This is what we call "hanging in there."—T.B.S.] ◀

Periovulatory Synchronization of Behavior in Male and Female Rhesus Monkeys. Rhesus monkeys, like many other primates, do not restrict their sexual activity to the ovulatory period. Richard P. Michael and R. W. Bonsall[4] (Atlanta, Ga.) used an operant conditioning technique, in which the female pressed a lever for access to her male partner, to obtain an independent, objective measure of female sexual motivation and relate it to circulating levels of ovarian hormones. It is difficult to assess the female's sexual mo-

---

(4)   Nature 265:463–465, Feb. 3, 1977.

tivation in testing pairs of monkeys without contamination by the threat of male aggression.

A total of 1,440 tests were done on 17 animal pairs during 63 menstrual cycles. Ejaculations were maximally frequent at the end of the 1st half of the cycle and minimal in the middle of the 2d half. The shortest access time occurred during reverse cycle days 18–16 and the longest times near the

Fig 38.—Changes in plasma steroids (estradiol, progesterone and testosterone) of female rhesus monkeys in periovulatory period. Changes in females' access times were synchronized with expected time of ovulation *(solid horizontal bars)*, when males' ejaculations were at their maximum. The 33 cycles were aligned on day of estradiol peak (day 0). Vertical bars show SEM. *N*, number of plasma samples; *n*, number of behavior tests (5 females, 5 males, 9 pairs, 252 tests). (Courtesy of Michael, R. P., and Bonsall, R. W.: Nature 265:463–465, Feb. 3, 1977.)

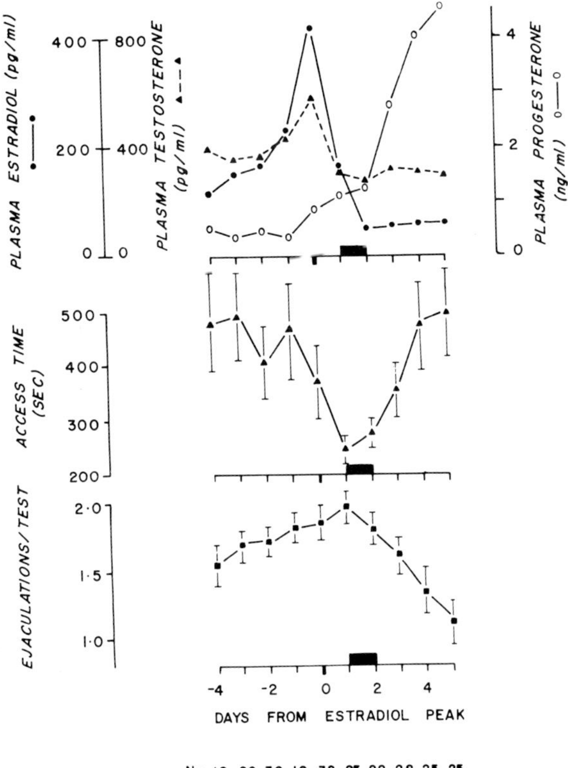

start and end of the cycle. Access times for males were not correlated with access times for food rewards on the same day or with access times when a female was the reinforcement. Hormonal data obtained from 5 females during 33 menstrual cycles are given in Figure 38. Both the highest ejaculation frequency and the fastest access time occurred 1 day after the estradiol peak. On that day, all males always succeeded in ejaculating and all females always pressed for access to their partners.

Administration of gonadal steroids to ovariectomized rhesus monkeys has shown that changes in sexual behavior of the pair can be induced by ovarian hormones. The midcycle plasma estradiol peak, besides triggering the gonadotropin surge responsible for ovulation 24–48 hours later, may also synchronize and maximize the female's sexual motivation and the male's ejaculatory performance. Neuroendocrine mechanisms underlying this behavioral synchrony clearly have a selective advantage by optimizing the chances for successful fertilization and thus survival in this highly evolved primate species in which sexual behavior serves more than a purely reproductive function.

▶ [Some explanations are necessary here. First, the female, separated by a partition from the male, *really* wanted the male's company; she had to press the lever 250 times before the partition was automatically raised. Access time is the interval from when the female is put into the cage to when the partition rises. Clearly, by the beginning of ovulation, the female could hardly wait. Note that there are preceding peaks not only of estradiol but of testosterone. In any event, it is extremely clear that gonadal hormones strikingly influence behavior of females as well as that of males. What about the influence of one sex on the other? Look ahead. — T.B.S.]

Pheromonally Induced Sexual Maturation in Females: Regulation by Social Environment of the Male was demonstrated by Joseph R. Lombardi (North Carolina State Univ.) and John G. Vandenbergh[5] (North Carolina Dept. of Mental Health, Raleigh). Social stresses due to high population densities may be important factors regulating mammalian populations under natural conditions, possibly through increasing adrenal function and reducing gonadal function. Reproductive function is inhibited in both juvenile and adult females as primary correlates of increasing population density. A pheromone in male mouse urine stimu-

---

(5)   Science 196:545–546, Apr. 29, 1977.

lates puberty in females. Social factors that alter gonadal function in the male have now been found also to alter the activity of the male urinary pheromone.

Cohabitation of dominant and subordinate males and of juvenile with adult males was used to alter testicular function in mice. The uterine weight of prepuberal females was measured after applications of male urine to the oronasal groove. Urinary pheromonal activity of subordinate mice was significantly less than that of dominant mice. Essentially no differences were found in uterine weight between females given urine from subordinate males and those treated with water. Subordinate mice had heavier adrenals and lighter testes than did dominant males, but no significant difference in seminal vesicle weights was observed. Pheromonal activity in maturing males increased with age under all cohabitation conditions, but significant suppression of pheromonal activity was found in urine from female-exposed mice. The appearance of pheromonal activity in the urine of mice housed with adult males was significantly delayed compared with that in males housed with comparably aged females. Coincident with the suppression of pheromonal activity was the production of litters by the stimulus females.

Social factors capable of suppressing gonadal function in male mice also reduce their capacity to stimulate sexual maturation in females pheromonally. The suppression of female maturation by other adult or juvenile females, in combination with the reduced capacity of stressed young and low-ranking adult males to overcome this inhibition, may be used as a model partly to explain suppressed fertility in populations where males are abundant. Androgen-dependent priming pheromones of the male may play an integrative role in controlling fertility in a population as a function of population density.

▶ [In the 1977 YEAR BOOK (p. 14) we commented that the contraceptive effect of phytoestrogens on quail was "an elegant example of endocrinologic ecology." Here is another.

Pheromones are important, not only between the sexes, but between the generations, as shown next. — T.B.S.] ◀

Bile, Prolactin and the Maternal Pheromone. The maternally behaving lactating rat emits a pheromone in her feces that strongly attracts young. Under certain conditions, nulliparous females and adult males behave maternally, coming to build a nest, lick, retrieve and crouch in a nursing posture when with young, a procedure known as concaveation. Howard Moltz and Lois C. Leidahl[6] (Univ. of Chicago) studied concaveated animals to determine whether they also emit the pheromone. Animals were provided with fresh litters of foster pups at 24-hour intervals, advancing in age during the study period.

The concaveated females began emitting the pheromone when their foster young reached age 16 days, as in lactating females. Concaveated males did not emit the pheromone, even when given injections of prolactin or castrated or both. Injections of estradiol benzoate and prolactin were also ineffective. Bile was tried because the pheromone is known to be synthesized within the cecum and because males have lower levels of hepatic prolactin receptors than females. Males given cecal injections of bile from females that had been lactating for 21 days (21-day bile) were preferred by pups, and the feces of these males attracted test young as effectively as the feces of females that had been lactating for 3 weeks. The effect was not seen in males given bile from animals lactating for 5 days or those given 21-day bile plus ergocornine hydrogen maleate, a potent prolactin inhibitor.

New prolactin receptor sites may be formed in the liver during the interval before pheromone emission begins in females. The increase in prolactin binding may lead to an increase in total bile acids or to a change in the ratio of one primary bile acid to another, altering the chemistry of the cecum so that fecal material comes to contain the pheromone. Further work is needed to determine what changes actually occur in bile to support pheromonal release and to identify the pheromone.

▶ [In both phylogenetic and ontogenetic terms, prolactin may be looked on as the concaveating hormone, and here we are treated to a fine example of this thesis at multiple levels. There is an investigative march from the behavioral effect of feces to the influence of hepatic prolactin receptors.

In passing, there are nice words and there are ugly words. Concaveation is a nice word; deafferentation is an ugly word.

What of hormone levels in aberrant sexual behavior? Look below.— T.B.S.] ◀

(6) Science 196:81–83, Apr. 1, 1977.

Psychologic Development and Blood Levels of Sex Steroids in Male Identical Twins of Divergent Sexual Orientation. Data relating sex hormones to sexual orientation have been inconclusive. Richard C. Friedman, Flemming Wollesen and Ruth Tendler[7] (Columbia Univ.) observed equivalent blood testosterone and estradiol levels in 2 monozygotic male twins of divergent sexual orientation. The twins, aged 25 years, include a homosexual who lives in a city with his male lover and a heterosexual who lives with his wife and children in a suburb. Psychologic development diverged from early childhood. The homosexual twin recalled first being romantically attracted to a young man at age 5 years. Masturbatory fantasies and dream content have been exclusively homosexual. Minnesota Multiphasic Personality Inventory (MMPI) scores of the homosexual (X) and heterosexual (Y) twins are given in the table. There were no differences in blood testosterone or estradiol levels between the 2 subjects. Twin X had a higher androstenedione value than his brother.

These genetically identical males used different mechanisms of coping with psychologic conflict from early childhood, but blood testosterone and estradiol levels were similar. There was no indication that the sexual orientation of the twins is related, as either cause or effect, to the blood hormone levels. The subjects did not appear to be distressed at the time of blood sampling. The reason for the discrepant androstenedione values is unclear.

► [This is as controlled an experiment as one could wish for to compare

---

MMPI SCORES AND RESPECTIVE RANKS

Scale	Twin X	Twin Y
Hypochondriasis	85 (6)	49 (9)
Depression	101 (3)	80 (1)
Hysteria	78 (8)	53 (8)
Psychopathic deviancy	74 (9)	76 (2)
Masculinity-femininity	94 (4)	57 (7)
Paranoia	82 (7)	59 (6)
Psychasthenia	105 (2)	73 (3)
Schizophrenia	120 (1)	65 (5)
Mania	88 (5)	45 (10)
Social isolation	73 (10)	66 (4)

---

(7)   J. Nerv. Ment. Dis. 163:282–288, October, 1976.

gonadal hormone serum concentrations in heterosexual and homosexual individuals. It provides additional evidence on the side of no difference in serum gonadal hormonal levels in males with differing sexual orientation. It also suggests that if there are genetic influences on sexual preferences, they can be totally overridden by environmental changes. While these two persons are identical twins, descriptions of their childhood clearly show that their interest and behavior differed markedly at a very early age. While, not unexpectedly, this phenomenon is rare, there are 11 such twin pairs recorded and, of the few hormonal studies performed, none was discordant.

I should also mention that the same authors (Am. J. Psychiatry 134:5, 1977) found no differences between the serum LH, testosterone estradiol and estrone levels of male homosexual and heterosexual subjects, and James et al. (Psychol. Med. 7:427, 1977) obtained similar results in treatment-seeking male homosexuals. What about females? Look ahead.— T.B.S.] ◄

Plasma Testosterone in Homosexual and Heterosexual Women. Nanette K. Gartrell (Harvard Med. School), D. Lynn Loriaux and Thomas N. Chase[8] (Natl. Inst. of Health) found that plasma testosterone levels in homosexual women are substantially higher than in heterosexual women of the same age. Twenty-one homosexual women were age matched with 19 heterosexuals; the respective mean ages were 26.8 and 26. No subject was taking birth control pills or other steroid preparations or was using marihuana frequently. All were in good general health, nullipa-

Fig 39.—Plasma testosterone and age in homosexual and heterosexual women. (Courtesy of Gartrell, N. K., et al.: Am. J. Psychiatry 134:1117–1119, October, 1977.)

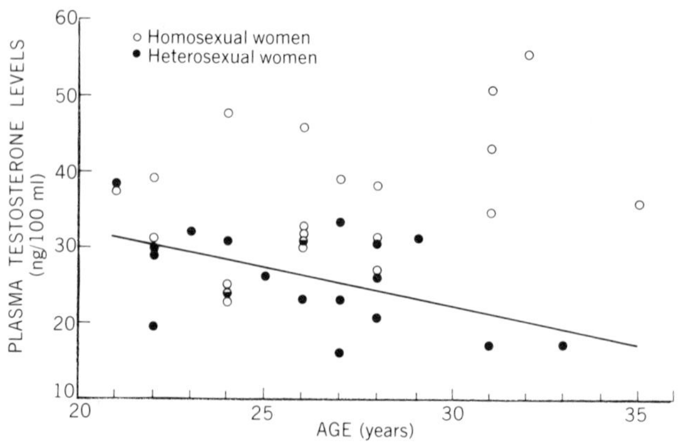

---

(8) Am. J. Psychiatry 134:1117–1119, October, 1977.

rous and free of menstrual irregularities and genital abnormalities. Plasma testosterone was measured by radioimmunoassay.

The mean testosterone was 26 ng/100 ml in heterosexual women and 36 ng/100 ml in the homosexuals, an average 38% difference. In the heterosexual group there was a significant inverse correlation between age and testosterone concentration (Fig 39), whereas the homosexual group exhibited a slight tendency in the opposite direction.

This study showed considerably higher plasma testosterone levels in homosexual than in heterosexual women and the lack of a significant inverse correlation between age and testosterone level in the homosexual group. There is currently no basis for speculating whether the endocrinologic differences may reflect a primary mechanism for, or a secondary response to, a particular sexual orientation.

▶ [Here the story seems different, as shown in Figure 39, and it doesn't fit well with previous reports (1976 YEAR BOOK, p. 331).

The reason for these discrepant findings between male and female homosexuals as compared with appropriate controls is, of course, speculative. In females, significant changes in testosterone may be easier to measure because basal levels are so much lower than in males. Also, it is theoretically possible that female homosexuals simply have a higher sex drive than their heterosexual counterparts and that this is reflected in higher testosterone levels. Similarly, the relatively elevated testosterone levels may reflect greater ongoing aggressive behavior. Finally, and least likely, there may be a relation between the high androgen levels and the sexual orientation itself of these women. — T.B.S.] ◀

Delayed Pituitary Hormone Response to LH Releasing Factor (LRF) and TSH Releasing Factor (TRF) in Patients with Anorexia Nervosa and with Secondary Amenorrhea Associated with Simple Weight Loss. The degree of blunting of the gonadotropin response to LRF in anorexia nervosa is related to the degree of weight loss. Robert A. Vigersky, D. Lynn Loriaux, Arnold E. Andersen, R. S. Mecklenburg and Judith L. Vaitukaitis[9] (Natl. Inst. of Health) analyzed responses to LRF and TRF both kinetically and quantitatively in 7 regularly cycling young women without endocrine disease and 40 patients aged 15–42 with secondary amenorrhea associated with weight loss. Twenty-one patients had a diagnosis of anorexia nervosa and 19 had secondary amenorrhea associated with simple weight loss

---

(9)   J. Clin. Endocrinol. Metab. 43:893–900, October, 1976.

QUANTITATIVE RESPONSE OF LH AND FSH TO 10 μg LRF

		Normal (N =7)	Anorexia nervosa (N = 21)	Simple weight loss (N = 19)
LH	Basal (mIU/ml)	7.9 ± 2.6*	3.9 ± 0.5†	8.3 ± 2.3
	Peak response (mIU/ml)	26.6 ± 2.2	22.0 ± 5.0	30.2 ± 5.0
	Per cent	380 ± 177	490 ± 165	502 ± 123
	Integrated (mIU/ml/min)	1,272 ± 318	2,080 ± 559	2,091 ± 570
FSH	Basal (mIU/ml)	15.3 ± 1.0	5.6 ± 1.1†	9.4 ± 1.2†
	Peak response (mIU/ml)	21.7 ± 1.4	16.9 ± 2.9	20.2 ± 2.5
	Per cent	39 ± 3.0	274 ± 54†	152 ± 43†
	Integrated (mIU/ml/min)	389 ± 115	1,419 ± 395†	1,692 ± 351†

*Values are mean ±1 SEM.
†P < 0.05 anorexia nervosa or simple weight loss versus normal.

(SWL). Gonadotropin levels were determined by radioimmunoassays after LRF and TRF were injected.

The results are given in the table. Basal gonadotropin levels were lower in the patients with anorexia nervosa than in those with SWL and the FSH content was lower in the SWL patients than in normal subjects. Quantitative LH responses were similar in the various groups but FSH responses were greater in both underweight groups than in the normal group. The times of the peak LH and FSH responses were delayed in patients with anorexia nervosa. The peak responses were correlated with the severity of weight loss in this group. The plasma TSH response to TRF was also delayed in the group with anorexia nervosa. The TSH and prolactin peaks after TRF were not correlated with the severity of weight loss. Plasma T_3 levels were significantly correlated with the severity of weight loss and with the time of the plasma TSH peak.

Responses to releasing hormones are quantitatively normal but abnormally delayed in patients with anorexia nervosa or SWL. The findings support the hypothesis that the endocrine changes seen in anorexia nervosa are consistent with hypothalamic dysfunction. Patients with SWL appear to be physiologically intermediate between those with anorexia nervosa and normal women.

▶ [Anorexia nervosa is a fascinating (and confusing) mixture of apparent hyperpituitarism and hypopituitarism. Basal plasma growth hormone and cortisol levels are often high, but responses to stimulation are often blunted. Serum triiodothyronine (T_3) levels are low and reverse T_3 levels are high. Here we see in the table that, whereas basal levels of LH and FSH are low, the response to stimulation with FSH is supranormal. Croxson and Ibbertson (J. Clin. Endocrinol. Metab. 44:167, 1977) found that there was a normal peak serum TSH after TRH administration, but that the fall in serum TSH was delayed—in effect, an overall hyperresponse. Wakeling et al. found that administration of estrogens to patients with anorexia nervosa reveals a persistence of negative feedback effects, but a loss of the subsequent positive feedback release of LH; Arrow et al. (Acta Endocrinol. (Kbh.) 85:673, 1977) performed a similar TRH stimulation study. They found higher than normal basal TSH levels and a normal peak response but a delayed initial response. They also reaffirmed what is mentioned above about the behavior of serum growth hormone and cortisol. Despair not! Not even a Moog synthesizer could put this welter of data together in a sensible way.

Now, the moment to exchange the hat of the professional endocrinologist for that of the "old clinician." In this article we are told about almost equal numbers of patients with anorexia nervosa and patients with simple weight loss. The differentiation was made on the criteria of Feigner et al. (Arch. Gen. Psychiatry 26:57, 1972). Included are such things as abnormal ideation about food and body image and a judgment by others, including physicians, that weight loss is inappropriately great. The patients with simple weight loss, then, were somewhat overweight and had fallen to what we generally consider to be a normal weight. Why did they have amenorrhea? In the past, it was not rare to see amenorrheic obese patients who were instructed that with weight loss, their periods would certainly return and, with weight loss, they often did. — T.B.S.] ◄

► ↓ Ambient confusion is often intensified by the new unisexual attitudes. The following article doesn't help. — T.B.S. ◄

Primary Anorexia Nervosa (Weight Phobia) in Males. Until recently it was widely thought that anorexia nervosa was by definition a disorder of females. It does occur in the male, though rarely, and the condition in males coincides closely with the female equivalent. M. K. Hasan and R. W. Tibbetts[1] reviewed 10 cases of primary anorexia nervosa in males treated in hospitals in Birmingham, England, over a 19-year period. No patient came on his own initiative to seek psychiatric help, and most consulted a physician only under considerable family pressure. Diagnostic criteria included avoidance of food, especially carbohydrates, with evidence of deceit about food intake or weight; weight loss beyond reasonable limits; and absence of an adequate explanation for the weight loss from either organic disease or primary psychiatric disorder.

In general the mother appeared to play the dominant role and to be the more approachable parent in these families. Three men deliberately smoked to great excess to curb their

---

(1) Postgrad. Med. J. 53:146–151, March, 1977.

appetites. One became secondarily dependent on alcohol. No patient had evidence of clinical epilepsy. An interest in providing food for others was common. Restlessness and overactivity were beyond the degrees expected, and affective disturbance was common and included frank depression. Three patients expressed suicidal ideas, but not in a serious manner. Serious organic disease was considered strongly in 3 cases. Two patients' fathers had died of gastric carcinoma. Sexual activity was substantially below that expected, but there was no firm evidence of homosexuality. Low testosterone values were found in 1 case. Five patients overate intermittently and 3 induced vomiting. Treatment was by operant conditioning in a flexible format; chemotherapy was mainly at a symptomatic level. The 9 surviving patients were followed for a mean of 27 months. One patient has relapsed and 2 are in precarious condition. One patient is frankly maladjusted, whereas 4 are entirely normal psychiatrically.

This condition appears to be the male counterpart of primary anorexia nervosa in the female. The etiologic picture seems to include an obsessional personality, skewed parental relations, self-consciousness about being overweight and apprehension of the threat of manhood, with particular reference to the heterosexual role. The disorder appears to be primarily psychogenic, although perhaps occurring in those with some physiologic predisposition.

► [It is likely that if the endocrine studies alluded to previously were carried out in these males, similar results would be obtained, because it is clear, at least to me, that the changes all derive primarily from inanition (Olusi: Clin. Chem. 74:261, 1977).

Anyway, unlike physicists, endocrinologists are reluctant to violate the principle of parity. We have fertile eunuchs and sterile studs, we have identical twins, one of whom is homosexual, we have lesbians with high serum testosterone levels and we have males with anorexia nervosa.—T.B.S.] ◄

Case of Cyclopia with D Trisomy. Cyclopia is a rare congenital defect in which the orbits have merged to form a single, central cavity with one eye. A proboscis-like structure is present above the orbit. Eight of 17 cases with chromosomal analysis had D trisomy and autoradiographic and G-banding studies in 3 of these showed that the extra chromosome was a no. 13. Richard L. Neu, James F. Grant and

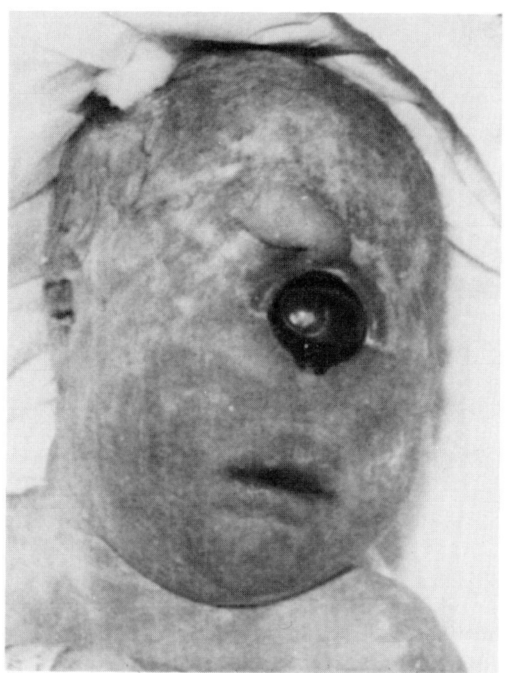

Fig 40. — Proposita shortly after birth. (Courtesy of Neu, R. L., et al.: Am. J. Obstet. Gynecol. 127:212–213, Jan. 15, 1977.)

Lytt I. Gardner[2] (State Univ. of New York Upstate Med. Center) report what is believed to be the ninth case of D trisomy-associated cyclopia.

Infant, the outcome of a first pregnancy, was born at term after an uneventful pregnancy, weighing 1,875 gm. She died within minutes after birth. A cyclops facial deformity was present, with a central orbital opening containing a fused globe (Fig 40). A superior nasal proboscis was also noted. Polydactylism was present. The infant's neck was short. Autopsy showed a large interventricular defect, a patent foramen ovale and ductus and marked pulmonary congestion. There was a cecum in the right upper quadrant, a large, cystic right kidney, a short blind ureter and a grossly deformed brain. All peripheral blood metaphases examined had a 47

---

(2)   Am. J. Obstet. Gynecol. 127:212–213, Jan. 15, 1977.

XX +D chromosome complement. Insufficient material was available for banding studies.

It is likely that this was a case of trisomy 13. The frequent finding of the extra D chromosome in cyclops does not mean that it alone is the cause, but it does appear to be involved in producing the phenotype. Perhaps cyclops should be classified into a group with the extracephalic anomalies characteristic of trisomy 13, causally related to the extra chromosome, and other cases due to as yet unidentified genetic and nongenetic factors.

► [Wince. – Ed.] ◄

Y Chromosomal Genes in a Phenotypic Male with a 46 XX Karyotype. Most theories of male differentiation in the apparent absence of a Y chromosome suggest the conservation in one form or another of male-determining (Y chromosomal) genes. Harvey Dosik, Stephen S. Wachtel, Farida Khan, Gabriel Spergel and Gloria C. Koo[3] (New York) report serologic and cytologic evidence of the presence of Y chromosomal genes in a putative XX man.

Man, 46, admitted with painless hematuria, had undergone normal external genital and vocal changes of puberty at age 15, but with a sparse growth of facial hair and breast enlargement. He married at age 26 and reported having had normal sexual relations. The patient was 178 cm tall, weighed 78 kg and appeared normal. The hair distribution was feminine, and bilateral gynecomastia was present. The testes were 1 cm in diameter and hard. Both inguinal rings contained small hernial sacs. The prostate was small. An ejaculate contained no sperm. Urinary 17-ketosteroids were 9.1 mg/24 hours and 17-hydroxysteroids, 10.8 mg/24 hours. Plasma follicle-stimulating hormone was 41.9 mIU/ml, luteinizing hormone was 17.5 mIU/ml and testosterone was 0.05 μg/100 ml. Testicular biopsies showed hyalinized tubules, Leydig cell proliferation and no spermatogonia. Exploration showed no internal female genitalia. The parents and siblings of both sexes were reportedly normal.

A single normal Barr body was identified in about a quarter of buccal mucosal cells on two occasions. Studies of phytohemagglutinin-stimulated lymphocytes indicated a 46 XX karyotype. One chromosome 17 had an enlarged short arm in up to 80% of metaphases, and in some cells it appeared satellited. An apparent Y chromosome was seen in 1 of 201

(3) J.A.M.A. 236:2505–2508, Nov. 29, 1976.

lymphocytes studied. There was no evidence of heterochromatin on the additional piece. Chromosome 17 was normal in skin fibroblasts. A serologic assay for H-Y antigen, a cell surface component associated with the Y chromosome, showed the presence of Y chromosomal genes in this patient. Standard cytologic techniques revealed the presence of a minor population of XXY cells, as well as cells bearing an abnormal chromosome 17 among the blood leukocytes.

This patient may have two cytogenetic abnormalities, either one explaining the XX male condition, mosaicism and Y-to-autosome translocation. It is not clear, however, whether the minor population of Y-bearing cells observed in the leukocytes could produce detectable levels of H-Y antigen.

► [Remember how exciting it was to learn that one could look at individual chromosomes and that man did, in fact, have 46 of them? That was only the first stage. The microscopic dissection goes on with immunologic and fluorescence techniques. Among the dicta that are emerging is that, regardless of the crude chromosomal picture, a man is not a man without some Y chromosomal material in him. This is supported by the present article as well as others (1977 YEAR BOOK, p. 340). The present authors find consonant results (J. Clin. Endocrinol. Metab. 43:1234, 1976) in patients with true hermaphroditism. —T.B.S.] ◄

Klinefelter's Syndrome: Experiences with 24 Patients. T. J. Humphery, S. Posen and J. H. Casey[4] (Sydney) studied 24 of the 85 patients seen during 1960–74 with a karyotypic diagnosis of Klinefelter's syndrome (table). Only 9 of the 24 patients grew up in "satisfactory" family situations. Fifteen patients were delinquents and 4 others were described as dependent, manipulative subjects who were habituated to alcohol, analgesics or other drugs. Eleven major episodes of physical trauma were recorded in 8 patients. No significant association with nonendocrine disorders was found. The patients, as a group, had long limbs (Fig 41). Fifteen patients had a female distribution of body hair and 16 had breast enlargement. In all but 1 patient the greatest testicular diameter was 2 cm or less. The penis was normal in size in 11 patients. The mean general intelligence level was 79.4.

No cases of mosaicism were found. Eleven of 12 testicular specimens showed no sperm precursors, as well as varying

---

(4)   Med. J. Aust. 2:779–782, Nov. 20, 1976.

FEATURES OF PATIENTS IN PRESENT SERIES

Patient No.	Age at Presentation (years)	Mode of Presentation	Results of Psychological and Interview Assessment
1	17	Delinquency	Dull-normal, poor reader.
2	16	Delinquency	Dull; hardened, aggressive criminal.
3	16	Delinquency	Dull-normal; rural ghetto background.
4	15	Delinquency	Marked literary deficit; self-confessed compulsive thief.
5	17	Delinquency	Dull; linguistic handicap; psychopathic tendencies.
6	15	Delinquency	Illiterate; moody; impulsive.
7	17	Delinquency	Mildly handicapped; poorly socialized.
8	14	Delinquency	Poor reader.
9	14	Delinquency	Retarded; naïve; immature.
10	24	Delinquency	Poor verbal and social reasoning; tradesmen's assistant.
11	16	Delinquency	Dull; gross educational deficit.
12	18	Delinquency	Dull; enuresis; poor social ability.
13	16	Delinquency	Illiterate.
14	13	Delinquency	Average; sullen and withdrawn; little insight.
15	16	Delinquency	Average ability; ambition to be cook.
16	19	Head injury	Dull; roams Australia; schizophrenic.
17	25	Head injury	Dull; dependent; manipulative; schizophrenic.
18	39	Sterility	Happily married; skilled workshop manager.
19	46	Renal calculus	Unskilled caretaker with considerable responsibility.
20	39	Gynaecomastia	Dull; menial shop worker protected by family.
21	39	Sterility	Self employed; well socialized rural manager.
22	37	Sterility	Stable; married toolmaker.
23	30	Analgesic abuse	Dependent; manipulative; schizophrenic.
24	46	Gout	Analgesic abuse; died in renal failure; no recognizable gonadal tissue at autopsy.

degrees of tubular hyalinization and fibrosis. Plasma androgen levels were below the normal male range in 10 of 21 patients and in the lower part of the range in 11. The serum LH level was above the normal range for adult males in 16 of 20 patients. Five of 6 patients had serum FSH levels more than 5 times the upper limit of normal. Testosterone administration resulted in high plasma androgen values in all 9 patients tested. Seven of 11 patients exhibited abnormal

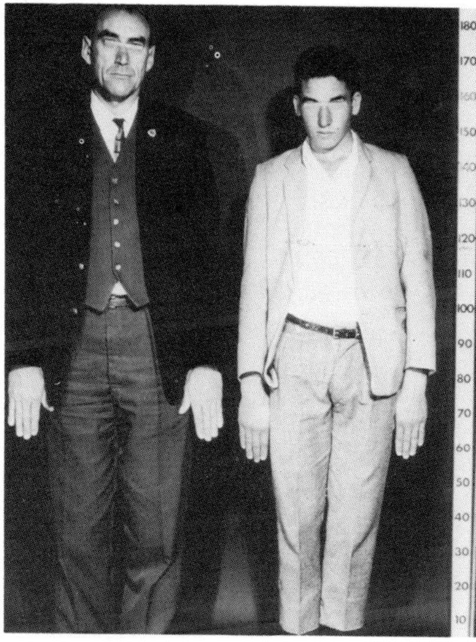

Fig 41.—Delinquent patient, aged 17, with his escort. Note disproportionately long arms and ill-fitting standard-issue trousers. (Courtesy of Humphery, T. J., et al.: Med. J. Aust. 2:779–782, Nov. 20, 1976.)

carbohydrate metabolism. Results of 2 of 12 EEG studies were clearly abnormal and 5 showed mild, nonspecific changes. An autopsy of a patient who died of renal failure at age 54 showed ischemic and fibrotic kidneys and completely fibrotic testes.

This study confirmed relative nonsuppressibility of LH secretion by androgens in Klinefelter's syndrome. High plasma estradiol levels may be responsible for gynecomastia in these patients. Beneficial effects from androgen therapy have been claimed in Klinefelter's syndrome, but undesirable sequelae may occur in these socially deviant subjects. The situation does not readily lend itself to a long-term controlled study.

► [These authors titled their article appropriately when they used "experiences." Yes, the extremities in Figure 41 look quite long and the skull in patients with Klinefelter's syndrome may be peculiar (1977 YEAR BOOK, p. 329), but it is also true that 4 children with Klinefelter's syndrome being followed from birth are all "well proportioned and remarkably handsome" (1976 YEAR BOOK, p. 340). Yes, more than half of the patients here were referred for delinquency, and aberrant behavior in XXY men has been noted before (1977 YEAR BOOK, p. 328), but a number of my patients function very well as good, mature, industrious members of society who have for some years enjoyed the blessings of androgen therapy. Recently, Tennes et al. (Pediatrics 59:574, 1977) have reported their experience with 12 boys with Klinefelter's syndrome. Some of these children were found to be "tall, inactive, poorly organized in motor functions, placid and delayed in language," but "these deviations from normal were relatively mild."

Smals (Acta Endocrinol. (Kbh.) 83:829, 1976) found that the elevated basal plasma levels of LH and FSH could be raised to levels considerably higher than the normal responses after the infusion of LH-releasing hormone to patients with Klinefelter's syndrome. Furthermore, if the infusion were continued for 8 hours the plasma testosterone concentration increased significantly. These authors (ibid. 84:72, 1977) also found these patients to have a decreased TSH reserve. On the other hand, Carter et al. (Br. Med. J. 1:212, 1977) have found a patient with Klinefelter's syndrome with associated hypogonadotropic hypogonadism. Finally, Doll (J. Urol. 116:675, 1976) and Isurugi (Cancer 39:2041, 1977) both describe patients with Klinefelter's syndrome who developed seminomas. Each believed that his was the first reported case. — T.B.S.] ◄

The following review articles are recommended to the reader:

Forest, M. G., et al.: Hypothalamic-pituitary-gonadal relationships in man from birth to puberty, Clin. Endocrinol. (Oxf.) 5:551, 1976.

Glenn, J. F.: Testicular feminization syndrome, Urology 7:569, 1976.

van Niekerk, W. A.: True hermaphroditism, Am. J. Obstet. Gynecol. 126:890, 1976.

Polyhormonal Disorders

High Level of a Nerve Growth Factor in the Serum of a Patient with Medullary Carcinoma of the Thyroid Gland. The frequent association of familial-type medullary carcinoma of the thyroid (MCT) with adrenal medullary involvement, mucosal neuromas, diffuse ganglioneuromatosis and neurofibromatosis is thought to result from a common defect of the neuroectodermal cell system. Mario Bigazzi, Roberto Revoltella, Silvio Casciano and Eliana Vigneti[5] report finding abnormally high levels of a factor, probably circulating human nerve growth factor (NGF), in the serum of a patient with this hereditary syndrome. Variations in the factor correlated with the progression of the tumor.

Woman, 41, presented after surgery for a MCT of the spindle cell type with metastases in the neck nodes. Café-au-lait spots were present on the shoulders. A typical marfanoid habitus was present in several relatives and a brother had a nodule in each thyroid lobe as well as nocturnal flushes and hypertension. Symptoms of sympathetic overfunction had been present for 8 years and resolved after removal of the tumor. The serum calcitonin was 12 ng/ml 5 months after surgery. Metastases in the lungs and bones subsequently were found; the serum cortisol was above 970 nmol/L and its nyctohemeral rhythm was lost. Pathologic bone fractures and diarrhea then developed and the patient died 2 years after presentation.

The bioassay results obtained at the time metastases developed are shown in Figure 42. Good correlation was found in the radioimmunoassay, proving immunologic cross-reactivity between human and mouse NGF. The serum level of NGF was 10–560 ng/ml, a result similar to that obtained in the bioassay. The older son of the patient had an abnormally high level of serum factor in both tests, though he had a normal calcitonin response in the calcium infusion test.

Although the material present in this patient's serum was

<hr>

(5) Clin. Endocrinol. (Oxf.) 6:105–112, February, 1977.

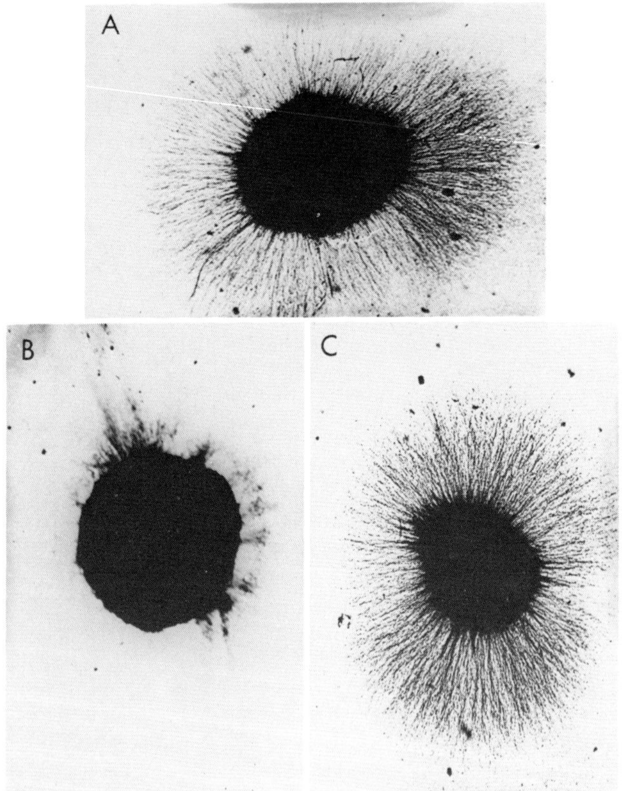

Fig 42.—Microphotographs of 8-day-old chick sensory ganglia cultured in vitro for 16 hours in semisolid medium in the presence of **A,** mouse submaxillary gland NGF at an optimal concentration of 10 ng/ml; **B,** serum of normal controls; **C,** serum of MCT patient, serum dilution 1/90. (Courtesy of Bigazzi, M, et al.: Clin. Endocrinol. (Oxf.) 6:105–112, February, 1977.)

not proved to be NGF, it was shown to be close immunologically to mouse NGF and was very potent biologically. In the mouse, the principal source of NGF seems to be the submaxillary glands. The present patient showed a correlation between high levels of serum NGF-like activity and the development of widespread metastases. A nerve growth factor may be related to the diffuse neural overgrowth sometimes associated with MCT. The presence of a high level of NGF in the serum of the patient's son suggests that abnormal levels could precede the thyroid tumor.

▶ [This is an excellent contribution. First, it helps to remind you that, as shown so dramatically in Figure 42, the discovery of growth factors grew out of (no pun intended) the ability to maintain intact cells in vitro. There is bone growth factor, known more familiarly as somatomedin. There is also epidermal growth factor, easily extracted from mouse submaxillary glands (1973 YEAR BOOK, p. 37), and ovarian growth factor from the pituitary (1975 YEAR BOOK, p. 11). Nerve growth factor resembles insulin and proinsulin (1973 YEAR BOOK, p. 38).

Second, you all are acquainted with type 2A of this syndrome (Bartley et al.: Med. J. Austral. 2:173, 1976) in which there is present, in addition to the medullary carcinoma of the thyroid and multiple pheochromocytomas, many mucosal neuromas and a marfanoid habitus. In the patients described here, marfanoid features were present in relatives and it is a reasonable presumption that the mucosal neuromas stem from the excessive NGF secreted by the tumor.

Third, there is a spate of publications on the subject of multiple endocrine neoplasia (MEN). They include a review of the Mayo Clinic experience by Carney et al. (Am. J. Clin. Pathol. 66:279, 1976). Variant patterns of MEN are reported by Berg et al. (Acta Med. Scand. 200:321, 1976) and Hansen et al. (ibid., p. 327). The Mayo Clinic group also emphasized the frequency in symptoms of ganglioneuromatosis (Carney et al.: N. Engl. J. Med. 295:1287, 1976), whereas Mulder and Su (Dtsch. Med. Wochenschr. 102:479, 1977) found the pentagastrin stimulation test to be an effective diagnostic marker. Samaan et al. (Ann. Intern. Med. 86:585, 1977) tell of the coincidence of medullary carcinoma and astrocytoma, whereas Pohl (Wien. Klin Wochenschr. 89:481, 1977) furnished the first report of type 2 MEN in identical twins, one of whom had a pheochromocytoma.

Finally, Calmettes (Biomedicine 27:52, 1977) reports the presence of carcinoembryonic antigen in patients with medullary carcinoma of the thyroid with a positive correlation of serum levels of the antigen and calcitonin. This last brings to mind an astonishing article, recently published (Lips et al.: Lancet 1:16, 1978), in which a common precursor protein of molecular weight of 65,000 was found in a number of ectopic hormone-producing tumors, including medullary carcinoma of the thyroid, insulinoma, parathyroid carcinoma, gastrinoma and renal carcinoma. The technique is ingenious and the hypothesis as an explanation of all ectopic hormone production is, if true, highly original. It goes like this: "The primary gene product of all cells thought to descend from the neural crest is a large protein containing several potential specificities; the specific hormone or hormones liberated from this protein are determined by enzyme systems in the differentiated cell, probably associated with the endoplasmic reticulum." In an addendum, the authors mention that this common precursor molecule also contains carcinoembryonic antigen. If these findings are confirmed, we probably can provide an "instant symposium" for the 1979 YEAR BOOK.

Already I have trouble conceiving of a single common precursor molecule. It would have to contain a plenitude of hormones. For some new ones, look ahead. —T.B.S.] ◀

Medullary Thyroid Carcinoma: Ectopic Production of Peptides with ACTH-like, Corticotropin-Releasing Factor-like and Prolactin Production-Stimulating Activities. Jan C. Birkenhäger, G. Virginia Upton, H. Jaqueline Seldenrath, Dorothy T. Krieger and Armen H. Tashjian Jr.[6] studied a patient with medullary thyroid carcinoma, galactorrhea and Cushing's syndrome, who had laboratory findings of pituitary-dependent Cushing's syndrome rather than of the classic type of ectopic ACTH syndrome. Cushing's syndrome appeared to be due to ectopic production of corticotropin-releasing factor-like material by the tumor. The tumor also contained a prolactin production-stimulating factor that could explain the galactorrhea.

Woman, 45, presented with facial roundness and reddening, skin darkening and an increase in body hair in the past year and

Fig 43.—Thyroid tumor-neuroendocrine interactions. *PRL-SA*, prolactin production-stimulating activity. One unit *(U)* is defined as that amount required to double rate of prolactin production per 24 hours by pituitary cells in culture. All values for ACTH were determined by bioassay; tumor content was measured after trypsin treatment. (Courtesy of Birkenhäger, J. C., et al.: Acta Endocrinol. (Kbh.) 83:280–292, October, 1976.)

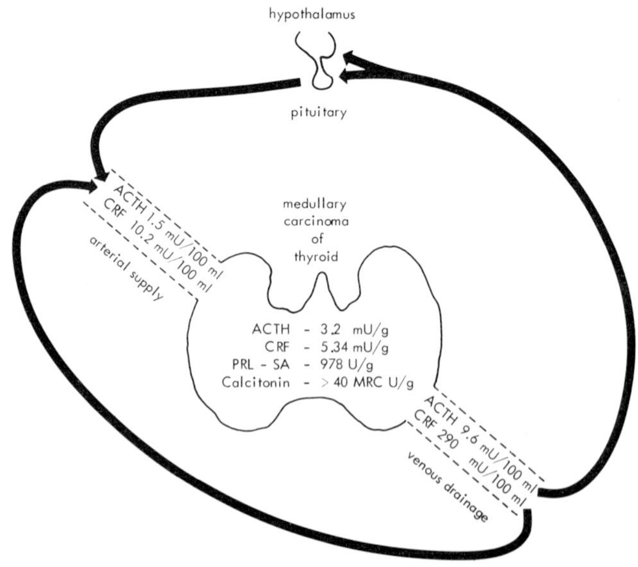

(6)   Acta Endocrinol. (Kbh.) 83:280–292, October, 1976.

galactorrhea for 3 months. She had moon facies, moderate bilateral proptosis, blood pressure of 160/100 mm Hg, truncal obesity and increased hair growth. A left thyroid nodule was palpated. The oral glucose tolerance curve was diabetic. The sella was normal in size. The plasma calcitonin concentration was 32 ng/ml and responded to calcium infusion, though not to glucagon infusion. The concentration was 10.4 ng/ml 2 weeks after total thyroidectomy. The serum parathyroid hormone value was high. The cortisol secretion rate was 65 mg/24 hours; plasma cortisol was suppressed by intravenous dexamethasone. Basal plasma immunoreactive ACTH concentrations were 220–320 pg/ml. Symptoms of cortisol excess and the galactorrhea abated rapidly after operation. Biologically active ACTH was detected in tumor extracts only after trypsin digestion. Tumor extracts also contained prolactin production-stimulating activity. The tumor was a typical medullary thyroid carcinoma.

Thyroid tumor-neuroendocrine interactions are outlined in Figure 43. Both the Cushing's syndrome and the galactorrhea in this patient were related to the presence of the major tumor mass. Galactorrhea was presumably due to stimulation of prolactin synthesis and its excessive release from the pituitary, induced by prolactin production-stimulating material in the medullary thyroid carcinoma.

► [This is an extraordinary patient even though ACTH and CRF-secreting tumors have been reported before (1972 YEAR BOOK, p. 341; and 1977 YEAR BOOK, p. 361). Talk about the conversion of "big ACTH" to "little ACTH" does fit with a hypothesis of the common precursor parent for multiple hormones. The prolactin-stimulating factor is new in this context. Estrogens are unlikely candidates here. Melatonin?

I should add that Toshihiro (J. Clin. Endocrinol. Metab. 44:440, 1977) found corticotropin-releasing factor in a patient with an ectopic ACTH-producing cancer of the colon. — T.B.S.] ◄

Polyendocrine Adenomatosis: Prolactin Pituitary Adenoma Associated with an Intrathyroidal Parathyroid Adenoma. J. Tourniaire, J. Trouillas, P. Maillet, L. David, D. Pallo, V. Tran Minh and C. Bressot[7] report the first documented case of prolactin cell adenoma in Wermer's syndrome.

Woman, 20, had a family history of stomach ulcers and renal lithiasis. Menarche occurred at age 13. At age 18, amenorrhea followed an accident which resulted in a leg fracture and a scalp injury. No estrogen treatment had been given. The only clinical abnormality was bilateral galactorrhea, elicited by pressure on the breasts. A prolactin cell tumor was identified by electron microsco-

---

(7) Ann. Endocrinol. (Paris) 38:1–11, Jan.–Feb., 1977.

py and confirmed by immunocytology. Intensive development of the Golgi complex and parallel band disposition of ergastoplasm indicated great cellular activity.

Cobalt irradiation of the pituitary (4,500 R) was administered for 1 month, but amenorrhea persisted and galactorrhea was only slightly diminished. Prolactinemia remained elevated (2,000 mU/ml); it was not stimulated by thyrotropin releasing hormone or checked by L-dopa. Thyrotropin deficiency persisted, and the gonadotropin response to luteinizing hormone-releasing hormone was moderately decreased (100 μg intravenously).

Oral bromocriptine was instituted (5 mg/day). Six months later, galactorrhea had disappeared, but amenorrhea persisted. Prolactinemia diminished from 120 ng/ml to 44 ng/ml. Clomiphene citrate for 5 days (50 mg/day) resulted in regular menses.

Hyperparathyroidism was diagnosed by the blood calcium levels and right ureteral lithiasis by intravenous urography. Exploratory cervicotomy with excision of three parathyroid glands and thoracotomy failed to reveal any parathyroid adenoma. A right ureterotomy performed for renal colic was followed by selective catheterization of thyroid veins and determination of parathyroid hormone levels. A repeat cervicotomy was negative. Total right thyroid lobectomy and isthmectomy revealed an intralobar parathyroid ad-

Fig 44.—Intrathyroidal parathyroid adenoma. Microscopic topography. (Courtesy of Tourniaire, J., et al.: Ann. Endocrinol. (Paris) 38:1–11, Jan.–Feb., 1977.)

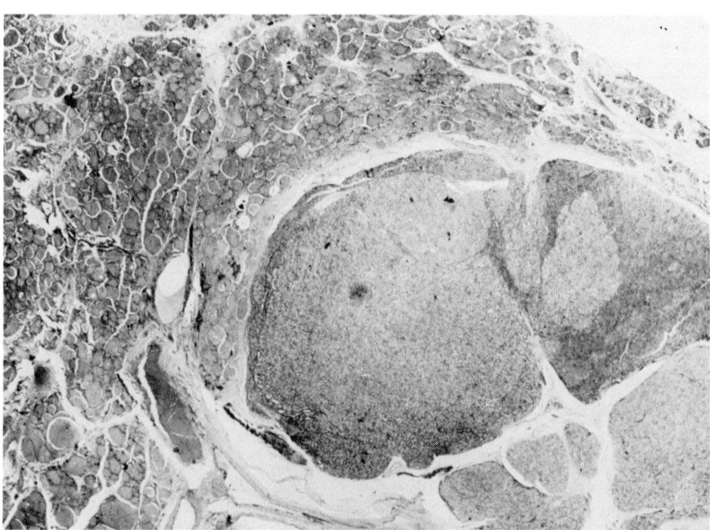

enoma. The nodule was 1.5 cm in diameter, encapsulated and well separated from the surrounding thyroid parenchyma (Fig 44).

Postoperative hypoparathyroidism required continuous treatment with calcamine (3 mg/day) and calcium (1 gm/day).

This patient's course illustrates the failure of combined neurosurgical and cobalt radiation treatment in such cases. Intrathyroid localization of a parathyroid adenoma is an exceptional occurrence, which explains the overly laborious discovery of this adenoma. The patient's genealogy is compatible with the theory of dominant autosomal transmission of Wermer's syndrome.

▶ [This article was selected for two reasons: (1) the nice figure (Fig 44) and (2) to share with you the authors' anguish in hunting down the parathyroid adenoma. Through my retrospectroscope, I would have advised that the biopsied parathyroid glands *not* be removed until the diagnosis was clearly confirmed or, if removed, be autotransplanted.

What endocrine disorders would be the farthest removed from this patient's problems? Why, the prolactin deficiency found in a patient with pseudohypoparathyroidism (Carlson et al.: N. Engl. J. Med. 296:140, 1977), of course. — T.B.S.] ◀

Plasma Prostaglandin E in Patients with Cancer with and without Hypercalcemia. The E prostaglandins induce hypercalcemia in animal tumor models in vivo and have been reported to be increased in the urine of hypercalcemic patients with nonhematologic neoplasms. R. Paul Robertson, David J. Baylink, Stewart A. Metz and Kenneth B. Cummings[8] (Univ. of Washington) determined circulating levels of immunoreactive prostaglandin E (iPGE), calcium and immunoreactive parathyroid hormone (iPTH) in 21 patients with various neoplasms, excluding those receiving radiotherapy, chemotherapy or treatment for hypercalcemia. Seven patients received 25 mg indomethacin orally every 6 hours to reduce elevated serum calcium values. Three also received 600 mg aspirin every 6 hours. Three patients with primary hyperparathyroidism were also studied.

Eleven of the 21 patients with malignant tumors were hypercalcemic; they had a variety of tumors with and without skeletal metastases. Four hypercalcemic patients and 1 normocalcemic patient had mean iPGE levels above the normal mean + 2 SD. Elevations of calcium and iPGE were unrelated to the presence or absence of skeletal metastases.

---

(8)   J. Clin. Endocrinol. Metab. 43:1330–1335, December, 1976.

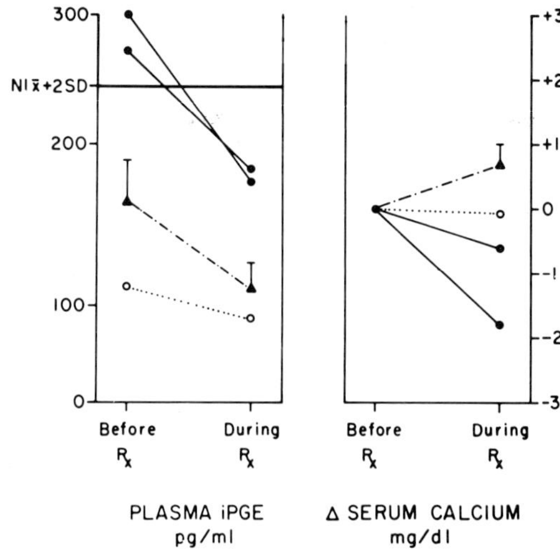

Fig 45.—Changes in circulating iPGE and calcium in patients with neoplasia treated with indomethacin given orally. Solid horizontal line represents upper limit of normal for iPGE (x̄ + 2 SD). Treatment lasted 3–8 (6 ± 1, x̄ ± SE) days. Mean of values obtained several days before treatment and value on last day of treatment are given. Solid circles denote 2 patients with neoplasia and elevated iPGE; solid triangles represent 4 patients with neoplasia and normal iPGE; open circles refer to 1 patient with parathyroid adenoma. (Courtesy of Robertson, R. P., et al.: J. Clin. Endocrinol. Metab. 43:1330–1335, December, 1976.)

Extracts of liver metastases from 3 hypercalcemic patients with iPGE elevations contained fivefold to 18-fold greater amounts of iPGE than did control liver specimens or a normal-appearing specimen from a hypercalcemic tumor patient. With 2 exceptions, serum iPTH levels were undetectable or below the normal mean. The hyperparathyroid patients had markedly elevated serum iPTH values; their plasma iPGE levels were below the mean of the normal group. Changes in iPGE and calcium levels in treated patients are shown in Figure 45. Plasma iPGE declined in 6 of 7 hypercalcemic patients treated with indomethacin, but serum calcium fell only in the 2 patients who had elevated plasma iPGE values before treatment.

Plasma iPGE elevations are found in some cancer patients, especially those with hypercalcemia, and this marker may identify those patients who will respond to indomethacin therapy.

► [This report reflects an interesting turnaround. It was once clear to all that hypercalcemia in patients with ectopic hormone-producing tumors was due to excessive PTH production. Now, one could easily gain the impression that prostaglandin E is the major, if not only, culprit. Very similar results have been reported by Demmers et al. (Cancer 39:1559, 1977). Where has all the PTH gone? Well, for one thing, many patients with ectopic ACTH production had "*inappropriately* high serum PTH levels" (Riggs: J. Clin. Invest. 50:2079, 1971). Maybe the PTH levels were inappropriately high because they were not suppressed by hypercalcemia induced by prostaglandin E.

Prostaglandins do other things. Jaffe and Condon found elevated levels of prostaglandin E in patients with carcinoid tumors, those with medullary carcinoma of the thyroid and a patient with the Verner-Morrison syndrome. The last patient had elevated levels of vasoactive intestinal peptide as well. — T.B.S.] ◄

Ectopic Production of Chorionic Gonadotropin and Its Subunits by Islet Cell Tumors: Specific Marker for Malignancy.

C. Ronald Kahn, Saul W. Rosen, Bruce D. Weintraub, Stefan S. Fajans and Phillip Gorden[9] measured human chorionic gonadotropin (hCG) and its subunits in 76 patients with islet cell tumors and found the tumor markers not only to be present in a high proportion of patients with functioning islet cell carcinomas but to be specific indicators of malignancy. All patients had surgical exploration and 33 were found to have malignant tumors. No tumor was found in 2 patients with Zollinger-Ellison syndrome. Hormone levels and concentration of hCG-α and hCG-β were determined by independent radioimmunoassays.

Eight of 14 patients with malignant insulinoma had increased serum levels of hCG-α and only 3 had elevated levels of hCG-β. Immunoreactive hCG was elevated in 2 of the 8 patients in whom it was measured. Four of 8 patients with malignant gastrinomas had elevated hCG-α levels, whereas only 1 had an elevated hCG-β level. None of 41 patients with benign insulinoma had elevated hCG, hCG-α or hCG-β levels. Six patients with nonfunctional malignant islet cell tumors had normal plasma levels of hCG subunits. The marker prevalence in 27 patients with functioning islet cell tumors was 63%. Subunits of hCG were found in extracts of all four malignant tumors examined, including 1 case with normal serum levels (table). Plasma placental lactogen was not detected in 13 patients with malignant or 39 with be-

---

(9) N. Engl. J. Med. 297:565–569, Sept. 15, 1977.

COMPARISON OF hCG SUBUNIT CONCENTRATIONS IN SERUM
AND TUMOR EXTRACTS

PATIENT CATEGORY	TUMOR TYPE	SERUM		TUMOR EXTRACT*	
		hCG-α	hCG-β	hCG-α	hCG-β
		ng/ml		*ng/g of tissue*	
Male or premeno-pausal female	None (controls)	<2.5	<2.0	—	—
	Benign insulinoma	1.5	<0.5	<0.3	<0.3
	Malignant insulinoma:				
	Case 1	2.0	<0.5	9.0	7.3
	Case 2	4.3	5.3	1.1	4.0
	Case 3	15.0	22.7	9.5	55.2
Postmenopausal female	None (controls)	<7.0	<3.0	—	—
	Malignant insulinoma	15	<0.5	27.9	<2.0

*Tumors were homogenized in 10 vol of acid-ethanol and extracted at 4 C for 12–18 hours; no attempt was made at quantitative recovery. The extracts were dialyzed against 0.05 M ammonium acid carbonate, lyophilized and resuspended in 1 vol of buffer approximately equal to the wet weight of the tumor.

nign islet cell tumors. Carcinoembryonic antigen was minimally elevated in 3 of 5 serums from patients with islet cell carcinomas; α-fetoprotein was elevated in 2 of 8 serums from such patients.

Chorionic gonadotropin and its subunits are specific and prevalent markers for islet cell carcinoma. Ectopic secretion does not occur in the same tumor types when they are benign. The findings support the derepression hypothesis, which predicts that ectopic proteins would appear only in cells that have undergone malignant transformation.

▶ [I recently was called on to discuss a male patient who had testicular choriocarcinoma. I reviewed the literature and was impressed by studies such as the one reported here. The prime mover in this area has been Doctor Vaitukaitis and her colleagues (1974 YEAR BOOK, p. 418). Even carcinoma of the breast is not exempt, as shown by Tormey et al. (Cancer 39:2391, 1977), but a word of caution. A recent *Lancet* editorial questioned the specificity of this tumor marker, and Yoshimoto et al. (Science 197:575, 1977) present evidence that normal tissue of normal subjects may produce chorionic gonadatropin-like substances.

I wish to mention that there is a case report by Fairlamb and Boesen (Postgrad. Med. J. 53:269, 1977) in which they describe the association of gynecomastia with a gonadotropin-secreting carcinoma of the lung and successful treatment of the gynecomastia with an antiestrogen. I hold the privilege, as Editor, to take particular notice of any article for any reason. I do so in this instance because Dr. Evelyn Boesen is a former fellow. Hi, Evelyn! – T.B.S.] ◄

Acromegaly Caused by Pulmonary Carcinoid Tumors. Occasionally, carcinoid tumor and pituitary adenomas are but two parts of a widespread pluriglandular syndrome. A carcinoid tumor could be directly responsible for acromegaly through secretion of a growth hormone-like substance, or it could cause acromegaly indirectly through secretion of a growth hormone-releasing factor. P. H. Sönksen, A. B. Ayres, M. Braimbridge, B. Corrin, D. R. Davies, G. M. Jeremiah, S. W. Oaten, C. Lowy and T. E. T. West[1] (St. Thomas' Hosp. Med. School, London) recently encountered a patient with acromegaly and a bronchial carcinoid in whom the latter mechanism appeared to be the likeliest explanation.

Woman, 60, with recurrent attacks of right-sided pneumonia over 19 years, had classic clinical features of acromegaly and bilateral carpal tunnel syndrome. She was 14 years postmenopausal. The pituitary fossa was enlarged, and fasting plasma growth hormone (GH) levels were 156 – 260 mU/L and were not suppressed on glucose tolerance testing. An insulin tolerance test confirmed insulin resistance. Bronchoscopy showed an adenoma occluding the right lower-lobe bronchus, and biopsy revealed it to be a carcinoid tumor. Urinary excretion of vanilylmandelic acid and 5 hydroxyindoleacetic acid was normal. The right lower and middle lobes were removed. The plasma growth hormone was 6 mU/L postoperatively, and the patient has been well, with subjective and objective features of soft tissue regression. Glucose tolerance tests improved gradually postoperatively. Insulin tolerance testing a year postoperatively confirmed insulin sensitivity and showed a normal rise in plasma growth hormone and cortisol.

Records of a similar patient have been traced. In both cases, removal of the bronchial carcinoid cured the acromegaly. In the study case, the tumor was not secreting growth hormone, but apparently was producing a growth hormone-releasing substance. Growth hormone was not extracted from the tumor, and ultrastructural differences from pituitary somatotrophes were evident.

The association of bronchial adenomas with acromegaly is

---

(1)   Clin. Endocrinol. (Oxf.) 5:503 – 513, September, 1976.

well recognized. Bronchial carcinoids are almost certainly apudomas. Some cases of the pluriglandular syndrome may be secondary to small bronchial carcinoid tumors producing as yet unidentified substances which stimulate the growth and hyperactivity of other endocrine tissue. Every effort should be made to detect such tumors, since the syndrome may remit if the carcinoid tumor is completely removed.

▶ [On the surface, this is just another case of a peculiar polyglandular syndrome, but it is not. This may be an instance of a *very* peculiar polyglandular syndrome. There is suggestive, but not conclusive, evidence to support the notion that the carcinoid tumors made a somatotropin-releasing hormone of some sort, driving the pituitary to excessive growth hormone secretion. — T.B.S.] ◀

Plasma Arginine Vasopressin in Syndrome of Antidiuretic Hormone Excess Associated with Bronchogenic Carcinoma. A syndrome of inappropriate antidiuretic hormone secretion (SIADH) has been described in association with a variety of states, particularly oat cell bronchogenic carcinoma. The syndrome is said to occur in 1.6% of patients with bronchogenic carcinoma. Paul L. Padfield, James J. Morton, Jehoiada J. Brown, Anthony F. Lever, J. Ian S. Robertson, Martin Wood and Ruth Fox[2] (Glasgow) used a new radioimmunoassay for plasma arginine vasopressin (AVP) to evaluate 31 patients with bronchogenic carcinoma, 17 of whom were referred because of a plasma sodium value below 125 mM/L and osmolality relations suggestive of SIADH. Studies were also done on 18 inpatients with psoriasis and 16 healthy subjects. Nine patients were restudied after a period of fluid restriction and 1 after another 9 days of free access to fluid.

Plasma osmolality in patients with SIADH was significantly lower than in those with bronchogenic carcinoma but without SIADH. Both groups had values significantly below those of normal subjects. Plasma AVP values were generally elevated in patients with SIADH (Fig 46). Concentrations in patients with carcinoma but no overt SIADH were above those in normal subjects, but all but two values were in the upper normal range. In all carcinoma patients, plasma AVP showed significant negative correlation with plasma osmolality. Dilutions of plasma extracts from carcinoma patients paralleled the standard curve in most in-

---

(2) Am. J. Med. 61:825–831, December, 1976.

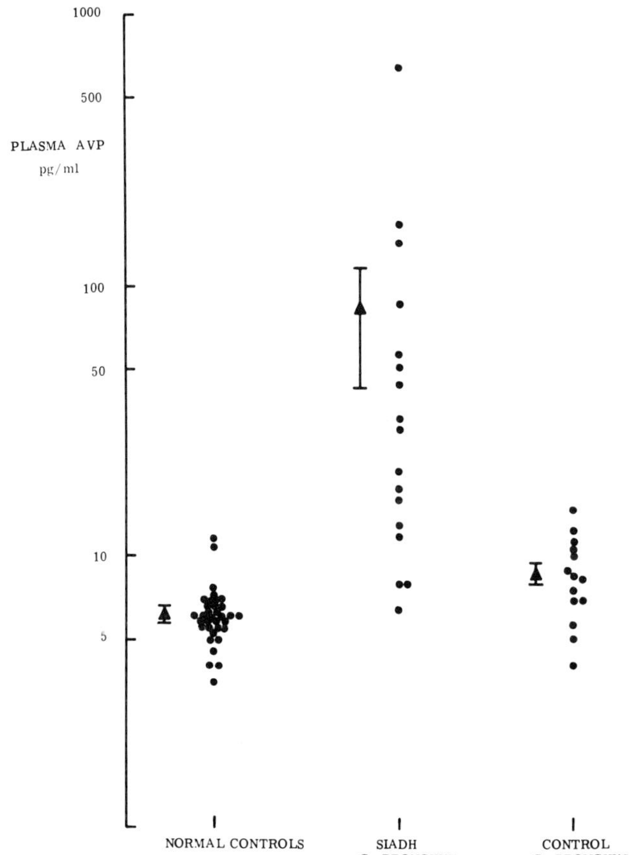

Fig 46.—Comparison of plasma AVP among groups. Means and standard errors are indicated. (Courtesy of Padfield, P. L., et al.: Am. J. Med. 61:825–831, December, 1976.)

stances. Fluid deprivation led to marked increases in serum sodium and urea and plasma osmolality and a moderate increase in urine osmolality. Significant weight loss and a decrease in plasma volume were also observed. Plasma AVP increased in 7 of 9 cases, despite initially high levels in 6.

Patients with SIADH have excess circulating AVP, and patients with bronchogenic carcinoma but no overt SIADH tend to have relatively high levels. The appearance of overt

SIADH in patients with bronchogenic carcinoma appears to herald a terminal stage of illness. The possibility that differences from normal in circulating vasopressin levels would be accentuated by forced hydration is being investigated.

► [This is more to a clinician's liking. The absolute elevation in serum arginine vasopressin levels is more clear-cut than the usual apologetic mention of "levels in the normal range but still inappropriately high for the plasma osmolality," or some such. Similar results have been reported by Haefligur et al. (Schweiz. Med. Wochenschr. 107:726, 1977) and the syndrome was described by Kaye and Ross (Postgrad. Med. J. 53:274, 1977) in a patient with a carcinoma of the bladder. — T.B.S.] ◄

Adrenocortical Carcinoma and Hypoglycemia: Evidence for Production of Nonsuppressible Insulin-like Activity by the Tumor. The plasma level of an insulin-like peptide, NSILA-s or a closely related peptide, is elevated in about a third of patients with extrapancreatic tumors and hypoglycemia. T. Hyodo, K. Megyesi, C. R. Kahn, J. P. McLean and H. G. Friesen[3] report data on a patient with adrenocortical carcinoma and hypoglycemia in whom elevated NSILA-s-related peptides were demonstrated in serum and in tumor tissue extracts.

Man, 42, presented with abdominal pain and a right upper quadrant mass and was found to have a large unresectable tumor adherent to the inferior vena cava. A biopsy specimen was consistent with adrenocortical carcinoma, although urinary steroid levels were normal. Radiotherapy and cytotoxic drug therapy were ineffective and hypoglycemia developed 4 years after presentation. Plasma immunoreactive insulin levels were normal and growth hormone levels were low. Treatment with diazoxide and glucagon was not helpful and the patient died after a hypoglycemic episode, with a 2000-gm right adrenal tumor and 75% involvement of the liver with metastases.

Increased insulin-like activity was found in an insulin radioreceptor assay and in a fat cell bioassay. With a NSILA-s-multiplication stimulating activity radioreceptor assay, the level of NSILA-s-related peptides was four times normal. Acetone-ethanol extracts of tumor were fourfold to 20-fold more active in this assay than unaffected tissues. Acid-ethanol extracts showed the same general pattern, but material was detectable only in the more sensitive receptor assay not in the insulin radioreceptor assay or fat cell bioassay.

---

(3)   J. Clin. Endocrinol. Metab. 44:1175–1184, June, 1977.

Elevated levels of NSILA-s-related peptides may play an important pathogenetic role in some patients with tumor hypoglycemia. The peptides appear to be produced by the tumor itself. Great variability in extraction methods and a lack of specific and sensitive assays in the past may explain the difficulty found in detecting the insulin-like peptide.

▶ [Did you know that in 1930, the same year in which Doege described the association of a large mediastinal fibrosarcoma with hypoglycemia (Ann. Surg. 92:955, 1930), Anderson (Am. J. Med. Sci. 180:71, 1930) had already described this variant, that is, adrenocortical carcinoma and hypoglycemia. I didn't know it either, but learned about it from Scandellari et al. (Diabete Metab. 2:191, 1976), who describe still another patient.— T.B.S.] ◀

The VIPoma: Further Confirmation of VIP as the Hormonal Agent in the WDHA Syndrome. The hormone responsible for the watery diarrhea, hypokalemia, achlorhydria (WDHA) syndrome has not been completely established, although two workers have independently confirmed vasoactive intestinal peptide (VIP) as the agent involved. Charles F. Shield, III, and Roderick C. Haff[4] (Lackland AFB) report data on a patient, followed-up for 2 years, in whom many of the proposed agents were assayed.

Man, 39, with a 1-year history of increasing watery diarrhea and persistent diarrhea for 3 weeks, had a serum potassium value of 2.7 mEq/decaliter. An extensive workup for malabsorptive syndrome, endocrine syndromes and infectious processes gave negative results. Gastric analysis showed achlorhydria. The diarrhea persisted despite massive fluid and electrolyte replacements, and an episode of hypokalemic uremia occurred. An extrinsic mass effect on the greater gastric curvature and transverse colon was noted and angiography showed a hypervascular 20-cm lession in the tail of the pancreas (Fig 47). Distal hemipancreatectomy, splenectomy, midtransverse colectomy and colocolostomy were carried out. The patient has since been asymptomatic for a 2-year follow-up period. Examination of serums and tumor specimens for gastrin, VIP and prostaglandins E and F showed pathologic levels of VIP alone in the preoperative serum and tumor specimens.

Reports of secretin, glucagon and gastric inhibitory peptide as the polypeptides responsible for the WDHA syndrome could be explained by contamination of these polypeptide preparations with VIP. Bloom found islet cell tumors and elevated serum VIP levels in 3 of 5 patients with

---

(4) Am. J. Surg. 132:784–786, December, 1976.

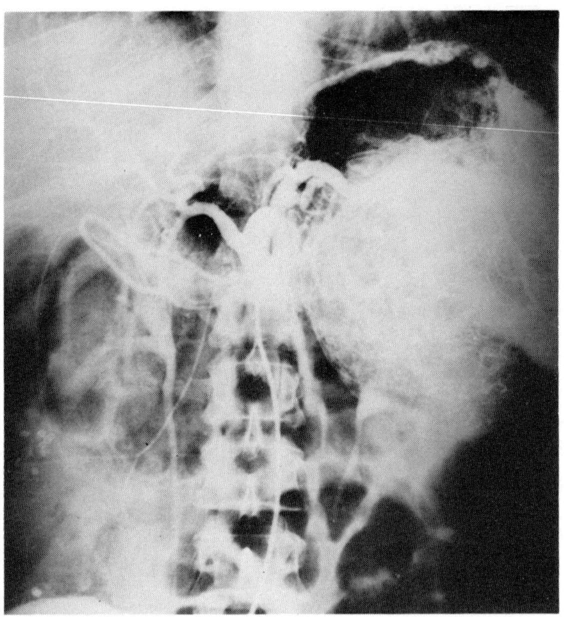

Fig 47.—Splenic artery angiogram. Large hypervascular pancreatic tumor was present. (Courtesy of Shield, C. F., III, and Haff, R. C.: Am. J. Surg. 132:784–786, December, 1976.)

chronic diarrhea symptoms. Standardization of the VIP assay will result in increased diagnosis of this disease state before its fulminant clinical presentation.

► ["VIPoma." It sounds like a disease contracted by a careless snake handler. But who are we to slow the march of science? Figure 47 shows an astonishing vascularity. The numerous vessels remain distinct so that what is seen is not merely a tumor blush.

A patient with this syndrome also had episodic hypercalcemia (Holdaway: Aust. N. Z. J. Med. 7:63, 1977) and a patient similar to the one presented here was described by Cryer and Hill (Cancer 38:2217, 1976). Improvement was noted after streptozotocin therapy. This patient and that of Judge et al. (Arch. Pathol. Lab. Med. 101:262, 1977) also produced gastrin. Finally, for those who think that ectopic hormone production is beginning to make sense, let me say that Jansen-Gomans and Engelhardt (Pediatrics 59:710, 1977) report a VIP-producing ganglioneuroblastoma occuring in the neck of a 1-year-old boy. —T.B.S.] ◄

Two Cases of Multiple Hormone-Producing Small Cell Carcinoma of the Lung: Coexistence of Tumor ADH, ACTH and β-MSH. The ectopic ACTH syndrome and the syndrome of inappropriate antidiuretic hormone (ADH) secretion due to nonendocrine tumors have been well documented in recent years. Yukio Hirata, Shigeru Matsukura, Hiroo Imura, Toshihiro Yakura, Satoshi Ihjima, Chiaki Nagase and Motohiko Itoh[5] report 2 cases of small cell carcinoma of the lung associated with the ectopic production of ADH, ACTH and melanocyte-stimulating hormone (β-MSH).

CASE 1.—Woman, 63, presented with anorexia and vomiting and was found to have hyponatremia and hypo-osmolar plasma associated with hypernatriuresis and hyperosmolar urine. The findings were consistent with inappropriate ADH secretion. An undifferentiated small cell lung carcinoma metastatic to supraclavicular nodes and the mediastinum was found. Despite intensive chemotherapy, the patient's condition deteriorated, and she died 4 months after hospitalization.

CASE 2.—Man, 66, presented with a persistent cough and right-sided backache. A left hilar mass was noted at roentgenographic examination. The findings were consistent with inappropriate ADH secretion before a left pneumonectomy was performed. An oat cell carcinoma was present in the lung. Histochemically, the tumor cells were argentaffin negative and argyrophil positive. The patient died 5 months after admission.

The presence of bioactive and immunoreactive ADH was demonstrated in the tumors of both patients. Significant amounts of bioactive and immunoreactive ACTH, as well as immunoreactive β-MSH, were found. The biologic, immunologic and gel chromatographic properties of the ectopic hormones were very similar to those of hormones of pituitary origin. The effect of excessive ADH secretion dominated the clinical picture in both cases; manifestations of the ectopic ACTH-MSH syndrome were minimal.

Multiple hormone production without clinically overt sequelae of excess hormone appears not to be uncommon in small cell (oat cell) carcinoma of the lung. Failure to detect an ADH-neurophysin complex in the present cases might be due either to diminished cross-reactivity of the antiserum used with the complex or to dissociation of noncovalent linkages in the acid condition.

▶ [A conjoint secretion of ACTH and β-MSH is hardly surprising these days. The addition of inappropriate ADH secretion is something new, al-

---

(5) Cancer 38:2575–2582, December, 1976.

though an almost identical patient was described by Coscia (Am. J. Med. 62:303, 1977) 3 months later.

In this area too, the specificity of ectopic hormone for neoplastic tissue can be questioned. Bloomfield (Clin. Endocrinol. (Oxf.) 6:95, 1977) has found ACTH-like materials in all lung tumors of carcinoid or oat cell type. Furthermore, they find ACTH-like materials in nontumorous lung tissue in patients with lung cancer. Hmm. See the comment following the article by Kahn et al., in this chapter.

Don't go away yet. Ectopic ACTH production has been reported in patients with prostatic oat cell carcinoma (Wenk: Cancer 40:773, 1977) apudoma of the esophagus (Tateishi: Virchows Arch. [Path. Anat.] 371:283, 1976), carcinoma of the cervix (Jones et al.: Cancer 38:1629, 1976), salivary gland adenocystic carcinoma (Sugawara: Arch. Intern. Med. 137:102, 1977), pheochromocytoma (Arch. Pathol. Lab. Med. 101:31, 1977) and liver (Hindsworth et al.: Clin. Endocrinol. (Oxf.) 7:45, 1977). This last patient was remarkable in that he secreted "big ACTH" (? common precursor protein) and calcitonin as well. – T.B.S.] ◄

Autoimmune Vitiligo: Detection of Antibodies to Melanin-Producing Cells. The presence of thyroid, adrenal and gastric parietal cell antibodies in many patients with both vitiligo and endocrine disease has suggested a common, perhaps autoimmune, origin. An increased prevalence of organ-specific autoantibodies has been found in several large series of patients with vitiligo. Kenneth C. Hertz, Laura A. Gazze, Charles H. Kirkpatrick and Stephen I. Katz[6] (Natl. Inst. of Health) describe 2 patients with vitiligo, alopecia universalis, mucocutaneous candidiasis and multiple endocrine insufficiencies in whom a circulating antibody to melanocytes, nevus cells and melanoma cells was demonstrated. A woman aged 34 had widespread candidiasis, total alopecia, hypoparathyroidism, pernicious anemia, primary ovarian failure, vitiligo and hypoadrenalism. A woman aged 18 had candidiasis of the nails, total alopecia, vitiligo, hypoparathyroidism, hypoadrenalism and primary ovarian failure.

Serums from both patients produced cellular fluorescence with all substrates but vitiliginous skin when examined by the in vitro complement-binding test for complement fixation, as evidenced by C3 deposit. The fluorescent cells were identical in location with melanocytes. Nevi showed staining of clusters and theques of nevus cells, and a metastatic melanoma showed fluorescent staining of sheets of melanoma cells. Complement binding occurred through activation

---

(6) N. Engl. J. Med. 297:634–637, Sept. 22, 1977.

of the classic pathway. The serum factor appeared from ultracentrifugation and specific immunoabsorption studies to be an IgG.

The findings constitute evidence for an antimelanocyte antibody in certain patients with vitiligo. The antibodies bind to intracellular rather than to cell surface antigens, raising the question of whether they are functionally active in vivo or represent an epiphenomenon secondary to melanocyte injury with exposure of cytoplasmic antigens. Their role in the origin of vitiligo and in the endocrinopathies that occur in this syndrome is unclear. The findings, however, should renew interest in the possibility that at least some cases of vitiligo represent an autoimmune phenomenon.

▶ [Nice! The well-known connection between vitiligo and autoimmune multiple endocrine deficiency syndromes now has a reasonable explanation. The authors quite properly provide disclaimers in case it really doesn't work out that way.

Other variants on this theme are the combination of Hashimoto's thyroiditis, myasthenia gravis and idiopathic thrombocytopenic purpura (Segal and Weintraub: Ann. Intern. Med. 85:761, 1976) and hypogonadism, hypoparathyroidism, hypoadrenocorticism and hypothyroidism (Weinberg et al.: Am. J. Med. Sci. 272:215, 1976). — T.B.S.] ◀

A Syndrome of Immunoglobulin A Deficiency, Diabetes Mellitus, Malabsorption and a Common HLA Haplotype: Immunologic and Genetic Studies of 43 Family Members. A number of patients with isolated IgA deficiency have evidence of associated disease, including malabsorption. David H. Van Thiel, William I. Smith, Jr., Bruce S. Rabin, Stanley E. Fisher and Roger Lester[7] (Univ. of Pittsburgh) report the findings in 3 related persons with IgA deficiency and a unique form of malabsorption. These 3 patients were part of a 43-member kindred that manifested multiple immune-related diseases, including thyroiditis and a variety of antibodies to endocrine tissue. The syndrome consisted of IgA deficiency, diabetes, malabsorption and a common HLA haplotype. The proband exhibited life-threatening malabsorption, intestinal mucosal atrophy with inflammation, insulin-dependent diabetes and the major histocompatibility antigens HLA-A2, B8 and DW3. Other conditions present in the family included Graves' disease, vitiligo, hypocomplementemia, rheumatic fever, multiple sclerosis and a high frequency of antibodies to endocrine tissue.

---

(7) Ann. Intern. Med. 86:10–19, January, 1977.

These cases represent variable expressions of a genetically determined syndrome within a single family. Full expression of the syndrome includes life-threatening malabsorption; intestinal mucosal atrophy and inflammation; isolated IgA deficiency and polyendocrine autoantibody production; and insulin-dependent diabetes and multiple diseases associated with abnormalities of immune mechanisms. Since Graves' disease, diabetes and idiopathic Addison's disease have been described in association with HLA-B8 and DW3, the present findings suggest a single immune response gene or gene complex linked with HLA-B8 and DW3. The study patients had a marked increase in intestinal plasma cells, in contrast to many cases of isolated IgA deficiency or hypogammaglobulinemia. The mechanism by which immune response genes exert their effects is not clear.

▶ [An autoimmune pathogenesis for some patients with diabetes seems hardly contestable now, and this article does not weaken the thesis. Other variants include a description by Pulini et al. (Ann. Intern. Med. 85:749, 1976) of a patient with insulin resistance and acanthosis nigricans in whom antibodies to insulin receptors were demonstrated. Winter and Green (for president? — A pun that only those who are old enough to remember an ancient musical called *Of Thee I Sing* will understand) reported (J. Pediatr. 89:401, 1977) an increased prevalence of diabetes mellitus in patients with lymphocytic thyroiditis, whereas Poonai et al. (Obstet. Gynecol. 49:86s, 1977) seem to have had their hands full with a pregnant patient who had diabetes mellitus, Addison's disease and hypothyroidism. — T.B.S.] ◀

Sheehan's Syndrome of Hypothalamic Origin in Woman with Juvenile Diabetes Mellitus. Hypopituitarism may have a hypothalamic origin after irradiation and after trauma to the hypothalamus. Georg Herbai and Ivar Werner[8] (Univ. of Uppsala) attempted to stimulate the pituitary by hypothalamic releasing factors in a patient with clinically typical Sheehan's syndrome after gestational toxicosis; she also had juvenile diabetes which was ameliorated by development of the hypopituitary state.

Woman, 25, had acquired diabetes after a bacterial infection at age 7 and had been managed on insulin. She had conceived at age 23 and developed toxicosis, being delivered by cesarean section 2 months before term. Cerebral palsy developed in the child. The patient had frequent attacks of hypoglycemia after surgery and

---

(8)   Acta Med. Scand. 199:539–541, 1976.

EFFECT OF TSH-RELEASING FACTOR (TRH), LH-RELEASING FACTOR (LRH) AND VASOPRESSIN ON TSH, LH AND PLASMA CORTISOL LEVELS*

		Time (min)								
		−10	0	10	20	30	40	60	80	120
TRH (200 μg)	Serum TSH (μU/ml)									
	Exp. 1		9.5	24	25		14			
	Exp. 2	7.3	9.0	16	19		14			8.2
LRH (100 μg)	Serum LH (ng/ml)		0.7	0.9	1.9	1.5	1.8	2.9	1.3	1.5

		Time (h)		
		0	2	5
Vasopressin (10 IU)	Plasma cortisol (μg/100 ml)			
	Exp. 1	10.0	27.8	15.2
	Exp. 2	11.5	21.6	17.4

*All experiments were made during investigation period before substitution therapy. Drugs were injected intravenously at zero time.

her insulin requirement fell from 100 to about 30 IU/day. Total amenorrhea, muscle weakness, loss of libido and loss of axillary and pubic hair also occurred. The patient became sensitive to cold and showed leg edema, some loss of memory and low blood pressure. Low doses of cortisone and thyroxine were given for 2 years after delivery. Examination showed signs of hypothyroidism and absent secondary sex characteristics. Laboratory findings were typical of anterior pituitary insufficiency. The results of releasing-factor tests are given in the table. She was given insulin, hydrocortisone, thyroxine, ethinyl estradiol and norethisterone and she rapidly became practically free of symptoms on this regimen. Secondary sex features reappeared and a normal sex life was resumed. Laboratory values were essentially normal 3 months after the start of substitution therapy. The patient felt well 2 years later and had no signs of pituitary insufficiency.

A hypothalamic form of postpartum pituitary insufficiency occurs. Treatment is by combined substitution with different target-organ hormones, as in other forms of the syndrome. The development of long-acting hypothalamic releasing-factor preparations will probably soon permit a new type of management and this may make a distinct etiologic diagnosis important.

▶ [Strange but plausible! Vaguely related to this is the report of Chandra (Acta Endocrinol. (Kbh.) 84:80, 1977), who found a diabetic patient in whom hypothyroidism, probably due to thyrotropin-releasing hormone deficiency, was also present and Olson and Winternitz (South. Med. J. 70: 411, 1977) describe another 3 patients with hypopituitarism and diabetes. − T.B.S.] ◀

The following review articles are recommended to the reader:

Cole, P. C., and Cramer, D.: Diet and cancer of endocrine target organs, Cancer 40:434, 1976.

Cooperman, A. M.: Gastrointestinal hormones and apudomas, Cleve. Clin. Q. 44:83, 1977.

Taylor, S.: Thyroid medullary carcinoma, Ann. R. Coll. Surg. Engl. 59:374, 1977.

Telenius-Berg, M.: Diagnostic studies in medullary carcinoma of the thyroid, Acta Med. Scand. [Suppl.] 201:597, 1977.

Tischler, A. S., et al.: Neuroendocrine neoplasms and their cells of origin, N. Engl. J. Med. 296:919, 1977.

Volpé, R.: The role of autoimmunity in hypoendocrine and hyperendocrine function, Ann. Intern. Med. 87:86, 1977.

The Parathyroid Glands, Calcitonin and Calcium Metabolism

Multicellular Origin of Parathyroid "Adenomas." Most cases of primary hyperparathyroidism are associated with enlargement of a single gland or with chief cell hyperplasia, but the relative frequency of these entities is unclear. It has been postulated that adenomas do not arise spontaneously, but rather result from prolonged hyperplasia in response to unknown stimuli. Philip J. Fialkow, Charles E. Jackson, Melvin A. Block and Kenneth A. Greenawald[9] studied four parathyroid adenomas from 3 women with heterozygosity *(Gd^B/Gd^A)* for the X chromosome-linked enzyme glucose-6-phosphate dehydrogenase (G-6-PD) to determine the number of cells from which the growths arise. A unicellular origin would be compatible with a rare oncogenic event and a multicellular origin with hyperplasia.

Three black women with primary hyperparathyroidism who were heterozygous at the G-6-PD locus were studied. All were found to be hypercalcemic at routine screening. One patient had previously had a kidney stone and 2 had x-ray evidence of renal calculi. Two patients had a single enlarged parathyroid, removal of which corrected the hypercalcemia. One had multigland involvement, and hypercalcemia was corrected by removal of two enlarged parathyroids. Both B and A isoenzymes were found in each "adenoma" in proportions similar to those found in normal tissues, suggesting multicellular origin of the lesions.

Parathyroid hyperplasia and adenomas may be similar biologically, but the finding of both enzyme types does not necessarily indicate a multiple-cell origin for the tumor. Other possibilities include admixture with nonneoplastic

---

(9)   N. Engl. J. Med. 297:696–698, Sept. 29, 1977.

cells and activity of both X chromosomes in each tumor cell. Perhaps in parathyroid adenomas hyperplasia results from stimuli not yet identified. Ultimately, the cells in one gland may become autonomous and suppress the activity of the other glands.

▶ [No wonder we have difficulty telling parathyroid adenomas from hyperplasia! — W.G.R.] ◀

Parathyroid Adenomas and Glands in Normocalcemic Hyperparathyroidism: A Light Microscopic Study. In a previous article by Johansson et al., the outcome after parathyroid surgery in 84 patients with recurrent kidney stones and suspected normocalcemic hyperparathyroidism was described. The best clinical results were obtained in those with parathyroid adenomas. L. Grimelius, S. Ejerblad, H. Johansson and I. Werner[1] (Uppsala Univ.) relate the histopathologic findings of the parathyroid glands to the clinical course in the 84 patients (55 men and 29 women, aged 20–75 years at the time of operation). All had a history of renal stones, and all had serum calcium levels in the upper normal quartile. Most patients had hypercalciuria. All 4 glands were explored, and biopsy specimens of at least 2 glands were examined. In hyperplasia, the 3 largest glands were removed, with part of the 4th if enlarged. When all glands appeared normal in size, the 3 largest were extirpated. The mean postoperative follow-up was 3.5 years.

A solitary adenoma was found in 17 patients and 2 adenomas in each of 2 patients. No patient had symptoms of renal stone postoperatively. Dark chief cells predominated in 7 adenomas and light chief cells in 6. In all adenomas most parenchymal cells contained glycogen. In 39 patients the parathyroids were hyperplastic. Ten patients had recurrent renal stóne disease postoperatively. Chief cell hyperplasia was present in all cases. Small fibrotic areas were seen in about one third of glands in the "cured" group but only occasionally in the relapsed group (Fig 48). Normal histogic findings were noted in 26 patients; 12 relapsed after operation. Small fibrotic areas predominated in the subgroup of patients who were "cured."

A higher glandular and parenchymal cell weight, a predominance of light chief cells and small fibrotic areas appear

---

(1) Am. J. Pathol. 83:475–484, June, 1976.

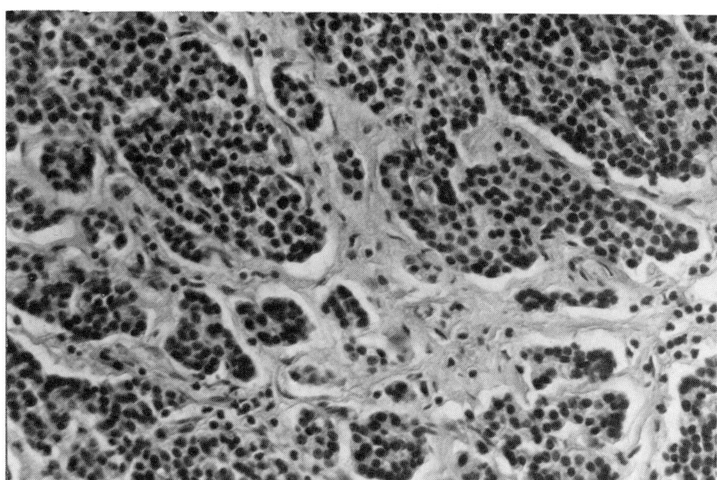

Fig 48.—Parathyroid gland with slight hyperplasia (mean weight, 60 mg). The dark chief cells predominate. Some partly fibrotic areas, mainly perivascular, are seen. This patient did not relapse. Hematoxylin-eosin; reduced from ×120. (Courtesy of Grimelius, L., et al.: Am. J. Pathol. 83:475–484, June, 1976.)

to be favorable for the outcome of surgery on hyperplastic parathyroid glands. The pathogenesis of the fibrotic areas is unclear; they may be the sequel of an earlier inflammation. Patients with normal glands may have incipient hyperplasia, "idiopathic hypercalciuria," renal calcium loss or intestinal hyperabsorption of calcium.

▶ [I've always been nervous about the diagnosis of normocalcemic hyperparathyroidism, although it must occur somewhere along the spectrum of normalcy to primary hyperparathyroidism. In this study, I do not find it surprising that the patients with adenomas had the best response.—W.G.R.] ◀

Hypercalcemia in Patients with Known Malignant Disease. Hypercalcemia is common and potentially lethal in patients with nonendocrine malignancies. In many cases the cancer may be responsible through bone metastasis or the production of a hypercalcemic humoral factor, but hyperparathyroidism may coexist. N. A. Samaan, R. C. Hickey, M. R. Sethi, K. P. Yang and S. Wallace[2] (M. D. Anderson Hosp., Houston) evaluated 89 patients in a cancer institu-

---

(2) Surgery 80:382–389, September, 1976.

tion who had hypercalcemia. Three patients had previously had unsuccessful neck exploration for parathyroid adenoma. Parathyroid hormone was measured by radioimmunoassay. Immunoreactive parathyroid hormone (iPTH) was identified in nonendocrine cancer tissue in 2 cases.

All patients repeatedly had serum calcium concentrations of 10.5 mg/100 ml or above and phosphorus concentrations below 3.5 mg/100 ml. Peripheral iPTH was elevated in 75% of patients, and 83 patients had elevated iPTH values in the cervical or mediastinal veins. Seventy-nine of these patients had primary benign hyperparathyroidism; the serum calcium concentration returned to normal after surgery. The parathyroid tumor was correctly lateralized in 73 cases. Nearly a third of the patients had a history of cancer elsewhere but were free from clinical recurrence or metastasis. Six patients had large amounts of iPTH in the venous bed of the tumor compared with the arterial supply. Four patients had familial multiple endocrine adenomatosis. Three had parathyroid cancer.

Primary benign hyperparathyroidism should be considered if hypercalcemia occurs in patients who have had successful treatment of malignancy. Selective venous catheterization of the neck may help differentiate pseudohyperparathyroidism and may localize the parathyroid lesion. Because of the lethality of hypercalcemia, operative search for benign coexistent parathyroid disease is indicated when the issue is unclear. From catheterization and tissue extract studies, ectopic-type iPTH can be identified as the humoral substance in pseudohyperparathyroidism, unrelated to bone destruction by cancer. Hyperparathyroidism may be the first clue to a familial multiple endocrine syndrome.

► [This says something to the effect that common things occur commonly and it behooves one to look for them. — W.G.R.] ◄

Effect of Methandrostenolone on Postmenopausal Bone Wasting as Assessed by Changes in Total Bone Mineral Mass. Postmenopausal osteoporosis often results in significant morbidity. It is thought to be due to an inadequate bone mass present before menopause, an excessive loss of bone after menopause or both. Treatment has been less than satisfactory. Charles H. Chesnut III, Wil B. Nelp, David J. Baylink and John D. Denney[3] (Seattle) used serial

---

(3) Metabolism 26:267–277, March, 1977.

measurements of total body calcium (TBC) to evaluate the effects of the synthetic anabolic steroid methandrostenolone on long-term calcium balance in 26 osteoporotic postmenopausal women aged 55–75 years. The presence of atraumatic vertebral compression fractures or vertebral osteopenia, or both, was a selection criterion. Groups of 13 patients received the steroid or a placebo in a double-blind manner. Study patients received 5 mg methandrostenolone daily for 3 of every 4 weeks. The TBC was measured by neutron activation analysis.

Ten study and 6 control subjects completed the 26-month protocol. The study patients had an average 2% gain in TBC over an average of 2.4 years, whereas placebo patients had an average of 3.1% loss over 2.3 years; the final changes differed significantly (Fig 49). Only 1 study patient lost TBC, and increases of up to 8% were observed. In the overall study, there was a 1.8% gain in TBC in the 13 treated patients and a 3% loss in the placebo patients. One patient in each group had a fracture. All patients had normal serum glutamic-oxaloacetic transaminase values at the end of the study. No fluid retention, hirsutism or menstrual bleeding was observed in the study patients.

These data strongly suggest that the long-term use of

Fig 49.—Percentage change in TBC in all patients participating in the study, mean ± SE. The number of patients remaining in the study is shown in parentheses. (Courtesy of Chesnut, C. H., III, et al.: Metabolism 26:267–277, March, 1977.)

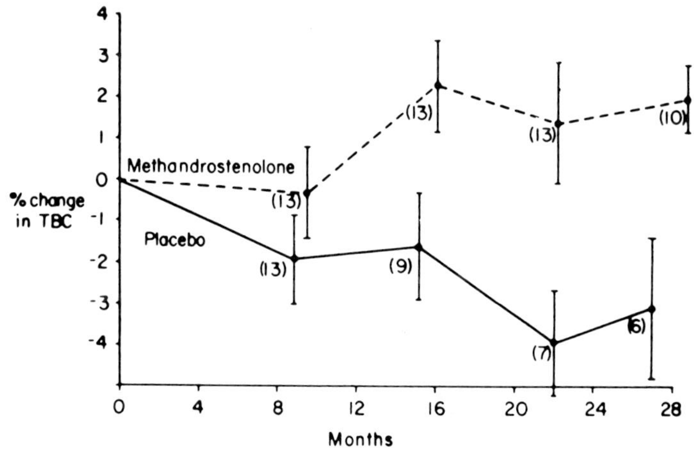

methandrostenolone in postmenopausal osteoporosis prevents bone loss in women with postmenopausal bone wasting. The possibility that it increases bone mass above initial levels is less certain. Possibly, the use of this agent in combination with others would produce additive effects. Any drug that arrests bone loss could be more effective if instituted before severe skeletal depletion has occurred.

► [Results are seemingly comparable to those obtained with estrogen therapy. After some experience with fluoride and calcium treatment of osteoporosis, I'd appreciate hearing about something that effectively *increases* bone mineral content. (See the following article.) — W.G.R.] ◄

Combination Therapy for Osteoporosis. It is possible that any treatment for osteoporosis that results in either increased bone formation or reduced bone resorption will eventually lead to compensatory changes with a failure to increase skeletal mass and thus lead to the concept of combined treatment of osteoporosis. John F. Aloia, Italo Zanzi, Ashok Vaswani, Kenneth Ellis and Stanton H. Cohn[4] attempted to increase skeletal mass in osteoporosis by combined therapy with human growth hormone (hGH), calcium supplements and salmon calcitonin (sCT). Four women and 1 man with a mean age of 60 who had primary osteoporosis with multiple vertebral compression fractures and back pain were treated. Calcium glubionate was given in a daily dose of 1,032 mg throughout the study and a low-hydroxyproline diet containing 500 mg calcium and 900 mg phosphorus was maintained. Patients received daily subcutaneous injections of hGH, alternated with 100 MRC units of sCT. The mean dose of hGH was 4 units, which was doubled after 4 months and continued for another 6–12 months. Serum parathyroid hormone (iPTH) assay, photon absorptiometry and total body neutron activation analysis were carried out before and after therapy.

No patients had worsening of pain but 1 had a rib fracture. There were no complications at the injection site. Fasting hyperglycemia was noted in only 1 patient. There were no appreciable changes in plasma calcium or phosphorus levels. With the exception of 1 patient who had a marked reduction in tubular phosphorus resorption during treatment and an increase in serum iPTH, urinary calcium ex-

---

(4)   Metabolism 26:787–792, July, 1977.

cretion increased and tubular calcium reabsorption declined on sCT treatment days. Urinary phosphate excretion decreased and tubular phosphorus resorption increased on hGH treatment days. Four of 5 patients had more than a 3% increase in total body calcium during treatment. With the exclusion of the patient who became hyperparathyroid, the mean increase in total body calcium for the high-dose hGH period was 6.5%. Urinary hydroxyproline did not change significantly during treatment. No significant changes in photon absorptiometric values for the radius were observed.

These findings, though preliminary, are quite encouraging and suggest not only that loss of skeletal mass can be diminished in osteoporosis but also that increments in skeletal mass may be achieved. Controlled trials of combination therapy of osteoporosis should be carried out.

▶ [Osteoporosis stubbornly resists attempts to reverse it. Here in a Herculean effort a modest effect was achieved that required total body neutron activation analysis to show it. One hopes the calcium retention was not extraskeletal, as no effect was seen in the radius by a photon absorption technique that should be demonstrable at this percentage increase of bone calcium. – W.G.R.] ◀

Effect of Long-Term Calcitonin Therapy on the Clinical Course of Osteogenesis Imperfecta was studied by E. Rosenberg, R. Lang, V. Boisseau, S. Rojanasathit and L. V. Avioli[5] (St. Louis). The encouraging results reported for short-term calcitonin treatment of osteogenesis imperfecta prompted an evaluation of the response to long-term treatment. Six patients with the "congenita" and 4 with the "tarda" variety of osteogenesis imperfecta were studied. They were placed on 800-mg calcium, 1,200-mg phosphorus, low-hydroxyproline diets during inpatient study and then received 1 – 2 MRC units of synthetic salmon calcitonin (SCT) per kg subcutaneously, 3 times weekly, for up to 3 years. Fasted patients were challenged with 0.0125 mg SCT before and after the cessation of SCT therapy to assess their biologic response to calcitonin.

The yearly fracture incidence decreased in 3 of 4 "tarda" patients during SCT therapy. Treatment resulted in lower serum calcium levels, and serum phosphate levels also declined in several patients. The alkaline phosphatase became normal in the 3 "tarda" patients with initially elevated lev-

---

(5)   J. Clin. Endocrinol. Metab. 44:346 – 355, February, 1977.

els. Acid phosphatase returned to or below normal in the 2 "tarda" patients with initially elevated levels. Parathyroid hormone levels were within or below the normal range both before and after chronic SCT therapy. Urinary hydroxyproline fell to normal in 3 of 5 children with the "congenita" form who had initially increased levels. Diaphyseal bone mass was decreased in untreated patients with the "congenita" form of disease and increased during treatment in the "tarda" patients. No relationship was found between the duration of treatment, antibody binding capacity and patient response to SCT.

The preliminary findings suggest that long-term treatment with SCT may prove beneficial in the prepubescent "tarda" form of osteogenesis imperfecta. Further study of a large number of patients appears warranted.

▶ [These are hopeful observations that will require more controlled studies for confirmation. — W.G.R.] ◀

Cellular Immune Responses in Familial Medullary Thyroid Carcinoma. Medullary thyroid carcinoma is usually familial. The explanation for the variable rates of tumor progression observed once metastasis has occurred is unclear. Ross E. Rocklin, Robert Gagel, Zoila Feldman and Armen H. Tashjian, Jr.[6] (Boston) instituted a prospective study of the cellular immune response to tumor antigen in 46 members of a family with familial medullary thyroid carcinoma, including 18 patients with proved carcinoma (group I), 7 with proved thyroid C cell hyperplasia (group II), 12 genetically at risk for the disease (group III) and 9 considered not to be at risk (group IV). Human macrophage migration inhibitory factor was assayed, and plasma calcitonin was estimated by radioimmunoassay.

The mean migration inhibitory factor response of group I patients was significantly greater than that of normal controls. The other groups did not have mean values significantly different from the control mean on testing with tumor antigen. Responses to normal thyroid tissue were not significant in any patient group, and responses to streptokinase-streptodornase were similar in all groups. Lymphocyte proliferative responses to tumor and normal thyroid anti-

---

(6)   N. Engl. J. Med. 296:835–838, Apr. 14, 1977.

gens were comparable in the various groups, and responses to streptokinase-streptodornase were also comparable.

Two thirds of patients in this study with familial medullary thyroid carcinoma had in vitro tumor-specific reactivity as measured by lymphocytic production of macrophage migration inhibitory factor. Why asymptomatic relatives who presumably do not have the disease show cellular immune reactivity to tumor antigens is unclear. Whether the development of cellular immune reactivity to thyroid tumor antigen provides clinical protection against medullary thyroid carcinoma or its spread is unknown. Of interest are whether group III subjects will develop C cell hyperplasia or medullary thyroid carcinoma, and whether group I and group II patients with or without positive migration inhibitory factor responses differ in long-term survival.

► [An interesting concept seeking an explanation for biologic variability in tumor spread is presented here. — W.G.R.] ◄

Aluminum Absorption and Distribution: Effect of Parathyroid Hormone. There have been increasing reports of aluminum toxicity from environmental exposure, although aluminum has traditionally been considered as nonessential and nontoxic. A progressive encephalopathy has been observed in an aluminum ball-mill operator, patients with Alzheimer's disease and patients on long-term hemodialysis, in association with elevated brain aluminum concentrations. Commercial aluminum-containing antacids are commonly used for mild gastric upset and ulcers, exposing large numbers of subjects to potential toxicity. Gilbert H. Mayor, Joan A. Keiser, Dhirajlal Makdani and Pao K. Ku[7] (Michigan State Univ., East Lansing) sought a link between gastrointestinal exposure and tissue deposit of aluminum mediated by parathyroid hormone.

Groups of rats were fed a diet supplemented with 0.1% aluminum and were inoculated subcutaneously with 17 units of parathyroid extract twice weekly. Serum aluminum concentrations were determined in 39 long-term hemodialysis patients by atomic emission spectrophotometry. Absorption of aluminum was higher in parathyroid hormone-treated rats than in controls. The unsupplemented rat chow

---

(7) Science 197:1187–1189, Sept. 16, 1977.

was found to contain 119 mg aluminum per kg. Aluminum concentrations in kidney, muscle, bone, whole brain and gray matter were significantly higher in treated rats. No rat showed overt behavior changes during 25 days of observation. Parathyroid hormone and aluminum concentrations were positively correlated in the dialysis patients.

Both studies of dialysis patients and animal studies indicate that exogenous aluminum, in the presence of markedly elevated parathyroid hormone concentrations, can result in increased gastrointestinal absorption and altered tissue distribution of aluminum. The significant correlation of serum parathyroid hormone and aluminum in human subjects suggests that both Alzheimer's disease and dialysis encephalopathy may be explained in part by parathyroid hormone acting on orally ingested aluminum.

▶ [Are Koch's postulates fulfilled? — W.G.R.] ◀

Inhibitory Effects of Hypermagnesemia on the Renal Action of Parathyroid Hormone. Both hypercalcemia and hypermagnesemia suppress the release of parathyroid hormone (PTH), and the relative serum levels of these ions may modify the biologic activity of PTH at the level of the target organs. E. Slatopolsky, A. Mercado, A. Morrison, J. Yates and S. Klahr[8] (Washington Univ.) determined the role of hypermagnesemia in the renal response to PTH administration by measuring urinary phosphate and cyclic adenosine monophosphate (cAMP) excretion in normomagnesemic and hypermagnesemic dogs before and after PTH administration. The effect of magnesium on cAMP production and adenyl cyclase activity was studied in vitro with use of rat renal cortical slices. A dose of 100 units of PTH was given to normal and hypermagnesemic dogs, followed by administration of 1 unit per minute. Some animals had thyroparathyroidectomy before study, some normal dogs received sodium sulfate and some hypermagnesemic thyroparathyroidectomized dogs received dibutyryl cAMP intravenously.

Parathyroid hormone increased phosphate excretion markedly in normomagnesemia and increased cAMP. Phosphate excretion increased less markedly in hypermagnesemic animals with a mean serum magnesium of 4.4 mg/100

---

(8)   J. Clin. Invest. 58:1273–1279, November, 1976.

ml and fractional phosphate excretion increased much less than in normomagnesemic dogs. Identical results were obtained in thyroparathyroidectomized dogs. Sodium sulfate did not affect the phosphaturic effect of PTH. In vitro studies showed a progressive decrease in cAMP production in response to PTH as Mg^{2+} concentrations were increased in the incubation medium. Adenyl cyclase activity was greatly increased by magnesium, and the addition of PTH increased activity twofold. Hypermagnesemia did not block phosphaturic activity of dibutyryl cAMP.

Calcium and magnesium may participate in a double feedback mechanism, not only controlling PTH release but also altering the biologic activity of the hormone at the target organ level. Hypermagnesemia partially inhibits the phosphaturic response to PTH, primarily due to an impairment of PTH stimulation of cAMP production by the renal cortex. Other studies have suggested that the biologic action of PTH at the skeletal level is impaired in the presence of hypomagnesemia. Magnesium concentrations may, affect the renal response to PTH and also affect the action of the hormone at the level of bone.

► [The interrelationships of calcium and magnesium metabolism have been difficult to unravel. This study helps significantly. – W.G.R.] ◄

Evidence for a Defect in the Formation of 1α,25-Dihydroxyvitamin D in Pseudohypoparathyroidism. Resistance of the kidneys to parathyroid extract or hormone (PTH) in pseudohypoparathyroidism (PHP) has been attributed to a metabolic defect of the adenylate cyclase system in the renal tubules. Hypocalcemia has been attributed to a similar defect in the skeletal system but a number of patients have been described with PHP, secondary hyperparathyroidism and osteitis fibrosa cystica, suggesting a renal defect in 1α-hydroxylation of 25-hydroxyvitamin D. Tushar K. Sinha, Hector F. DeLuca and Norman H. Bell[9] report evidence that supports the idea that the abnormal calcium metabolism in PHP results from impaired synthesis of 1α,25-dihydroxyvitamin D. Three patients were studied. Serum PTH was determined by radioimmunoassay.

Each patient had an abnormally low serum calcium and an abnormally elevated serum PTH; 2 had no rise in urinary

---

(9)   Metabolism 26:731–738, July, 1977.

cyclic adenosine monophosphate in response to PTH. Each patient had short stature, a round face and short metacarpals. Two had mothers with pseudo-PHP. All 3 patients had high fecal calcium levels and 2 had elevated serum 25-hydroxyvitamin D levels. On treatment with 1 μg 1α,25-dihydroxycholecalciferol daily for 12 days, fecal calcium decreased, the serum and urinary calcium increased and serum PTH declined to or toward the normal range. These events were reversed after treatment was stopped. Serum phosphorus levels remained normal during treatment, whereas fecal phosphorus levels decreased in 2 patients during treatment. Urinary phosphorus was not altered by 1α,25-dihydroxycholecalciferol.

These findings support the hypothesis that decreased intestinal calcium absorption, hypocalcemia and secondary hyperparathyroidism in PHP result from a defect in the formation of 1α,25-dihydroxyvitamin D in the kidney and they indicate that 1α,25-dihydroxycholecalciferol is a useful specific means of treating the abnormal calcium metabolism in this disorder. There appears to be genetic heterogeneity with regard to PTH-responsive adenylate cyclase systems in various tissues in man.

▶ [Another kudo for 1α,25-dihydroxycholecalciferol! However the following article tends to muddy the waters a bit. — W.G.R.] ◀

Case of Idiopathic Hypoparathyroidism and Dietary Vitamin D Deficiency: Requirement for Calcium and Vitamin D for Bone, but not Renal Responsiveness to PTH. Parathyroid hyperplasia often does not correct the hypocalcemia present in vitamin D-deficient patients. Most studies of the interaction of vitamin D and parathyroid hormone have used parathyroidectomized vitamin D-deficient and hypocalcemic animals. Adi A. Gerblich, Saul M. Genuth and John G. Haddad, Jr.[1] studied a patient presenting with hypocalcemia who had both vitamin D deficiency and idiopathic hypoparathyroidism. The effects of the restoration of parathyroid hormone could be observed while the variables of circulating vitamin D and serum calcium were independently changed.

Woman, 62, presented with muscle cramps and difficulty breathing for 2 weeks. She had taken a complete vegetarian diet for 14

---

(1) J. Clin. Endocrinol. Metab. 44:507–514, March, 1977.

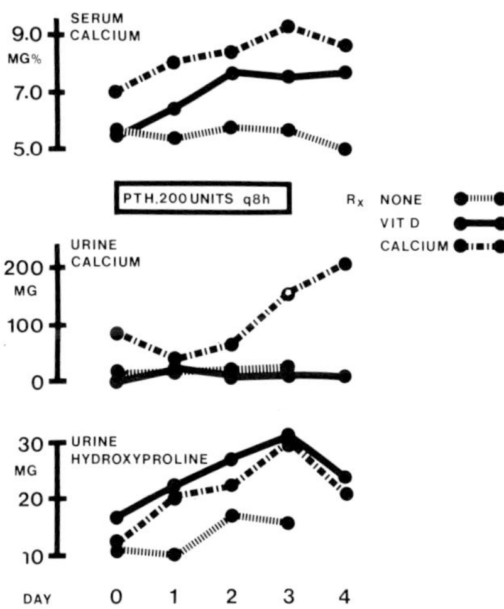

Fig 50.—Parathyroid extract, 200 units every 8 hours intramuscularly, was administered for 3 days before treatment, after and during constant calcium infusion to maintain a basal serum calcium level of 7 – 7.5 mg/100 ml and after 2 weeks of oral vitamin D at 1,000 units per day. Urine calcium and hydroxyproline results are expressed as mg/gm creatine excretion. Average creatinine excretion was approximately 800 mg per day. (Courtesy of Gerblich, A. A., et al.,; J. Clin. Endocrinol. Metab. 44:507 – 514, March, 1977.)

years. Acute respiratory distress and bilateral carpal spasm were noted. The thyroid gland was twice normal size, with bilateral nodules and generalized hyperreflexia present. The serum calcium level was 4.7 and the phosphorus level, 5.8 mg/dl. The patient improved on intravenous calcium gluconate; the serum calcium level gradually rose to 6.5 mg/dl. The average daily vitamin D intake was about 60 IU. A supplement of 150 mg calcium and 800 mg phosphorus was given and studies of responsiveness to parathyroid hormone were carried out over a 5-week period, with no adverse reactions. A daily dose of 50,000 – 100,000 units vitamin D has been required to maintain the serum calcium level above 8 mg/dl, as well as supplementary calcium.

Idiopathic hypoparathyroidism was confirmed in this patient. The results of parathyroid extract administration are shown in Figure 50. The largest rise in urinary phosphorus occurred during sustained calcium infusion, and an intermediate response was seen after serum 25-hydroxyvitamin D levels were returned to normal. Tubular phosphate reabsorption, initially over 99%, fell to 89% during vitamin D therapy and to 84% during calcium infusion therapy.

These findings support the view that vitamin D is required for the skeletal but not the renal actions of parathyroid hormone. For the human being, in the renal tubule as in bone, parathyroid hormone-stimulated translocation of calcium is not entirely prevented by vitamin D deficiency as long as adequate circulating calcium is available.

▶ [These observations tend to confirm the observations that vitamin D is necessary for the calcium-mobilizing effect of parathyroid hormone on bone. I suppose that this is a protective mechanism that mother nature has devised, for if parathyroid-stimulated mobilization of calcium from bone continued apace in the absence of vitamin D to assure a continued calcium absorption from the gut, we would eventually dissolve our bones and collapse to something resembling a bowl full of jelly. Ho! Ho! Ho!— W.G.R.] ◀

Autonomous Hyperparathyroidism: Possible Late Complication of Neck Radiotherapy. In most cases of autonomous hyperparathyroidism (HPT), the cause is unknown. L.-E. Tisell, S. Carlsson, S. Lindberg and I. Ragnhult[2] (Univ. of Göteborg), after encountering a few patients with autonomous HPT who gave histories of previous neck irradiation, undertook to determine whether there is any relation between previous exposure to irradiation and subsequent development of HPT. Data were reviewed on 170 patients operated on for autonomous HPT in the 4 years ending in 1974; 123 were females. The diagnosis was confirmed histologically in all cases but 1. Parathyroid adenoma was present in 150 patients, hyperplasia in 14 and mixed adenoma and hyperplasia in 5. Two patients had slight persistent hypercalcemia a few months after operation; 1 had a colonic cancer.

Radiotherapy had been delivered to the neck in 24 cases (14.1%). Eighteen patients had their first course of radiotherapy in childhood or early adult life, 15 for cervical tuberculous adenitis. Six patients were irradiated at ages 49–65 years, 5 for cervical spondylosis. Ten patients received more than one course of radiotherapy. Estimates of absorbed dose in the parathyroids in 19 cases ranged from 200 to 3,000 rad. Involvement of only a superior gland was present in 71% of 14 patients treated for tuberculous adenitis and in only 39% of unirradiated patients. Symptoms were similar in irradiated and unirradiated patients. Thyroid disease occurred

---

(2)   Acta Chir. Scand. 142:367–373, 1976.

simultaneously with HPT in 47% of unirradiated and 83% of irradiated patients. Four patients irradiated and 2 not irradiated had thyroid carcinoma. All 4 of the former had received their first course of x-ray therapy before age 14 years.

The findings indicate a possible relation between radiotherapy of the neck and development of HPT, but further studies are needed to confirm this association.

► [Another possible complication of radiation therapy at a young age is described here. I'm not aware of this having been seen in the large recall series of patients who are being examined for suspected thyroid carcinoma. — W.G.R.] ◄

Plasma 1,25-Dihydroxyvitamin D Levels in Patients Receiving Anticonvulsant Drugs. Alterations in vitamin D metabolism have been postulated to cause calcium and bone abnormalities in patients using anticonvulsant drugs, but intestinal vitamin D absorption is normal in these patients and hepatic conversion of vitamin D to 25-hydroxyvitamin D is increased. William Jubiz, Mark R. Haussler, Toni A. McCain and Keith G. Tolman[3] measured plasma 25-hydroxyvitamin D (25-(OH)D) and 1,25-dihydroxyvitamin D (1,25-$(OH)_2$D) in 12 control institutionalized patients, 5 normal ambulatory subjects, 6 patients receiving 4–6 mg Dilantin per kg daily; 7 patients receiving 2 or 3 mg phenobarbital per kg daily; and 12 patients receiving both Dilantin and phenobarbital in the same doses. Plasma 1,25-$(OH)_2$D was quantitated by a radioreceptor assay that used the chick intestinal receptor protein for 1,25-$(OH)_2$D and its binding to intestinal chromatin.

Serum calcium and phosphorus concentrations were lower and alkaline phosphatase values were higher in the patients given Dilantin, phenobarbital or both. Plasma levels of 25-(OH)D were generally lower in the drug-treated groups, but differences were significant only for the phenobarbital-treated patients. Levels of 1,25-$(OH)_2$D were normal in patients given both drugs and were apparently elevated in the groups given a single drug; only patients given phenobarbital alone had a significant increase. Institutionalized patients had a much wider range of circulating metabolite concentrations than the normal population.

The finding that changes in patients given both anticon-

------

(3)   J. Clin. Endocrinol. Metab. 44:617–620, April, 1977.

vulsants were less marked than those in patients given only one drug may represent acceleration of the hepatic metabolism of Dilantin by phenobarbital or vice versa. The decreased plasma 25-(OH)D levels associated with anticonvulsant therapy are probably due to increased catabolism of this sterol to inactive derivatives. Depressed circulating levels of 25-(OH)D may contribute to development of the metabolic abnormalities, but enough is still available to biosynthesize adequate amounts of $1,25\text{-}(OH)_2D$.

► [The first sentence of the last paragraph is an interesting speculation, i.e., two drugs not as bad as one because one decreases the effects of the other. — W.G.R.] ◄

Diphosphonate Therapy of Paget's Disease of Bone. Various treatments have been recommended for Paget's disease of bone and, recently, agents inhibiting increased bone resorption have been reported to be effective. R. Canfield. W. Rosner, J. Skinner, J. McWhorter, L. Resnick, F. Feldman, S. Kammerman, K. Ryan, M. Kunigonis and W. Bohne[4] (New York) evaluated the efficacy of treatment with disodium ethane-1 hydroxy-1, 1-diphosphonate (EHDP) in 75 patients. Forty-eight patients were treated with various doses for 6 months in a double-blind protocol and 27 received 10 or 20 mg EHDP per kg daily on a nonblind basis. In the double-blind study, patients received placebo or EHDP in doses of 2.5, 5, 10 or 20 mg/kg daily, orally, for 6 months. Patients given 10 mg/kg daily or less who continued to have elevated serum alkaline phosphatase and urinary hydroxyproline values subsequently received 20 mg/kg daily.

Nine of 10 patients given 20 mg EHDP per kg daily in the double-blind study had a fall in a urinary hydroxyproline to normal, and lower doses produced significant reductions. The serum alkaline phosphatase fell significantly in all treated groups, but more slowly than the urinary hydroxyproline. The average percent reductions in the patients on the open trial were virtually identical to those in the double-blind test who received 20 mg/kg per day. Some patients given higher doses had a rise in serum phosphate. Five of 12 placebo patients were improved symptomatically at 6 months but 2 were worse. Twelve of the 15 patients treated with 2.5 or 5 mg/kg daily were improved and none were

---

(4) J. Clin. Endocrinol. Metab. 44:96–106, January, 1977.

worse. Six of 21 patients in the open trial given 10 or 20 mg/kg daily were improved and 6 were worse. Some patients in the open trial acquired incapacitating new pain at sites of pagetic involvement, particularly the femur. Few radiographic changes were seen during the 6-month treatment period. Of the 49 patients followed for 18 months or longer, 21 have had a sustained remission of biochemical indices of disease for a year after discontinuing therapy, whereas 28 have required retreatment with EHDP. Nine patients had fractures through pagetic bone during follow-up. Diarrhea occasionally occurred in patients given higher doses of EHDP.

It appears that initial treatment of Paget's disease of bone with 5 mg EHDP per kg daily maximizes benefits while minimizing possible adverse effects.

► [The last sentence gives the "meat" of the conclusions. Speaking of meat reminds me of something my younger brother said when he was a young child and wanted a puppy. When offered a toy dog, he protested, "No, I want a *meat* puppy." – W.G.R.] ◄

Primary Hyperparathyroidism: Cause of Hypercalciuria and Renal Stones in Patients with Medullary Sponge Kidney. The discovery of a structural cause for urinary tract stone formation may inhibit the search for a metabolic cause, but if both causes are present, the latter may be more amenable to treatment. Dhanwada S. Rao, Boy Frame, Melvin A. Block and Alwyn M. Parfitt[5] (Henry Ford Hosp.) report 3 cases of concurrent medullary sponge kidney (MSK) and primary hyperparathyroidism. In 1 case, stone passage ceased for over 20 years after parathyroidectomy; in the other 2 cases, there was a substantial fall in urinary calcium excretion and stone formation has not recurred.

Woman, 31, seen for hypertension, reported recurrent left loin pain associated with hematuria. Blood pressure was 210/110 mm Hg. Serum calcium was 14.4, inorganic phosphate 2 and creatinine 1.2 mg/100 ml. Urinary calcium excretion was 254 mg/24 hours on a low-calcium diet, and phosphorus excretion was 460 mg/24 hours. Creatinine clearance was 60 ml per minute. A pyelogram showed typical findings of MSK with bilateral nephrolithiasis. Skeletal roentgenograms were unremarkable. Neck exploration revealed a left inferior parathyroid adenoma, which was removed. The serum calcium concentration fell to 9.4 mg/100 ml, and no epi-

(5) J.A.M.A. 237:1353–1355, Mar. 28, 1977.

sodes of loin pain, hematuria or stone passage occurred in the next 21 years. The most recent 24-hour urine sample contained 52 mg calcium in a volume of 2,230 ml. The serum creatinine concentration at this time was 2.9 mg/100 ml.

Medullary sponge kidney is usually discovered accidentally in the absence of stone formation. Small renal calculi may form in the medullary cysts, even without hypercalcemia or hypercalciuria, but persistent hypercalciuria is common and probably increases the risk of stone formation. The only other cause that might predispose to stone formation is primary hyperparathyroidism, 4 other concurrent cases of which have previously been reported. In the present case, the MSK appears to have determined the location of the stones, not their occurrence.

A complete metabolic workup for a metabolic cause should be done in all patients with stones, whether or not an anatomical abnormality such as MSK is present.

▶ [Another reminder for us not to have tunnel vision is provided here. — W.G.R.] ◀

Calcinogenic Factor in *Solanum malacoxylon*: Evidence that It Is 1,25-Dihydroxyvitamin D_3-Glycoside is presented by R. H. Wasserman (Ithaca, N.Y.), John D. Henion (Cornell Univ.), Mark R. Haussler and Toni A. McCain[6] (Univ. of Arizona). The biologically active form of vitamin D, 1,25-dihydroxyvitamin D_3 (1,25-$(OH)_2D_3$), has not previously been detected in plants but the ingestion of certain plants, such as *Solanum malacoxylon* from South America, by grazing animals causes calcinosis and pathologic features similar to hypervitaminosis D.

An aqueous extract of *S. malacoxylon* has been found to mimic the biologic properties of 1,25-$(OH)_2D_3$. The plant increases calcium absorption and inducts calcium-binding protein synthesis in chicks fed strontium to inhibit the kidney enzyme that is responsible for the formation of 1,25-$(OH)_2D_3$. The *S. malacoxylon* factor is water-soluble and had an apparent molecular weight exceeding 1,000, whereas 1,25-$(OH)_2D_3$ is preferentially soluble in organic solvents and has a molecular weight of 416. After glycosidic cleavage of the principle, the active lipophilic portion was purified by column chromatography and analyzed by combined gas

---

(6)   Science 194:853–855, Nov. 19, 1976.

chromatography and mass spectrometry. It was identified as $1,25\text{-}(OH)_2D_3$, confirming that this metabolite exists in the plant world and it probably accounts for pathologic calcifications in grazing animals ingesting *S. malacoxylon.*

The naturally occurring form of the *S. malacoxylon* factor appears to be a $1,25\text{-}(OH)_2D_3$-glycoside. Its discovery raises the question of whether this sterol hormone is present in other calcinogenic plants, such as *Cestrum diurnum* which is indigenous to the southeastern United States. The naturally occurring glycoside may offer therapeutic advantages over the synthetic sterol in the treatment of human disorders of calcium and phosphorus metabolism.

▶ [This plant was referred to in the 1977 YEAR BOOK (p. 77) and it was suspected that $1,25\text{-}(OH)_2D_3$ is the active principle. Here is the chemist's confirmation. I wonder what form of natural selection produced it.— W.G.R.] ◀

Functioning Lipoadenoma of the Parathyroid Gland. A unique parathyroid tumor, the lipoadenoma, was described in 1962. Philip J. Daroca, Jr., Richard L. Landau, Richard J. Reed and Mark D. Kappelman[7] (New Orleans) report the second case of functioning lipoadenoma of the parathyroid gland.

Man, 64, presented with nocturia, terminal dysuria, frequency and a decrease in the urinary stream. A moderately enlarged prostate was noted. The serum calcium level was 12.5 and the phosphorus level, 2.8 mg/100 ml; the alkaline phosphatase level was 78 mU/ml. Pyelography showed a trabeculated bladder containing a calculus. Neck exploration revealed a left upper parathyroid mass, which was resected, along with the slightly enlarged right lower gland. The serum calcium level eventually fell to 10.5 mg/100 ml. Vesicolithotomy and prostatectomy were subsequently performed for nodular glandular hyperplasia. When last seen the patient had a serum calcium level of 10.3 and a phosphorus level of 4.5 mg/100 ml. The tumor proved to be a lipoadenoma, with chief cells predominating. The preexisting gland contained a microscopic cyst and the right lower parathyroid contained several microcysts but was normal histologically. It was surrounded by considerable adipose tissue.

Lipoadenoma is a rare parathyroid tumor. The finely fibrillar myxomatous stromal tissue observed in these cases may represent an altered metabolic phase or a more primitive phase of adipose-tissue differentiation. Admixtures of

---

(7)   Arch. Pathol. Lab. Med. 101:28–30, January, 1977.

different phases of adipose tissue are seen in such diverse lesions as lipoblastomatosis, variants of well-differentiated liposarcomas and bronchial hamartomas.

▶ [My radiologist friends have shown me lipoadenomas of the adrenal glands. I was unaware of their occurrence in the parathyroid. — W.G.R.] ◀

Use of ^{131}I-Toluidine Blue in Radionuclide Imaging of Enlarged Parathyroid Glands. Radiolabeled toluidine blue is taken up selectively by the parathyroids of experimental animals. E. Normann, K. Rootwelt, D. Solheim and G. Sødal[8] (Oslo) report the results obtained with ^{131}I-toluidine blue scintigraphy of the parathyroid glands in 40 patients, including 27 with hyperplasia or adenomas, 3 with negative neck explorations and 10 patients not having operations, 3 of whom are thought to have hyperparathyroidism. A dose of 0.6 – 1 mCi ^{131}I, corresponding to 10 – 12 mg dye, was injected intravenously and Lugol's solution or potassium iodide was given for 6 days, starting the day before scintigraphy, to block thyroid uptake. Imaging was with a gamma camera with pinhole collimator; it was begun 1 – 2 minutes after radionuclide injection. Serum parathyroid hormone was determined by radioimmunoassay.

The location of enlarged parathyroids was predicted scintigraphically in 18 of 27 patients with hyperparathyroidism, but the correlation between scintiscans and operations was only partially correct in 4 patients. A correctly positive study is shown in Figure 51. In 1 patient both scintigraphy and neck exploration were negative. Six false negative scintigrams were obtained; the largest adenoma in this group weighed 2 gm. There were 2 false positive scintigraphic studies. Incorrect localizations were predicted in 3 patients, 2 of whom had lymph nodes corresponding to the "hot" areas on the scintiphotographs. Scintigraphy was negative in 9 of 10 patients not having surgery and falsely negative in 2 patients in this group.

Parathyroid nuclide imaging done with ^{131}I-toluidine blue correctly predicted the localization of enlarged parathyroid glands in over 50% of the present patients. The results compare favorably with those obtained with the use of ^{75}Se-selenomethionine. This agent represents an improvement as a scintigraphic agent for the parathyroids. Data manipulation

(8)   Ann. Chir. Gynaecol. 65:249 – 252, 1976.

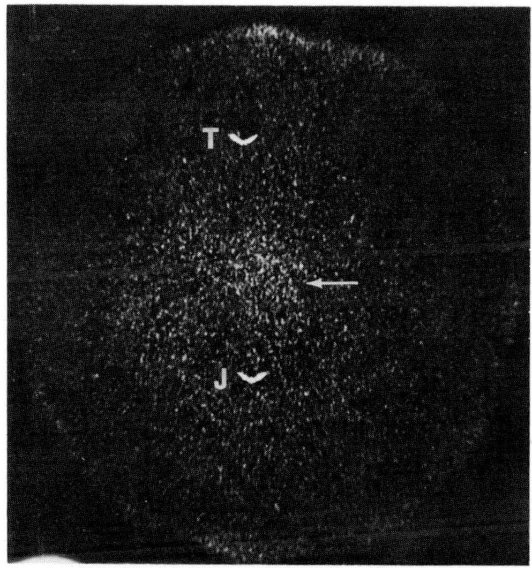

Fig 51.—Parathyroid scintigraphy with ^{131}I-toluidine blue in woman, aged 72, with serum calcium 6.1–6.8 mEq/L. An area with high radioactivity is seen on the left side of the neck. Here an adenoma weighing 7.5 gm was found at operation. *J*, jugular fossa; *T*, thyroid cartilage. (Courtesy of Normann, E., et al.: Ann. Chir. Gynaecol. 65:249–252, 1976.)

with field nonuniformity correction of the pinhole scintiphotographs and subtraction of background activity might improve the results, as might the labeling of toluidine blue with lower-energy gamma-emitting nuclides like technetium-99m or iodine-123. It might also be helpful to stimulate the parathyroids by glucagon-induced hypocalcemia, which might lead to a higher uptake of labeled toluidine blue by the glands.

► [Radionuclide imaging of parathyroid glands has received sporadic attention over the past decade. Our lack of success with ^{75}Se-selenomethionine localization was abysmal. This technique appears somewhat more promising, but needs considerable refinement. — W.G.R.] ◄

Family Studies in Patients with Primary Parathyroid Hyperplasia. It has been suggested that familial hyperparathyroidism may be a syndrome distinct from familial multiple endocrine neoplasias (FMEN) I and II. S. J. Marx, A. M. Spiegel, E. M. Brown and G. D. Aurbach[9] (Natl.

---

(9) Am. J. Med. 62:698–706, May, 1977.

Inst. of Health) screened the families of 25 patients treated for primary parathyroid hyperplasia in 1966–75. Thirteen subjects had 1 or more hypercalcemic relatives. In 4 families, 1 or more members had clear evidence of FMEN I. Two families were classified as having familial hypocalciuric hypercalcemia (FHH).

Autosomal dominant inheritance was evident in the kindreds with both FHH and FMEN I. Asymptomatic hypercalcemia was found in many young subjects, virtually all in kindreds with FHH. Clinical complications of hypercalcemia in this group were less frequent and generally milder than in FMEN I. Hypercalciuria was not present in the families with FHH. Hypercalcemia persisted after exploration in 4 of 13 subjects with FMEN I. Three appeared to have permanent hypoparathyroidism. Surgery was much less effective in subjects with FHH; 6 of 7 patients had persistent or recurrent hypercalcemia. All familial groups included some subjects without clearly increased peripheral plasma concentrations of parathyroid hormone. Five of 6 subjects with FMEN I but none of 6 with FHH had an increased plasma glucagon concentration. Three subjects with FMEN I had hypergastrinemia and Zollinger-Ellison syndrome. One subject in each group had an elevated serum prolactin value.

The findings support the classification of FHH and FMEN I as distinct syndromes with fundamentally different pathogeneses. The distinction is important, since hypercalcemic patients with FHH may be particularly unresponsive to subtotal parathyroidectomy but often have a mild clinical course. Renal and parathyroid abnormalities in FHH may be related to abnormalities of cell structure resulting in disordered calcium fluxes or to excessive or low levels of an unidentified humoral factor.

► [These authors quote studies indicating a 20–50% incidence of parathyroid hyperplasia as the cause of primary hyperparathyroidism. In our experience, this is much less common—occurring in, at most, less than 10% and more likely less than 5% of the patients we see who have primary hyperparathyroidism. The present study indicates that when primary hyperplasia is found it is probably a good idea to screen the families of such patients for hyperparathyroidism. In view of the poor results with surgery and the benign course whether or not to treat such patients is another matter. Perhaps one should leave stones "unturned."—W.G.R.] ◄

Postthyroidectomy Hypocalcemia: A Feature of the Operation or the Thyroid Disorder? The traditional view that postthyroidectomy hypocalcemia is due to surgical interference with the parathyroids has been challenged. T. J. Wilkin, T. E. Isles, C. R. Paterson, J. Crooks and J. Swanson Beck[1] (Dundee, Scotland) studied prospectively and serially the changes in serum calcium, inorganic phosphate (IP) and alkaline phosphatase (AP) that occurred in 54 patients with Graves' disease, 21 with serum AP levels above 14 King-Armstrong units (group I) and 33 with normal serum AP levels (group II). Seventeen controls who underwent partial thyroidectomy for simple nontoxic goiter (group III) were also studied. All group I and group II patients had been thyrotoxic and received carbimazole and triiodothyronine for 20–22 weeks before surgery. They were studied 1 week and 4–6 weeks postoperatively.

No clinical tetany occurred. Postthyroidectomy hypocalcemia, with a corrected serum calcium value below 2.15 mM/L, occurred in 5 of 12 group I patients, 9 of 20 group II patients and 7 of 15 group III subjects, always within 24 hours after surgery. Significant decreases in serum calcium and AP occurred in all groups on the 1st postoperative day. Serum IP also fell in all groups, but not significantly in group III. The changes were not due to hemodilution. Serum calcium returned to about preoperative levels by postoperative day 7 and in all groups after 4–6 weeks. No significant group differences in corrected serum calcium values were observed the day before or the day after operation.

This study produced no evidence that postthyroidectomy hypocalcemia is related to thyrotoxic osteodystrophy. The pattern of the biochemical changes observed is thought to be consistent with the release of thyrocalcitonin at surgery. The temporary nature of the changes and the return to preoperative values observed suggest that the fall in serum calcium concentration is a response to some factor associated with thyroid surgery rather than thyrotoxicosis. The possible role of thyrocalcitonin release in early postthyroidectomy hypocalcemia remains to be established.

▶ [The authors' hypothesis would have been helped greatly by some cal-

(1) Lancet 1:621–623, Mar. 19, 1977.

citonin measurements in these patients. Because of the relatively weak hypocalcemogenic effect of calcitonin, I am skeptical. However, if postoperative hypocalcemia is not due to surgical interference with parathyroid function or "hungry bones" or calcitonin, then what is it due to? – W.G.R.]

Anemia in Primary Hyperparathyroidism. Michael Boxer, Leonard Ellman, Richard Geller and Chiu-An Wang[2] (Massachusetts Genl. Hosp., Boston) recently encountered anemic patients with no apparent cause other than primary hyperparathyroidism, in whom the anemia resolved after parathyroidectomy. A review was made of data on all patients seen in 1962–75 with primary hyperparathyroidism that was well documented. Cases with a hematocrit below 38% for men and 35% for women were selected, where other causes of anemia were ruled out. Data on a total of 332 patients were reviewed and 5.1% of patients were found to have had a normochromic, normocytic anemia not related to blood loss, a deficiency state or uremia. No patient had neutropenia or thrombocytopenia.

Marrow biopsy specimens were available in 5 of the 17 study patients; 4 specimens showed significant fibrosis of the marrow cavity, whereas 1 showed minimal fibrosis. No diagnostic abnormalities were noted on the blood smears. Red blood cell indices were within normal limits in all cases. The presence of anemia correlated well with the severity of the hyperparathyroidism. The anemic patients had higher serum calcium and parathyroid hormone levels than those without anemia. A relationship with roentgenologic manifestations of primary hyperparathyroidism was also evident; bone cysts and subperiosteal bone resorption were more prevalent in the anemic group. All the anemic patients had exploratory neck surgery and 88% had parathyroid adenomas, compared with 77% of the operated nonanemic patients; the difference was not significant. Six of the 7 study patients followed 3–12 months after surgery showed complete correction of the anemia. The patient who remained anemic had further deterioration in renal function.

A normochromic, normocytic anemia may be a feature of primary hyperparathyroidism. The pathogenesis of the anemia remains obscure but myelofibrosis appears to be a factor. Perhaps elevated levels of parathyroid hormone

(2) Arch. Intern. Med. 137:588–590, May, 1977.

stimulate marrow fibroblasts. All patients followed showed improvement or resolution of their anemia after parathyroidectomy.

▶ [An interesting observation with interesting speculation as to the etiology is presented. I can't recall having seen any anemic patients with primary hyperparathyroidism, but perhaps I wasn't sensitized enough. — W.G.R.] ◀

Successful Transplantation of Frozen Parathyroid Tissue in Man is reported by Samuel A. Wells, Jr., J. Caulie Gunnells, Robert A. Gutman, John D. Shelburne, Arthur B. Schneider and Louis M. Sherwood.[3] Transplanted parathyroid tissue has functioned in experimental animals and in man and recently it became necessary to preserve human parathyroid tissue in a frozen state before autotransplantation. Five enlarged parathyroid glands were removed and chilled; one was diced and placed in 10% dimethyl sulfoxide, 10% autologous serum and 80% Waymouth's tissue culture medium and frozen at −196 C. Twenty-five pieces of tissue were subsequently thawed and transplanted into the brachioradialis muscle.

Man, 31, with medically unresponsive renal osteodystrophy and uremia, had been diagnosed as having pyelonephritis 10 years before. Five large parathyroid glands were removed and generalized clear cell hyperplasia discovered. After surgery the serum calcium fell from 10.5 to 5.5 – 6 mg/dl and dihydrotachysterol and calcium administration was required. The patient was symptomatic from hypocalcemia and required frequent calcium gluconate injections. Frozen parathyroid tissue was reimplanted 6 weeks after surgery. No improvement was evident in the next few months and chronic hemodialysis was instituted. The parathyroid hormone level in venous blood draining the graft bed was 2.7 ng/ml. A renal transplant procedure was performed with use of an HLA-identical sibling donor. Parathyroid hormone levels remained much higher in the arm with the graft bed. A biopsy specimen done nearly 2 years after tissue implantation showed the tissue pieces to be 3 – 4 times the size of the original implants. The histologic findings strongly suggested that the grafts were synthesizing hormone. The serum calcium is 9.5 mg/dl 30 months after parathyroid autografting. Dihydrotachysterol and oral calcium have been discontinued for 16 months and the patient is asymptomatic.

The ability to preserve parathyroid tissue viably in a frozen state is of advantage to the surgeon. The technique is of

---

(3)   Surgery 81:86 – 90, January, 1977.

use where only a single parathyroid neoplasm is present in a hyperparathyroid patient and the state of the remaining glands is uncertain. Cryopreservation appears to be useful clinically in preventing permanent hypoparathyroidism.

▶ [Another technologic tour de force! It is interesting also that although functional, the transplanted tissue couldn't do the job adequately until a new kidney was inserted into the patient. — W.G.R.] ◀

Chondrocalcinosis after Parathyroidectomy. Hyperparathyroidism is a well-established cause of secondary articular chondrocalcinosis and pyrophosphate arthropathy. Persistent hypercalcemia is considered the important factor in articular calcification in hyperparathyroidism. J. S. Glass and R. Grahame[4] (Guy's Hosp. Med. School) attempted to determine to what extent the natural history of chondrocalcinosis secondary to primary hyperparathyroidism is influenced by parathyroidectomy. Data on 57 patients having surgery for primary hyperparathyroidism in 1952–74 were reviewed. Thirty patients were evaluable with respect to preoperative and postoperative joint symptoms and 11 with respect to x-rays.

Relevant joint symptoms were recorded in 12 of 30 patients (40%). Only 2 of these patients improved significantly after operation, whereas 5 remained unchanged and 5 others worsened after parathyroidectomy. Most patients had nonspecific joint aches and pains; only 3 had true pyrophosphate arthropathy confirmed, all of them postoperatively. Plasma urate was elevated in 4 of 26 patients; 2 had renal impairment and 2 were receiving oral diuretics for hypertension. Chondrocalcinosis articularis was found in 14 of 35 patients with x-rays available. In none of 11 patients was there a discernible reduction in chondrocalcinosis postoperatively, but 4 patients had increased chondrocalcinosis and 5 acquired it after operation. The findings in 1 such case are shown in Figure 52.

Joint symptoms generally failed to improve after parathyroidectomy in these patients. Although parathyroidectomy is capable of reversing most of the clinical and biochemical features of primary hyperparathyroidism, this is not true of articular symptoms and chondrocalcinosis, both of which may persist or worsen after the operation. Patients having

(4)   Ann. Rheum. Dis. 35:521–525, December, 1976.

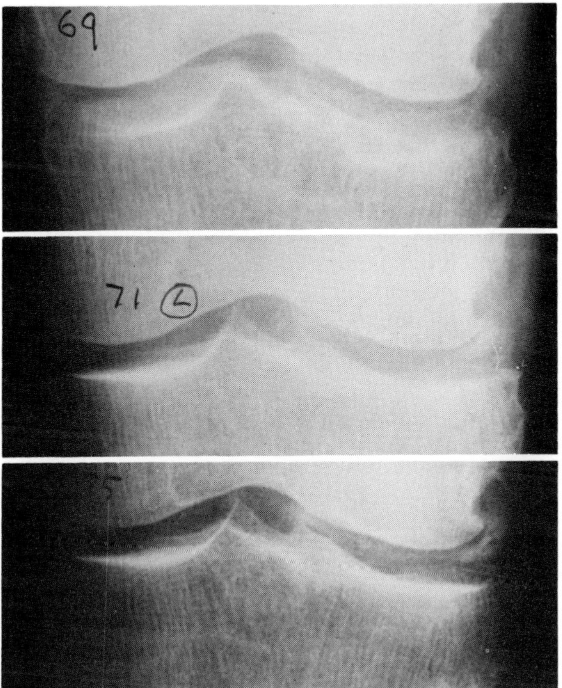

Fig 52.—Serial anteroposterior x-rays of right knee over 6 years show increasing calcification of both articular cartilage and fibrocartilage. (Courtesy of Glass, J. S., and Grahame, R.: Ann. Rheum. Dis. 35:521–525, December, 1976.)

parathyroidectomy for hyperparathyroidism and who have joint complaints should be warned of this possible occurrence.

▶ [Pyrophosphate arthropathy or pseudogout occasionally accompanies hyperparathyroidism and frequently is accompanied by chondrocalcinosis. The postoperative appearance of these joints (Fig 52) suggests that the inciting damage had already been done and couldn't be prevented by correction of the hypercalcemia. — W.G.R.] ◀

Rapid Identification of "Normal" Parathyroid Glands by Presence of Intracellular Fat. It is necessary to establish a correct diagnosis of primary hyperparathyroidism by examination of the parathyroids during surgical exploration. Sandford I. Roth and Michael J. Gallagher[5]

<hr>

(5)   Am. J. Pathol. 84:521–528, September, 1976.

describe a simple, rapid method for use at the time of surgery to distinguish between chief cell hyperplasia and adenoma. Two to four parathyroids were examined during operation in 60 patients explored for primary hyperparathyroidism. Frozen sections were cut from unfixed biopsy specimens and stained with Sudan IV in Hexheimer's acetone 70% ethanol mixture and aqueous toluidine blue. Forty-seven patients had a single adenoma removed. Nine patients who had primary chief cell hyperplasia involving all 4 glands had subtotal parathyroidectomies. In 4 cases, no pathologic parathyroid glands were found.

One to three "normal" glands from 51 patients showed numerous $0.5-1.5$-μ Sudan-positive intracellular granules in the chief cell cytoplasm. The cytoplasm of the oxyphil and chief cells of the glands of adenomas and chief cell hyperplasias was generally free from sudanophilic granules. Hyperplastic and adenomatous glands could not be distinguished. The serum calcium fell by $3-6$ mg/100 ml within $24-48$ hours of operation in all patients except those with only "normal" glands.

The routine use of fat stains on frozen sections of parathyroid glands during operation has permitted a confident distinction to be made between a chronically suppressed "normal" parathyroid gland and an abnormal gland, even when the gland was only partially involved in an early hyperplasia. The surgeon can in this way be given the information he requires to do the least surgical exploration and to remove the minimal amount of tissue necessary to cure the patient.

► [Seemingly, this is a useful procedure. I've been suggesting it to our pathologists but they seem to be dragging their "sudanophilic buttocks."—W.G.R.] ◄

Parathyroidectomy: Extent of Resection and Late Results. Some reports suggest that as many as 30% of patients have recurrent hypercalcemia after limited parathyroid resection for adenoma. T. J. C. Cooke, J. H. Boey, E. C. Sweeney, J. M. Gilbert and Selwyn Taylor[6] (Hammersmith Hosp., London) studied the long-term results of parathyroidectomy for primary hyperparathyroidism in 122 patients treated between 1955 and 1974. A total of 102 patients were followed for over 1 year, the mean follow-up being 6 years.

---

(6) Br. J. Surg. 64:153–157, March, 1977.

One surgeon performed most of the neck explorations. Seventy-three patients had a parathyroid adenoma, 26 had hyperplasia and 3 had carcinoma. Two in the hyperplasia group had "multiple adenomas."

An adenoma was not found at initial surgery in only 3 patients. In the other 70 patients, no hypercalcemia was observed after removal of the adenoma. Persistent or recurrent hypercalcemia was a problem in 9 patients with primary hyperplasia who had inadequate resection initially and also in the 3 patients with carcinoma. Hyperplasia was diagnosed as adenoma in 4 patients when the normal glands were not identified. In 4 patients, hyperplasia was correctly diagnosed, but subtotal parathyroidectomy was not done. Hypertrophy or further hyperplasia of the remnant was a possible cause of true late recurrence of hypercalcemia in 1 patient having subtotal operation.

Hypercalcemia noted within a year of parathyroidectomy is usually the result of a failure to diagnose hyperplasia or inadequate resection or to the failure to find an adenoma. Less commonly, persistent hypercalcemia may be due to parathyroid carcinoma. True recurrence of hypercalcemia is rare. Biopsy and frozen-section study of all glands is now done before deciding which glands should be excised. Subtotal resection may be reserved for patients in whom hyperplasia is demonstrated. Most patients with adenoma do not require subtotal resection, and its indiscriminate use carries unnecessary risks of producing permanent hypocalcemia in some patients.

▶ [I strongly agree with the last sentence. – W.G.R.] ◀

Vitamin D-Resistant Rickets Associated with Epidermal Nevus Syndrome: Demonstration of a Phosphaturic Substance in the Dermal Lesions. Nine cases of hypophosphatemic vitamin D-resistant rickets and osteomalacia associated with mesenchymal tumors have been reported in which excision of a bone or soft tissue tumor resulted in improvement of the bone lesions. Only 3 patients were children when symptoms began. It has been postulated that these tumors produce a phosphaturic substance leading to renal phosphate loss and, in turn, to the rickets. Lorenzo C. Aschinberg, Lawrence M. Solomon, Petros M. Zeis, Parvin Justice and Ira M. Rosenthal[7] (Univ. of Illinois) investi-

____
(7) J. Pediatr. 91:56–60, July, 1977.

gated the phenomenon in a boy with epidermal nevus syndrome.

Boy, 12, with severe rickets, had been seen at birth to have a large, verrucous, brown plaque on the temporoparietal area, face and ear, linear verrucous lesions on the legs, multiple, raised, melanocytic nevi, an area of hypopigmentation on the thorax, café au lait spots and several fleshy, vascular and fibrovascular tumors. Skeletal abnormalities were also present. Growth had always been below the 3d percentile. Active rickets was observed at age 5 years and did not respond to vitamin D in doses up to 750,000 IU daily. Added neutral potassium phosphate was also without effect. At age 9 the child was bedridden with pseudofractures and multiple deformities; subtotal parathyroidectomy produced no benefit. At age 12 he could not lift his head or sit without support, and the bones were extremely tender. Newer fibroangiomatous lesions had appeared. Serum calcium concentration was 9.6 mg/dl and serum phosphorus concentration, 1.3 mg/dl. Tubular phosphorus reabsorption was 35%. The serum parathyroid hormone value was normal. Several fibroangiomas were removed from the face and left leg, and pain was markedly reduced 4 weeks later, when the serum phosphate concentration was 3.9 mg/dl and tubular phosphorus reabsorption was 72%. Removal of a group of epidermal nevus lesions produced no further improvement in phosphorus reabsorption, but the rickets healed over the next 3 months. Corrective osteotomies were done at age 13, and the patient is currently ambulatory.

Part of the excised tissue was homogenized and injected into a puppy aged 6 weeks and induced excessive phosphaturia and a marked fall in tubular phosphorus reabsorption. Injection of skin homogenate produced no change in phosphate excretion.

A humoral substance elaborated in the dermal lesions apparently caused phosphaturia in this case. The substance is distinct from parathyroid hormone and calcitonin. Further studies in similar patients may lead to identification of a substance other than parathyroid hormone that is physiologically important in phosphorus homeostasis.

► [At last some light is shed on this peculiar disorder. – W.G.R.] ◄

Altered Copper and Zinc Metabolism in Primary Hyperparathyroidism. Aminoaciduria has been associated with untreated primary hyperparathyroidism and also with hypercupriuria and hyperzincuria in man and in animals. L. E. Malette and R. I. Henkin[8] (Natl. Inst. of Health) found such changes in patients with untreated hyperparathyroidism, resolving after surgical correction of the condition. Seventeen patients with primary hyperparathyroidism were studied. Of these, 13 were studied both before and after surgical treatment. The disease was severe in only 4 patients. Copper and zinc concentrations were determined by atomic absorption spectrophotometry in fasting blood and in 24-hour urine samples.

The urinary excretion of copper was significantly above normal in untreated patients, and the mean total concentration of copper in the serum was significantly greater than the normal mean. The urinary excretion of zinc was also significantly increased, but the serum zinc was not abnormal. Only 7 patients had elevated urinary levels of both copper and zinc, but only 2 had normal excretion of both metals. Glomerular function was normal in most patients, and most had no sign of renal tubular disease. No diseases previously associated with renal tubular defects were iden-

Fig 53.—Changes in urinary excretion of copper and zinc after surgical treatment of hyperparathyroidism. Values before surgery *(arrow)* represent the mean urinary excretion of copper and zinc for 3 preoperative days in Patient 1 *(open* and *closed triangles)* and Patient 2 *(open* and *closed circles),* respectively. Values after surgery are given each day for 11 consecutive days. Normal ranges are shown at left *(copper)* and right *(zinc).* (Courtesy of Malette, L. E., and Henkin, R. I.: Am. J. Med. Sci. 272:167–174, Sept.-Oct., 1976.)

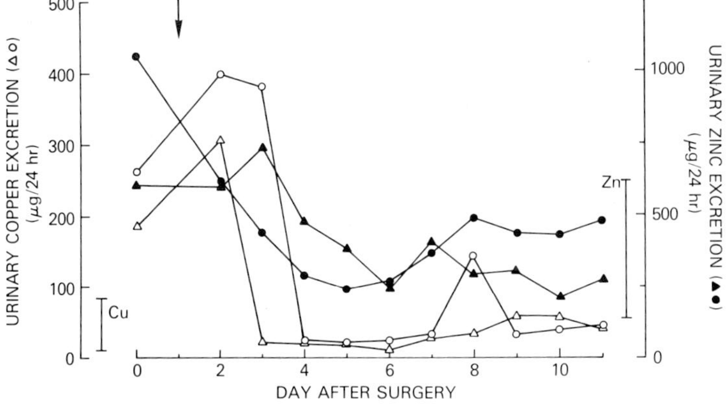

(8)   Am. J. Med. Sci. 272:167–174, Sept.–Oct., 1976.

tified. The cause of hyperparathyroidism did not correlate with changes in the urinary or serum levels of copper and zinc. Urinary copper and zinc levels increased significantly postoperatively, followed by a fall in excretion of the metals (Fig 53). Mean serum copper and zinc levels did not change postoperatively.

Possibly the increased metal excretion noted in patients with untreated primary hyperparathyroidism is the result of an aminoaciduria induced by parathyroid hormone excess. The increased urinary excretion of copper and zinc reflect the increased bone turnover commonly present in this disease. Measurements of copper and zinc excretion might be useful in following these patients after surgery. Further study of copper and zinc metabolism in hyperparathyroidism is warranted.

▶ [These are interesting observations. I just read a report that zinc therapy led to improvement in sexual function of patients on dialysis. This report led someone to comment that we are likely to see an increase in cases of zinc poisoning as a result.

I live in an old ethnic (Italian) neighborhood and am frequently amused by the "for men only" preparations that are advertised at the neighborhood pharmacy. Sure enough, the latest one is for a zinc tonic! — W.G.R.]

Paravertebral and Peripheral Ligamentous Ossification: Unusual Association of Hypoparathyroidism. J. E. Adams and M. Davies[9] (Manchester, England) report data on a man with idiopathic hypoparathyroidism and extensive paravertebral and ligamentous ossification.

Man, 62, was seen with a 6-week history of failing vision, with bilateral cataracts and diabetes mellitus. A 40-week illness involving facial paresthesias and rigidity and flexion of the hands and feet had occurred at age 18 and pain and stiffness had appeared in the back, neck, hips, elbows and shoulders 22 years before admission and had persisted. The patient had always been of small stature. He was 147 cm high and weighed 63 kg. The spine was immobile apart from slight movement at the thoracolumbar junction. Hip movements were absent apart from 45 degrees of flexion. Some nails were dystrophic. Bilateral posterior subcapsular cataracts were noted. The sedimentation rate was 50–90 mm per hour. The serum calcium was 5.9 mg/100 ml and the inorganic phosphorus, 4.3 mg/100 ml. No serum parathyroid hormone was immunoassayable. The serum phosphorus level declined on parathyroid extract infusion and phosphaturia was noted. Radiographs of the skull

---

(9) Postgrad. Med. J. 53:167–172, March, 1977.

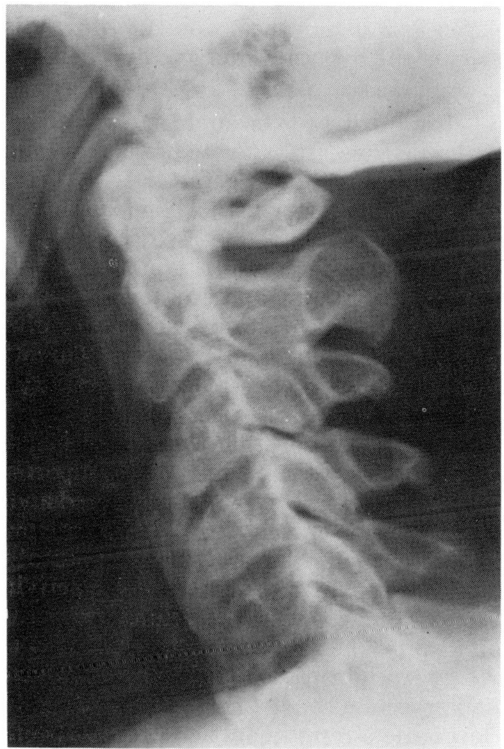

Fig 54.—Cervical spine with plaques of ossification lying anterior to the vertebral bodies. (Courtesy of Adams, J. E., and Davies, M.: Postgrad. Med. J. 53:167–172, March, 1977.)

showed basal ganglia calcification and ossification of pelvic ligaments and the hip capsules. Nearly complete spinal ankylosis was present (Fig 54). Ossification was present in the interosseous membranes of the forearms and at the elbows. Vascular calcification was noted in the feet. Growth arrest lines were present in the upper tibias and fibulas.

Four previously described patients with similar features were reviewed. All had hypoparathyroidism with paravertebral and ligamentous ossification, but normal sacroiliac joints. Evidence of erosive arthropathy or any disease known to be associated with ligamentous ossification was lacking. The mechanism of paravertebral and soft tissue calcification in hypoparathyroid patients is unknown, but it may be related as much to the chronicity of the disorder as to the severity of the hypocalcemia and hyperphosphatemia.

▶ [For those of you thinking as I did, HLA-B$_{27}$ wasn't present. — W.G.R.]

Big and Little Forms of Osteoclast Activating Factor. When blood leukocytes are activated, a potent bone-resorbing factor, osteoclast activating factor (OAF), is released into the medium. This factor is biochemically distinct from other humoral mediators of bone resorption such as parathyroid hormone, active vitamin D metabolites and prostaglandins. Gregory R. Mundy and Lawrence G. Raisz[1] (Univ. of Connecticut), with the technical assistance of James L. Shapiro, Janet G. Bandelin and Robert J. Turcotte, found that two distinct peaks of bone-resorbing activity are present in activated leukocyte culture supernates.

A bioassay for bone resorption that used release of ^{45}Ca from fetal rat long bones was done. When supernates from activated leukocyte cultures were concentrated and chromatographed, bone-resorbing activity eluted at the peak of big OAF between the molecular weight markers at 12,500 – 25,000 daltons. A separate peak of biologic activity, which has been called little OAF, was eluted from Bio-Gel P6 columns at 1,330 – 3,500 daltons. Big OAF was converted to little OAF by equilibration in 1M NaCl or 2M urea. Little OAF was self-associated back to big OAF by equilibration in buffers of low ionic strength. Little OAF has been purified more than 6,000-fold, so that bone-resorbing activity is maximal in a sample with a protein concentration of 80 ng/ml.

The bone-resorbing activity produced by phytohemagglutinin-activated leukocyte culture supernates is heterogeneous; two distinct peaks of activity can be distinguished by gel-filtration chromatography. The relationship of OAF to other lymphokines is not known. It is possible that OAF is an important mediator of bone resorption in both health and disease. Cultured neoplastic cells from patients with myeloma and other B cell lymphoproliferative disorders produce a bone-resorbing factor with chemical and biologic characteristics similar to those of OAF. Osteoclast activating factor is also a potential mediator of the bone resorption that occurs adjacent to areas of chronic inflammatory cell infil-

---

(1)   J. Clin. Invest. 60:122 – 128, July, 1977.

tration in such diseases as rheumatoid arthritis, periodontal disease and cholesteatoma.

► [It seems that one can make big OAFs of little OAFs and vice versa. Those of us interested in Paget's disease would like to have a better anti-OAF. – W.G.R.] ◄

Hypercalcemic Hyperparathyroidism in Hypophosphatemic Rickets. Fewer than 10 isolated case reports documenting the concurrence of hyperparathyroidism, hypercalcemia and vitamin D-resistant rickets unassociated with vitamin D intoxication have appeared. M. Kleerekoper, R. Coffey, T. Greco, S. Nichols, N. Cooke, W. Murphy and L. V. Avioli[2] (St. Louis) report the 10th case of this combination of disorders of mineral metabolism.

Woman, 25, seen for drainage of a Bartholin's cyst, had been studied at age 2 because of short stature, genu valgum and rickets. Vitamin D therapy had been instituted but intoxication occurred 2 years later and vitamin D was stopped. Treatment was later reinstituted in a dose of 1,300 units daily and the patient remained well for 6 years. She received 50,000 units daily with oral phosphate supplements between ages 12 and 16. Hypercalcemia then led to the withdrawal of vitamin D therapy. Tibial osteotomies were done at age 18 about 2 years after vitamin D had been stopped. Deteriorating renal function was noted at age 25 and the patient was hypertensive and moderately anemic. The serum calcium was 10.3 – 10.8 mg/dl and the serum inorganic phosphate, 2.3 – 3.2 mg/dl. Serum immunoreactive parathyroid hormone was consistently 1,000 μLEq/ml or above. The tubular phosphate resorption was 54%. A skeletal survey showed generalized demineralization and several lytic lesions. Calcific deposits were present in the cerebellar tentorium. A ^{99m}Tc-pyrophosphate bone scan showed generalized skeletal hyperactivity. Bone density at the radial midshaft was markedly reduced.

Neck exploration revealed a markedly enlarged right upper parathyroid gland which, like the normal-sized right lower gland, exhibited chief cell hyperplasia. A bone biopsy specimen showed severe osteitis fibrosa and a marked increase in osteoid content. A beneficial radiographic response was noted 9 months postoperatively.

Persistent hypercalcemia unrelated to vitamin D toxicity is a very uncommon complication of vitamin D-resistant rickets. The present case is the first in which vitamin D intoxication was excluded by documentation of normal serum

---

(2)   J. Clin. Endocrinol. Metab. 45:86–94, July, 1977.

levels of 25-hydroxycholecalciferol. This case probably represents the chance occurrence of two independent diseases. Many patients with vitamin D-resistant rickets, however, have mild secondary hyperparathyroidism and treatment efforts should be directed toward minimizing this complication.

▶ [This article reminded me of a patient of ours who had fibrous dysplasia of bone and hypophosphatemic rickets who later developed hyperparathyroidism. I suspect that more than the chance occurrence of these two diseases is involved. — W.G.R.] ◀

The following review articles are recommended to the reader:

Atkins, D., and Martin, T. J.: Metabolism of vitamin D, Ann. Clin. Biochem. 13:561, 1976.

Castleman, B., et al.: Parathyroid hyperplasia in primary hyperparathyroidism, Cancer 38:1668, 1976.

Knochel, J. P.: The pathophysiology and clinical characteristics of severe hypophosphatemia, Arch. Intern. Med. 137:203, 1977.

Paterson, C. R.: Hypocalcemia: Differential diagnosis and investigation, Ann. Clin. Biochem. 13:578, 1976.

Robertson, W. G.: Measurement of ionized calcium in body fluids. A review, Ann. Clin. Biochem. 13:540, 1976.

Russell, R. G. G.: Regulation of calcium metabolism, Ann. Clin. Biochem. 13:518, 1976.

Thomson, D. L., and Frame, B.: Involutional osteopenia: Current concepts, Ann. Intern. Med. 85:789, 1976.

Carbohydrate Metabolism and Diabetes

Ketoacidosis in Pancreatectomized Man. The importance of glucagon as a primary etiologic factor in the metabolic disturbance of diabetes has been questioned. Adrian J. Barnes, Stephen R. Bloom, K. George M. M. Alberti, Patricia Smythe, Frank P. Alford and Don J. Chisholm[3] studied the role of glucagon in early ketoacidosis by comparing the responses of pancreatectomized subjects and patients with juvenile-type diabetes to deprivation of insulin. Six dia-

Fig 55.—Plasma concentrations (mean ± SEM) of glucagon in 6 patients with juvenile-type diabetes and 4 pancreatectomized subjects after withdrawal of insulin. (Courtesy of Barnes, A. J., et al.: N. Engl. J. Med. 296:1250–1253, June 2, 1977.)

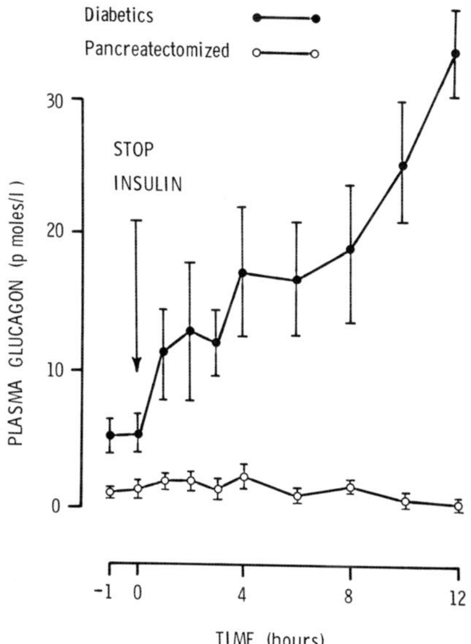

(3)   N. Engl. J. Med. 296:1250–1253, June 2, 1977.

betics and 4 totally pancreatectomized subjects were studied. The mean duration of juvenile-type diabetes was 24 years. All subjects were in good health at the time of study. An insulin infusion given in conjunction with a 12-hour fast was replaced by an infusion of saline alone for 12 hours. Plasma glucagon was determined by radioimmunoassay.

Basal glucagon levels in the two groups are shown in Figure 55 and changes in ketone bodies in Figure 56. The ratio of 3-hydroxybutyrate to acetoacetate rose significantly more in the diabetic patients. Both free fatty acids and glycerol increased during insulin deprivation in both groups. Increases in glucose were significantly greater in the diabetic patients. Blood alanine levels were higher in the surgical group both basally and during insulin deprivation. Pyruvate and lactate did not change during the study.

It appears likely that glucagon is not essential for the development of ketoacidosis and endogenous hyperglycemia. The presence of glucagon probably accelerated the onset and increased the extent of endogenous hyperglycemia in

Fig 56. – Changes in blood concentrations (mean ± SEM) of 3-hydroxybutyrate (A) and glucose (B) in 6 patients with juvenile-type diabetes and 4 pancreatectomized subjects after withdrawal of insulin. *Asterisks,* P < 0.05; *double asterisks,* P < 0.02. (Courtesy of Barnes, A. J., et al.: N. Engl. J. Med. 296:1250–1253, June 2, 1977.)

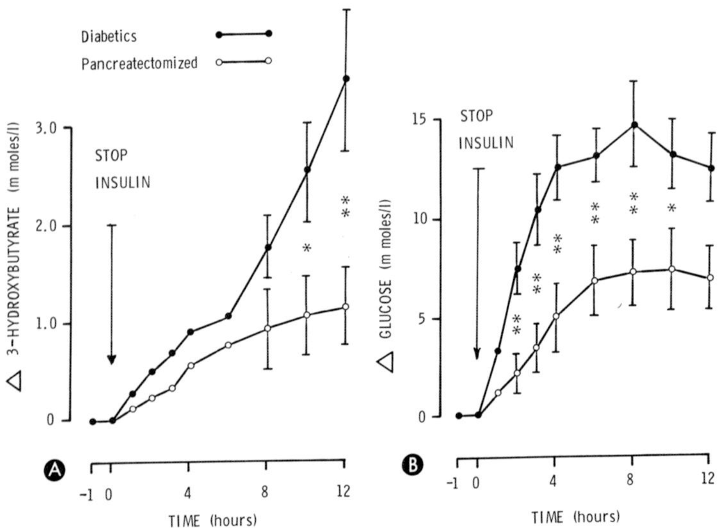

the diabetic patients. The increase may have resulted from enhancement of glycogenolysis or gluconeogenesis or both. In the absence of insulin, the actions of glucagon on lipid and carbohydrate metabolism may be relatively unopposed, and in this situation glucagon may accelerate the onset and progression of diabetic ketoacidosis.

▶ [Further evidence is provided here that glucagon plays some role, but not an essential one, in the genesis of diabetic ketoacidosis—a subject that has been a matter of some debate. — W.G.R.] ◀

Identification of Four Cell Types in Human Endocrine Pancreas by Immunoelectron Microscopy. Three types of secretory cells, the A, B and D cells, have been clearly identified in the pancreatic islets of mammals, and other cell types have been described in a few species. Recently somatostatin was localized in D cells. Human pancreatic polypeptide (hPP) has been detected by immunofluorescence in a few cells of human islets; these cells appear to contain small secretory granules. Georges Pelletier[4] (Univ. Laval) localized the various hormones by immune electron microscopy to correlate the different cell types of the human endocrine pancreas with specific secretory products. Studies were done in four human pancreata obtained at autopsy. Immunohistochemical studies were performed by using antiserums to the pancreatic hormones.

Four cell types, including one with 100 to 150-nm secretory granules that were more electron dense than the D granules, were easily recognized. Glucagon antiserum gave a reaction in A cells and insulin antiserum in the secretory granules of B cells. Somatostatin detection resulted in a strong reaction in typical D cells with large secretory granules. When tissue was immunostained for hPP, one to three cells in most islets exhibited a positive reaction. Small secretory granules were present in the reactive cells. Similar positively staining cells were occasionally observed in the exocrine pancreas. Absorption of the antiserum with bovine pancreatic polypeptide, which cross-reacts with anti-hPP serum, abolished the staining reaction. Immunostaining for gastrin produced no reaction in the different endocrine cell types.

The studies permit attribution of insulin secretion to the

---

(4) Diabetes 26:749–756, August, 1977.

pancreatic islet B cells, of glucagon to the A cells and of somatostatin to the D cells. Human pancreatic polypeptide has been identified in a fourth cell type and appears to be a hormone that is produced by hPP cells. No effect of hPP on the secretion of islet hormones has yet been described, although some influence of the peptide on the gastrointestinal tract has been observed.

► [The absence of gastrin reactive cells is surprising because gastrinomas are thought to arise from pancreatic islets. Perhaps they arise from other areas of pancreatic tissue. It appears that there are still no good clues as to the function of human pancreatic polypeptide. — W.G.R.] ◄

Fluctuations in Affinity and Concentration of Insulin Receptors on Circulating Monocytes of Obese Patients: Effects of Starvation, Refeeding and Dieting. Some obese patients have impaired binding of ^{125}I-insulin, and chronic caloric restriction improves the defect. Robert S. Bar, Phillip Gorden, Jesse Roth, C. Ronald Kahn and Pierre De Meyts[5] (Natl. Inst. of Health) examined insulin binding to circulating monocytes of obese patients under various dietary conditions in an attempt to clarify the mechanisms of insulin resistance in human obesity. Seven obese patients, aged 19–58, with a range of carbohydrate metabolic defects were studied in the basal, fed state, after 24–72 hours of starvation, after refeeding and after chronic diet. Initially patients were maintained on a 3,500-calorie, weight-maintaining diet for 3–7 days. Ten normal subjects aged 18–32 were also studied.

In the basal, fed state, the monocytes of 6 obese patients with clinical insulin resistance bound less insulin than normal subjects because of a decreased insulin receptor concentration. The single obese patient without clinical insulin resistance had normal insulin binding. In all patients, the total receptor concentration was inversely related to the circulating insulin level measured at rest after an overnight fast. A fast of 48–72 hours reduced circulating insulin and increased binding to normal levels, but only at low hormone concentrations. Increased receptor affinity for insulin without a change in receptor concentration was also noted. Refeeding resulted in a return to elevated plasma insulin levels, basal receptor affinity and depressed insulin binding as

---

(5)   J. Clin. Invest. 58:1123–1135, November, 1976.

observed in the basal, fed state. Chronic diet restored plasma insulin levels, insulin binding and receptor concentration to normal without a change in affinity.

These and previous findings suggest that the insulin receptor of human monocytes is more sensitive to regulation by ambient insulin than are the receptors of obese mice and cultured human lymphocytes. An insulin receptor appears to undergo in vivo modulation of its interaction with insulin by changing receptor concentration and by altering the affinity of existing receptors. By coordinating changes in receptor affinity and receptor concentration with other regulatory events within the cell, the target cell is capable of a broad range of responses to hormonal stimuli.

▶ [A nice demonstration is provided of the complexities of the "feed forward" mechanism of homeostasis. — W.G.R.] ◀

Myoinositol Metabolism in Diabetes Mellitus: Effect of Insulin Treatment. The physiologic significance of the urinary excretion of large amounts of myoinositol by human diabetics is unclear. A conditioned intracellular myoinositol deficiency in the peripheral nerve could be a factor in the pathogenesis of diabetic peripheral neuropathy in man. Rex S. Clements, Jr., and Richard Reynertson[6] (Univ. of Alabama) studied the effects of insulin treatment on myoinositol metabolism in 6 diabetics. Ten nondiabetic males were also evaluated. Respective mean ages were 41.2 and 25.9 years. Inpatients received a diet containing a determined amount of myoinositol. Studies were done with 2-^{3}H-myoinositol. Oral myoinositol tolerance was estimated by giving a dose of 3 gm myoinositol before and after the plasma glucose concentration was kept below 150 mg/dl for at least 24 hours by twice-daily injections of a mixture of NPH and crystalline insulins.

Myoinositol content of the diet and its distribution were similar in the diabetic and control groups. A significant elevation of plasma myoinositol was seen in the diabetic group, but plasma urea nitrogen was also elevated in the diabetics, and the two concentrations were linearly correlated with each other. Plasma myoinositol concentrations rose significantly during the day only in the diabetic group. Plasma myoinositol concentrations rose sharply on oral tolerance

---

(6)   Diabetes 26:215–221, March, 1977.

testing in the diabetics and were significantly above those in control subjects at all intervals. Insulin therapy restored oral myoinositol tolerance of the diabetics to normal. Urinary myoinositol excretion was significantly increased in uncontrolled diabetics and fell significantly after insulin therapy, though not to normal. Fecal myoinositol excretion was similar in the two groups. Urinary myoinositol and urinary glucose excretions were significantly correlated, as were urinary myoinositol excretion and plasma glucose concentration. The half-times of myoinositol disappearance were similar in diabetic and nondiabetic subjects. The half-time increased in all diabetics after treatment. The size of the rapidly equilibrating myoinositol pool in diabetics was less than half that of nondiabetics before treatment but returned to normal after insulin treatment.

This study showed a number of abnormalities in myoinositol metabolism in uncontrolled diabetics. Whether nerve myoinositol concentrations could be restored to normal by diet-induced elevation of the plasma myoinositol concentration is unknown. The possibility that oral myoinositol supplementation could improve peripheral nerve function of diabetics requires further study.

▶ [Improvement in motor nerve conduction velocity in diabetic rats whose diet contained 1% myoinositol forms the basis for the last sentence above. For an excellent discussion, see the article by Winegrad and Greene (N. Engl. J. Med. 295:1416, 1976). — W.G.R.] ◀

Effects of Pregnancy on Hemoglobin A$_{Ic}$ in Normal, Gestational Diabetic and Diabetic Women. Hemoglobin A$_{Ic}$ (Hb A$_{Ic}$), a normal minor variant of hemoglobin A, is elevated in diabetic subjects and markedly elevated in insulin-dependent diabetics. This hemoglobin is unique because of a carbohydrate moiety attached to the N-terminal amino acid, valine, of the beta chain by a Schiff base linkage. Herbert C. Schwartz, Katherine C. King, Alan L. Schwartz, Diana Edmunds and Robert Schwartz[7] studied the effect of pregnancy on the Hb A$_{Ic}$ level in women with normal and abnormal glucose tolerance. Sample chromatograms are shown in Figure 57.

The glucose linked to the β-chain of Hb A$_{Ic}$ interferes with the binding of 2,3-diphosphoglycerate, probably resulting in

(7)   Diabetes 25:1118–1122, December, 1976.

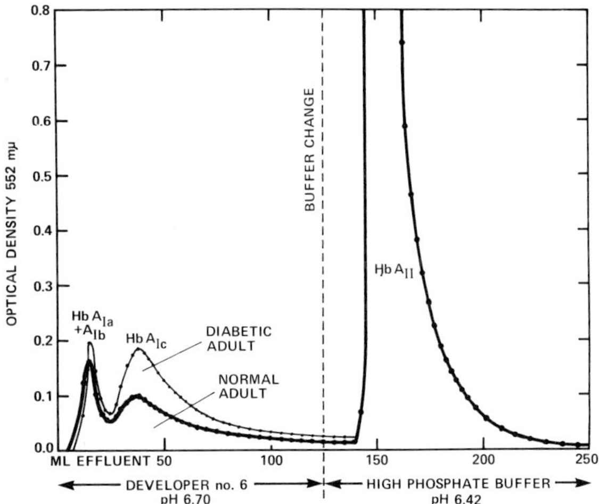

Fig 57.—Chromatography of human hemoglobin on Amberlite IRC-50. The hemoglobin A from a normal adult *(heavy line)* separates into a major component Hb A$_2$ and two "fast" minor peaks, one containing Hb A$_{Ia+b}$, the other Hb A$_{Ic}$. The minor hemoglobin components from an insulin-dependent diabetic adult *(fine line)* with an increased Hb A$_{Ic}$ have been superimposed. (Courtesy of Schwartz, H. C., et al.: Diabetes 25:1118–1122, December, 1976.)

an increased affinity of the hemoglobin for oxygen. Hemoglobin A$_{Ic}$ is increased to twice-normal levels in juvenile-onset insulin-dependent diabetes. The level was slightly elevated above that of normal females in pregnant normal, pregnant nondiabetic obese and gestationally diabetic subjects. A striking difference was found between nonpregnant diabetics and pregnant diabetics (12.8% and 8.5% of total hemoglobin, respectively). This difference was significant and was similarly significant when the pregnant diabetics were compared with the 4 diabetic females in whom the Hb A$_{Ic}$ was 12.7% of total hemoglobin.

The decrease in level of Hb A$_{Ic}$ found in diabetics pregnant more than 30 weeks may reflect a better state of diabetic control or a compensatory mechanism, or both, to protect the fetus by facilitating oxygen exchange from mother to fetus. Further studies are needed to elucidate the mechanism of the alterations of Hb A$_{Ic}$ noted in diabetes and pregnancy.

► [Hemoglobin A$_{Ic}$ has received considerable attention as a possibly better indicator of overall blood sugar control. Because it changes slowly and is responsive to long-term alterations in blood glucose, its level reflects average blood sugars over the preceding several weeks. One may speculate that the results seen in this study were due to better blood sugar control in the 3d trimester for one reason or another.

Recent evidence (Lancet 2:734, 1977) suggests that measurement of the combined A_1 hemoglobins (see Fig 57) may be just as useful and is easier to do. — W.G.R.] ◄

Successful Immunosuppressive Therapy in Insulin-Resistant Diabetes Caused by Anti-insulin Receptor Autoantibodies.

Koichi Kawanishi, Ko Kawamura, Yoshiaki Nishina, Akio Goto, Soji Okada, Toshihiko Ishida, Tadashi Ofuji (Okayama Univ.), C. Ronald Kahn and Jeffrey S. Flier[8] (Natl. Inst. of Health) report data on a patient with severe insulin-resistant diabetes accompanied by hypergammaglobulinemia and Sjögren's syndrome, who had a high titer of anti-insulin receptor antibodies. Immunosuppressive therapy resulted in disappearance of antibody titer and complete remission of the diabetes.

Woman, 45, had polyarthralgia, followed a year later by erythema of the cheeks and Raynaud's phenomenon and then increased thirst and polyuria. There was a history of pulmonary tuberculosis at age 19. The parotids were enlarged and several nodes were noted in the cervical, axillary and inguinal areas. The sedimentation rate was 120 mm/2 hours, the urinary sugar 2+ and the anti-DNA antibody titer 8.2%. The glucose tolerance test was abnormal, with high immunoreactive insulin and elevated C-peptide levels. Serum anti-insulin antibodies were not present. Initial treatment by glibenclamide was without effect (Fig 58) and glucose levels rose despite the administration of Rapitard insulin. Abnormal liver enzymes and hyperamylasemia developed. The serum γ-globulin level remained high. Biopsy of a cervical node showed benign lymph follicle hyperplasia. The percentage of B lymphocytes increased. Antinuclear antibodies became positive and Sjögren's syndrome was confirmed. The patient improved gradually on 440 units insulin daily, prednisolone and cyclophosphamide. Tuberculous meningitis developed when cyclophosphamide was discontinued because of increasing leukopenia, but responded to treatment. Normal insulin sensitivity was subsequently documented and cyclophosphamide treatment was again discontinued. Serum γ-globulin increased and immunosuppressive therapy was resumed.

Elevations of serum anti-insulin antibodies of up to 17.5% were documented despite chronic, large-dose insulin therapy. Antirecep-

---

(8) J. Clin. Endocrinol. Metab. 44:15–21, January, 1977.

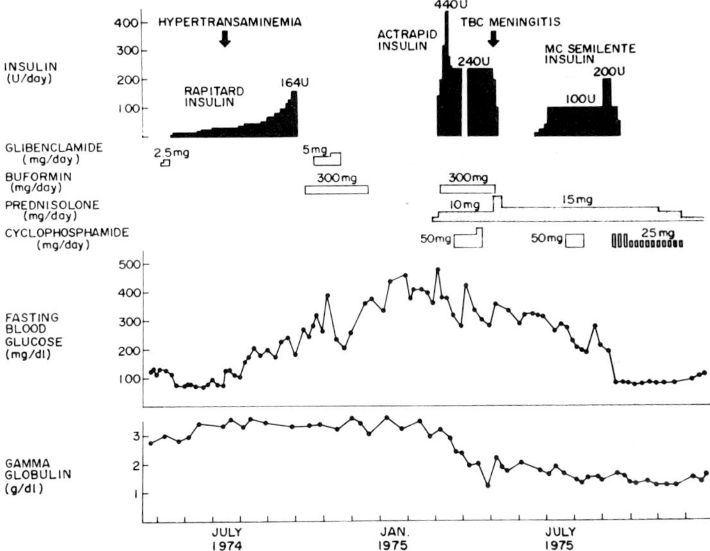

Fig 58. – Hospital course of the patient. (Courtesy of Kawanishi, K., et al.: J. Clin. Endocrinol. Metab. 44:15–21, January, 1977.)

tor activity was present in high titer before, but not after immunosuppressive therapy.

Diabetes resolved after 8 months of immunosuppressive therapy in this case, insulin sensitivity returned to normal and serum antireceptor antibodies disappeared. Glucose tolerance deteriorated after cyclophosphamide was withdrawn and the dose of prednisolone was reduced. A spontaneous remission seems unlikely in this case.

► [This form of diabetes was included in the 1977 YEAR BOOK. A useful treatment is described here. – W.G.R.] ◄

► ↓ The following four articles form an "instant symposium" on islet cell antibodies. – W.G.R. ◄

Pancreatic Islet Cell Antibodies in Diabetes Mellitus Correlated with Duration and Type of Diabetes, Coexistent Autoimmune Disease and HLA Type. Pancreatic islet cell antibodies (ICA) have been found in about half of young, recently diagnosed, insulin-treated diabetics, and an increased prevalence of the histocompatibility antigens B8 and W15 has been reported in insulin-treated or juvenile-onset diabetics. W. J. Irvine, C. J. McCallum, R. S. Gray, C. J. Campbell, L. J. P. Duncan, J. W. Farquhar, H. Vaughan and P. J. Morris[9] examined correlations among prevalence of ICA, age at onset of diabetes, duration and type of diabetes, sex, other evidence for organ-specific autoimmunity and HLA type in 952 diabetics. Studies were done on 628 insulin-treated diabetics, 217 treated by diet and oral hypoglycemic agents and 107 treated by diet alone. Islet cell antibodies were detected by the indirect immunofluorescence test. The standard NIH-Terasaki microlymphocytotoxicity test was used for HLA typing.

Antibodies were found in 38% of insulin-treated diabetics who had associated overt organ-specific autoimmune disease (AID) and in 22% of those who did not. They were also detected in 8% of diabetics treated with oral hypoglycemic agents, but not in those requiring diet alone and in only 0.5% of 434 controls. Islet cell antibodies were found in 6% of 522 patients with overt organ-specific AID who were not diabetic. They were present in the serums of 2% of 157 first-degree relatives of ICA-positive subjects. In insulin-treated diabetics, the prevalance of ICA was strongly dependent on duration of diabetes, falling from 60% in the 1st year after diagnosis to 5% at 10 – 20 years. No correlation with patient age at time of testing was apparent. Persistence of IC Ab for more than 5 years from the diagnosis of diabetes was associated with coexistent organ-specific AID and with HLA B8, A1 and A1 + B8.

The occurrence of ICA in diabetics who do not require insulin is correlated with a strong tendency for these patients subsequently to require insulin for metabolic control. The concept of an autoimmune form of diabetes is supported by the association of insulin-treated diabetes with organ-specific AID; a higher prevalence of thyrogastric antibodies in insulin-treated diabetics; and evidence for cell-mediated immunity to the endocrine pancreas in insulin-dependent but not in insulin-independent diabetics.

► [One question is "Do these antibodies produce destruction of islets or are they formed in response to destruction of islets by other agents?" – W.G.R.] ◄

---

(9) Diabetes 26:138 – 147, February, 1977.

Islet Cell Antibodies in Diabetes Mellitus. Antibodies of the IgG class reacting with normal human pancreatic islet cells have been described in diabetics with autoimmune polyendocrine disease and juvenile diabetics, but only rarely in maturity-onset diabetes or nondiabetic subjects. R. Lendrum, G. Walker, A. G. Cudworth, C. Theophanides, D. A. Pyke, A. Bloom and D. R. Gamble[1] studied the prevalence of islet cell antibodies (ICA) in diabetic and nondiabetic subjects and their relation to age, sex and the type and duration of disease. Studies were done in 829 insulin-dependent diabetics, 112 insulin-independent diabetics and 313 nondiabetic subjects. Serums were tested for ICA by immunofluorescence methods. High-titer ICA-positive serums were absorbed with bovine or porcine insulin.

Islet cell antibodies were found in 38% of insulin-dependent diabetics, the prevalence declining with an increasing duration of disease in both sexes (Fig 59). Islet cell antibodies were detected in 5.3% of insulin-independent diabetics.

Fig 59.—Prevalence of ICA in relation to duration of illness in 829 insulin-dependent diabetics. Average age of patients in each duration group is also shown. (Courtesy of Lendrum, R., et al.: Lancet 2:1273–1276, Dec. 11, 1976.)

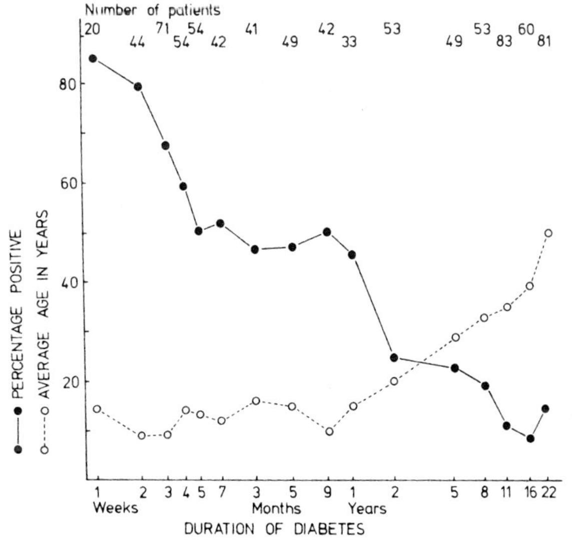

(1)   Lancet 2:1273–1276, Dec. 11, 1976.

The highest titer in this group was only 1:8. Islet cell antibodies occurred in 3 of 29 discordant identical co-twins of diabetics and in 3.7% of 107 1st-degree relatives of diabetic patients. Thyroid or gastric antibodies, or both, occurred in 23% of insulin-dependent diabetics and were twice as common in women as in men, their prevalence in both sexes increasing with age and with the duration of diabetes. Islet cell antibodies occurred in similar percentages of patients with and without thyrogastric antibodies, 33% and 39% respectively, and their prevalence fell at similar rates in both groups as the duration of disease increased. Absorption of three ICA-positive serums with insulin resulted in no change in the titers.

This study confirmed the strong association of ICA with insulin-dependent diabetes and showed a decline in their prevalence as the duration of disease increased. Islet cell antibodies appear to have a different prevalence pattern than other autoantibodies and may possibly be a simple by-product of islet cell destruction rather than the cause of an autoimmune destructive process. The autoimmune phenomena in diabetes may be triggered by an extrinsic agent, and ICA may provide clues about such agents.

▶ [I - C - A possible relationship to the genesis of diabetes. – W.G.R.] ◀

Pancreatic Islet Cell Antibody as a Marker for Asymptomatic and Latent Diabetes and Prediabetes. Pancreatic islet cell antibody (ICA) is most common in newly diagnosed insulin-dependent diabetes, the prevalence declining with increasing duration of diabetes. W. J. Irvine, R. S. Gray and C. J. McCallum[2] (Univ. of Edinburgh) performed glucose tolerance tests in ICA-positive subjects not previously recognized as diabetic. Studies were done in 36 subjects, including 31 with organ-specific autoimmune disorders, 4 first-degree relatives of ICA-positive diabetics and 1 apparently normal subject. None had clinical evidence of diabetes. Thirty-three subjects had oral and 3 had intravenous glucose tolerance tests.

Thirteen patients had multiple organ-specific autoimmune disorders. Of the 36 subjects, 10 had a diabetic tolerance test, 5 of whom had fasting blood glucose levels above 5.6 mM/L. Four subjects had lag-storage tolerance tests; 2 of

---

(2) Lancet 2:1097–1102, Nov. 20, 1976.

these had a history of thyrotoxicosis. Two subsequently acquired insulin-dependent diabetes; 22 had normal glucose tolerance tests. Mean antibody titers were similar for the diabetic and nondiabetic ICA-positive subjects. All but 1 of the 31 subjects who were antibody positive at the time of tolerance testing were positive 2 weeks to 11 years previously. Titers remained quite constant in some cases and rose and fell over the years in others. There was no correlation between the titer, change in titer or duration of ICA or the presence of HLA-B8, BW15 or CW 3 and the results of glucose tolerance testing.

In addition to serving as a marker for asymptomatic and latent diabetes and prediabetes, the presence of ICA in the serum may define a new group of potential diabetics with normal glucose tolerance tests. Many subjects have organ-specific autoimmune disorders but some are first-degree relatives of ICA-positive subjects. About 0.5% of the general population also have ICA in their serums. Idiopathic Addison's disease was particularly prevalent in the present series. The recognition that such a patient is at risk of acquiring diabetes is of major clinical importance.

► [And this is something perhaps better not known to your prospective insurance agent. — W.G.R.] ◄

Separate Autoantibodies to Human Pancreatic Glucagon and Somatostatin Cells. The presence of cells containing glucagon, insulin and somatostatin has been demonstrated in mammalian islets, and human pancreatic polypeptide (hPP) has been suggested to exist in a fourth cell type. Gian Franco Bottazzo and Richard Lendrum[3] (London) found autoantibodies reacting with discrete cell populations in normal human pancreatic islets by immunofluorescence. Study was made of serums from 1,279 subjects, collected during a study of the prevalence of islet cell antibodies (ICA). A double-immunofluorescence technique used antiserums to pancreatic glucagon, insulin, somatostatin and hPP.

Granular cytoplasmic fluorescence of individual islet cells was produced by 17 serums. In the double-staining system, 13 of 17 serums contained antibodies reacting specifically with glucagon cells; the other 4 reacted with somatostatin cells. These antibodies were directed against intracellular

---

(3)   Lancet 2:873–876, Oct. 23, 1976.

components, not against the hormones themselves. Both types of antibody occurred independently of the ICA described in diabetes. The antibodies reacting with glucagon cells belonged to the IgG or IgM classes. Those to somatostatin belonged to the IgG class or, in 1 instance, to the IgG and IgA classes. Antibodies to glucagon cells were not associated with a particular type of diabetes and were also found in 2 nondiabetic subjects. Two insulin-independent diabetics, 1 "chemical" diabetic and 1 presumably nondiabetic patient had antibodies to somatostatin cells.

The findings suggest selective damage to individual cell types in the pancreatic islets and raise the possibility of corresponding hormone deficiency syndromes. The possibility that somatostatin (D cell) autoantibodies reflect somatostatin deficiency warrants detailed clinical and metabolic studies of patients in whom they are found. Similar approaches may reveal antibodies directed against other peptide-secreting cells, such as those in the gastrointestinal tract. Antibody markers may be useful for further defining the normal physiology and the consequences of destruction of these cells.

► [An interesting finding and corresponding hypothesis are offered here. — W.G.R.] ◄

Genetic Susceptibility in Diabetes Mellitus: Analysis of the HLA Association. A. G. Cudworth and J. C. Woodrow[4] (Univ. of Liverpool) analyzed the results of HLA typing in 288 patients with insulin-dependent diabetes and an age at onset of 30 years or below. Fifty patients with insulin-dependent, late-onset diabetes and 100 with insulin-independent disease were also typed. The 375 controls consisted mainly of normal blood donors from the same geographic area. The two-stage microlymphocytotoxicity method was used for HLA typing; 23 specificities were determined.

Increased frequencies of HLA B8 and BW15 were confirmed in the juvenile-onset group. The relative risks for B5, B7 and BW35 were particularly low. The relative risk of having both B8 and BW15 for diabetics compared with controls was 5.4. There was no evidence of an increase in the frequency of A1 independent of that of B8. Combination of

---

(4)   Br. Med. J. 2:846–848, Oct. 9, 1976.

the data with those from two other centers confirmed the increase in frequency of B8, and the increase in the frequencies of BW15 and B18 became highly significant. The prevalence of B8 in patients with late-onset, insulin-dependent diabetes was significantly increased, and there were suggestive but insignificant increases in BW15 and B18 in this group. No abnormalities were found in late-onset, insulin-independent diabetics. There was no significant evidence of heterogeneity for age at onset of juvenile-onset diabetes and particular HLA phenotypes.

A reasonable interpretation of current evidence is that there is one major HLA-linked diabetogenic gene, which, because of linkage disequilibrium with the B locus, is non-randomly distributed in relation to the whole series of B locus antigens. The mode of action of the HLA-linked diabetogenic gene in insulin-dependent diabetes is speculative. Possibly there is an HLA-linked gene in insulin-dependent diabetes, irrespective of age at onset, which permits interaction of a virus with specific cell membrane antigens, resulting in direct virus invasion and destruction of the beta cells. Alternatively, the interaction between the virus and the membrane receptor may result in neoantigen formation, with consequent antibody-mediated beta cell destruction.

► [The HLA story is not complete for diabetes. Recent evidence suggests that antigens of the D system may be more specific. — W.G.R.] ◄

HLA System in Japanese Patients with Diabetes Mellitus. An increased frequency of HLA B8 or BW15, or both, has been found in white diabetic patients with juvenile-onset diabetes or insulin dependency, but race specificity is an important characteristic of the human leukocyte antigen (HLA) system. A. Kawa, M. Nakazawa, S. Sakaguchi, S. Nakamura, Y. Kono, H. Hazeki and T. Kanehisa[5] (Kagoshima Univ.) examined the HLA system in 78 Japanese patients with diabetes mellitus and 57 healthy control subjects. Twenty patients had juvenile-onset diabetes, and 28 were on insulin therapy. Sixteen patients had a family history of diabetes. Patients were HLA-typed by Terasaki's method.

Increases in HLA A9, B5 and BW40 were found in the Japanese, but A1, A3 and B8, which were found in the white

---

(5)   Diabetes 26:591–595, June, 1977.

patients, were almost absent in the Japanese. An increase in J-1 and a decrease in B5 seemed to be present in juvenile-onset diabetics, but late-onset diabetics did not differ from controls with respect to J-1. A significant increase in J-1 was also noted in patients with a positive family history of diabetes. Only 2 of 20 juvenile-onset patients compared to 28 of 58 control subjects, had HLA B5, but the difference was not significant.

Juvenile-onset diabetes in Japanese is characterized by a positive association with J-1, a Japanese specific subclass of BW22, and by a possible negative association with B5. These findings suggest that juvenile-onset diabetes is a disease entity in itself and different in origin and pathogenesis from adult-onset diabetes mellitus. The significance of a tendency to a decreased frequency of HLA B5 in juvenile-onset diabetics is difficult to interpret.

▶ [Here it is seen that the HLA association in diabetic Japanese differs from that of diabetic whites. – W.G.R.] ◀

Rat Insulin Genes: Construction of Plasmids Containing the Coding Sequences. Great progress has been made in understanding the role of insulin in normal glucose homeostasis and in diabetes, but little is known of the control of insulin gene expression in normal and pathologic states. Axel Ullrich, John Shine, John Chirgwin, Raymond Pictet, Edmund Tischer, William J. Rutter and Howard M. Goodman[6] (Univ. of California, San Francisco) isolated the coding region of the insulin gene by cloning in bacterial plasmids the complementary DNA (cDNA) synthesized in vitro from rat insulin messenger RNA (mRNA). The plasmids were found to contain the coding region for most of the translated portion of the gene for rat insulin I and the segment coding for the A chain of rat insulin II.

The general scheme used to isolate the plasmids is shown in Figure 60. A method allowing the extraction of intact, translatable mRNA from sources rich in ribonuclease was utilized. Polyadenylated RNA was isolated by chromatography on oligodoxythymidylate-cellulose and transcribed into cDNA with the use of avian myeloblastosis virus (AMV) reverse transcriptase and $dT_{12\text{-}18}$ as primer. An improved cloning method involves the ligation of chemically synthe-

---

(6)   Science 196:1313–1319, June 17, 1977.

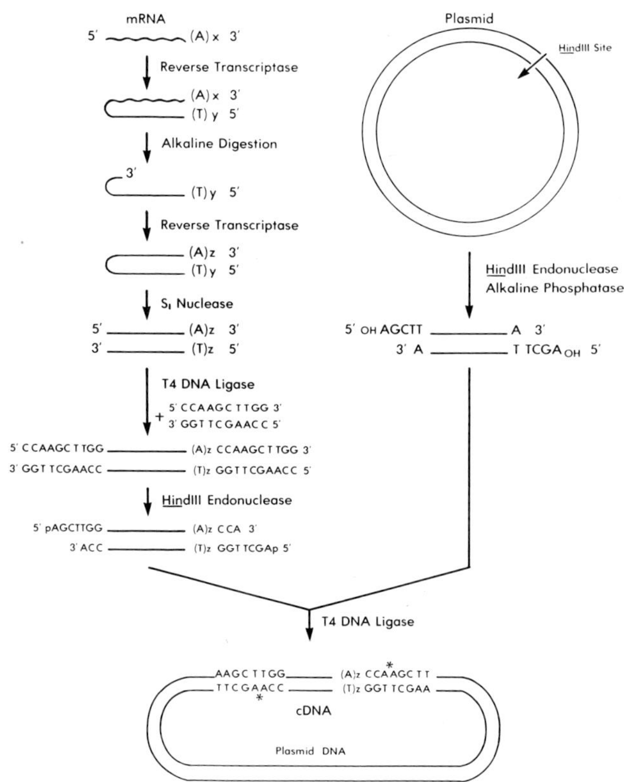

Fig 60. — Schematic diagram for insertion of cDNA into bacterial plasmids with the use of chemically synthesized restriction site linkers. The asterisks in the recombinant plasmid indicate the position where a phosphodiester bond has not formed because of the absence of a 5' terminal phosphate. The example shown here is for the Hind III decanucleotide. In certain cases, the Eco RI octanucleotide (5')TGAATTCA(3') was used; in these cases, insertion was made into the Eco RI site of the plasmid. (Courtesy of Ullrich, A., et al.: Science 196:1313–1319, June 17, 1977.)

sized restriction site linkers to cDNA and cleavage with the appropriate restriction endonuclease to produce cDNA molecules with cohesive termini for ligation to similarly cleaved plasmid DNA. The bacterial plasmid pMB9 was used. Mixtures of recombinant cDNA-pMB9 were used to transform the EK2 host *Escherichia coli* ₓ1776.

Three plasmids contain cloned sequences representing the complete coding region of rat proinsulin I, part of the preproinsulin I prepeptide and the untranslated 3' terminal region of the mRNA. A fourth plasmid contains sequences derived from the A chain region of rat preproinsulin II. The findings show the utility of molecular cloning in analyzing gene structures. The clones containing insulin gene segments should be very useful in studying regulation of insulin mRNA biosynthesis and its expression in bacteria.

▶ [And now 1984 is only 6 years away. — W.G.R.] ◀

Carbohydrate Metabolism and Insulin Resistance in Myotonia Dystrophica. Glucose intolerance and hyperinsulinism are among the more prominent biochemical findings in myotonia dystrophica (MD). If peripheral insulin resistance is the cause of the hyperinsulinism and is an integral part of the disease, it should be demonstrable in all affected subjects. Such resistance might also impair use of other common dietary hexoses. Gerald J. M. Tevaarwerk and Arthur J. Hudson[7] (Univ. of Western Ontario) investigated insulin responses in 5 women and 9 men, aged 22–72, with MD. Three patients were members of three consecutive generations in one family. The degree of disability varied greatly, though no subject was bedridden. Insulin levels in response to tolbutamide, glucagon, arginine and leucine were determined. Tolerance tests were also done in 25 healthy adults and 5 adults with chemical diabetes who were of normal weight.

Oral xylose tolerance tests showed normal absorption in 7 of 8 patients. Glucose tolerance tests in 12 patients showed elevated 2-hour plasma glucose values and delay in the peak plasma glucose value. Insulin levels were elevated during the test in all patients. Both glucose and insulin areas were significantly elevated in MD patients. Responses to fructose tolerance testing were generally normal but insulin values were increased and were significantly different from those in normal subjects. Galactose levels after an oral load were less in MD patients than in normal subjects and plasma glucose elevations were greater in the MD patients; serum insulin levels were also above normal. Sensitivity to exogenous insulin was reduced in MD patients compared with normal subjects, and the clinical reaction to hypoglycemia was milder. The rise in insulin after glucagon was signif-

---

(7)   J. Clin. Endocrinol. Metab. 44:491–498, March, 1977.

icantly greater in MD patients than in normal subjects. Insulin responses to tolbutamide, arginine and leucine were nearly double those in normal subjects. Sorbitol excretion was comparable in MD patients and normal subjects.

Impaired glucose tolerance and hyperinsulinism in MD appear to be due to peripheral insulin resistance that affected most if not all tissues including the liver. Excessive insulin responses to glucagon, tolbutamide and arginine are probably due to compensatory beta cell hyperresponsiveness. Cellular resistance to insulin may be important in the pathogenesis of MD, reflecting an alteration in insulin receptor-binding sites on tissues, a defect in receptor-binding-initiated enzymatic activity or impairment at a subsequent stage of intermediary metabolism.

▶ [Along our current line of thinking, these patients should have a receptor disorder. I suspect it's been sought, but I can't recall having seen such a study. — W.G.R.] ◀

Anti-insulin Antibodies and Late Diabetic Complications. The occurrence of late diabetic complications in patients not given insulin and the uncertainty about the specificity of histoimmunologic techniques have cast doubt on the significance of insulin-anti-insulin antibody complexes in the production of vascular complications of diabetes. O. Ortved Andersen[8] (Gentofte, Denmark) evaluated 274 insulin-dependent juvenile diabetics, 108 of whom had one or more late diabetic complications. The age of onset of diabetes was under 40 years in all cases. Plasma insulin-binding capacity (IBC) was determined in 265 patients.

The highest insulin requirement was reached after 10 – 15 years of treatment. Within groups of patients treated for varying periods, there were no significant differences in the duration of insulin therapy between those with and those without complications. In patients without complications, insulin requirements were significantly reduced as a function of duration of treatment. Elderly patients had a slightly lower insulin requirement than younger ones after several years of treatment. In a comparison of insulin requirements after about 10 years of treatment, patients who later had complications had significantly higher requirements than those who did not have complications. No difference in mean

---

(8)   Acta Endocrinol. (Kbh.) 83:329–340, October, 1976.

plasma IBC was found between patients without complications treated for a shorter or for a longer period. Patients with complications, especially an early onset of proliferative retinopathy or nephropathy, tended to have higher plasma IBC values than patients without complications, but the difference was not significant. Patients with complications had high titers significantly more often than those without complications.

These findings support the view that insulin-anti-insulin antibody complexes may aggravate the severe complications of diabetes. The significant elevation of insulin requirements found early in treatment in patients who later have complications may indicate that the anti-insulin antibody titer was elevated at the time. Further clinical and ultrastructural, histoimmunologic data are needed on patients in whom the anti-insulin antibody titer can be followed from the start of treatment.

▶ [This study addresses the question of whether or not diabetic complications may be a manifestation of immune complex disease secondary to chronic insulin therapy. The results could also be interpreted with the idea that high insulin action resulting in poorer control of blood sugar then leads to more complications. Also, lower insulin requirements could mean that there was some residual beta cell function. I doubt that any one of these tells the whole story of pathogenesis of diabetic complications.—W.G.R.] ◀

Decrease in Postprandial Insulin and Glucose Concentrations by Guar and Pectin. It has been suggested that fiber-depleted diets containing refined carbohydrates may be factors in the development of diabetes and that the benefit of unrefined carbohydrate foods is due to the smaller rises in blood sugar that occur after ingesting them compared with equivalent amounts of refined carbohydrates. David J. A. Jenkins, Anthony R. Leeds, Miguel A. Gassull, Bernard Cochet and K. George M. M. Alberti[9] (London) studied the blood glucose responses to various carbohydrate-containing meals to which were added either guar flour (a storage polysaccharide) or pectin (a structural polysaccharide or "dietary fiber") or both. Studies were done in 11 healthy men and 2 women aged 19–33. Four subjects received a liquid control meal with which guar flour was homogenized in the test situation, and 8 received a breakfast

---

(9)   Ann. Intern. Med. 86:20–23, January, 1977.

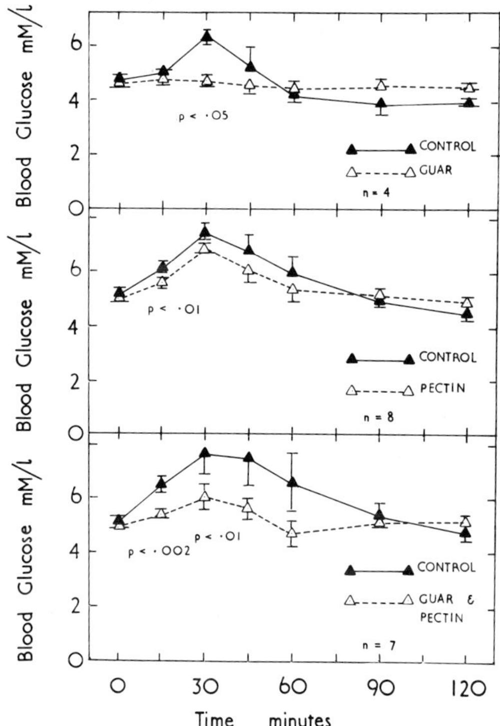

Fig 61. – Blood glucose levels (mean ± SEM) in 4 subjects after the test with guar and control liquid test meal *(upper panel),* in 8 subjects after the test with pectin and control solid test meal *(middle panel)* and in 7 subjects after the test with guar and pectin and control solid test meal *(lower panel).* (Courtesy of Jenkins, D. J. A., et al.: Ann. Intern. Med. 86:20 – 23, January, 1977.)

test meal with 10 gm pectin added. Seven subjects received a guar flour-containing bread in addition to pectin, after a 14-hour fast. Blood samples were analyzed for glucose and serum was separated for insulin assay.

Blood glucose levels after the various meals are shown in Figure 61. No significant rise in blood glucose followed the addition of guar flour to the liquid test meal, and the mean insulin response followed a similar pattern. The addition of pectin resulted in lower blood glucose levels. When both guar and pectin were present in the meal, the glycemia was markedly reduced and insulin levels were significantly below those of control subjects.

These studies provide some evidence that the presence of unabsorbable carbohydrate may reduce the rise in blood glucose and insulin that follows a meal containing carbohydrate. Their properties may be due to their effect on the rate of diffusion of digestion products, on the release of gastrointestinal hormones, which in turn affect insulin secretion, and on the release of hormones of the endocrine pancreas. It is possible that this effect will be seen with other unabsorbable noncarbohydrate gelling agents. This action of unavailable carbohydrates may prove useful in the dietary control of diabetics by reduction of their insulin requirements. If excessive postprandial rises in blood sugar contribute to the development of diabetes in man, the present findings support the hypothesis that fiber-depleted diets may be one contributory factor in the causation of diabetes.

► [Fiber is to the 1970's what polyunsaturates were to the 1960's. I would emphasize the "if" at the beginning of the last sentence of the article. For a little attempt at humor, I submit the following original limerick.

> If you believe that your eating of sugar
> Is like at your temple holding a Luger,
> Then put in your food plan
> Generous helpings of bran,
> And avoid clogging your jugular.

(You can see that I had trouble finding a word that rhymed with "sugar." Perhaps I should have used "sucrose.") – W.G.R.] ◄

Gastric Inhibitory Polypeptide (GIP) in Maturity-Onset Diabetes Mellitus. The pathophysiologic role of the enteroinsular axis in diabetes is speculative, partly because of uncertainties regarding the nature of the enteric signal potentiating insulin release. Gastric inhibitory peptide is perhaps the leading candidate for an intestinal hormone mediating the enteroinsular axis. Samuel E. Crockett, Ernest L. Mazzaferri and Samuel Cataland[1] (Ohio State Univ.) determined serum glucose, insulin and GIP concentrations during oral glucose tolerance tests in 35 adult diabetics who, as a group, were obese and retained the capacity to secrete substantial quantities of insulin. Forty-five normal subjects were also investigated. Subjects took 300 gm carbohydrate daily for 3 days and fasted overnight before ingesting 75 gm glucose. Serum GIP was determined by use of an antibody to

---

(1)   Diabetes 25:931–935, October, 1976.

porcine GIP. Serum immunoreactive insulin (IRI) was determined by radioimmunoassay.

The diabetics were older and more obese than the normal subjects. Serum glucose concentrations were significantly higher in the diabetics at all intervals. Fasting serum IRI concentrations were also higher in the diabetics, but peak serum insulin values did not differ substantially in the two groups, and total integrated incremental insulin concentrations were similar. Fasting and stimulated serum GIP values were higher in the diabetics, as was the total integrated incremental GIP. Both normal-weight and obese diabetics had elevated total integrated incremental GIP concentrations. On matching for age, total integrated GIP was more than twice as great in diabetics as in nondiabetics.

The role of GIP in the pathogenesis of diabetes is uncertain. In view of current hypotheses regarding the role of hyperglucagonemia in diabetes and of observations that GIP stimulates the release of glucagon in vivo, GIP may be important in the pathogenesis of diabetes. Alternatively, the elevated GIP concentration may merely reflect the diabetic state.

► [I'll cast my vote for the alternative. And I think I'll resist punning on GIP! — W.G.R.] ◄

Luteinizing Release Hormone Tests in Impotent Diabetic Males. Sexual impotence is 2 – 5 times more common in diabetic than in nondiabetic men, but no abnormalities of androgen production have been found in impotent diabetic men, and testosterone therapy usually fails to correct the impotence. A. D. Wright, D. R. London, G. Holder, J. W. Williams and B. T. Rudd[2] (Birmingham, England) assessed pituitary-gonadal function by luteinizing hormone-releasing hormone (LHRH) tests in 12 impotent diabetic men under age 60 years. They had had persistent impotence for at least 6 months and for a mean of 4.7 years. All had had insulin-treated diabetes longer than impotence. None had intercurrent illness or was on steroid therapy. Renal disease, when present, was mild. Nine patients of similar ages who had normal sexual function were also studied, as were normal men aged 21 – 40 years. The impotent and control diabetics had similar serum testosterone, sex hormone-

---

(2) Diabetes 25:975 – 977, October, 1976.

binding globulin capacity (SHBGC) and basal and incremental gonadotropin values. The SHBGC was lower in the diabetics than in the normal subjects, and serum FSH increments were more variable in the diabetics; 3 patients had exaggerated responses. Serum LH responses to LHRH were lower in diabetics than in normal subjects. The reduced SHBGC and LH increment were unrelated to patient age, duration of diabetes, serum testosterone or serum FSH increment. The 3 patients with exaggerated FSH responses had had diabetes for over 18 years.

Testicular function appears to be normal in impotent diabetic men. The impotence does not appear to correlate with any endocrine abnormality. Peripheral vessels were normal in all but 1 of the patients. Peripheral neuropathy was the most frequent clinical complication of diabetes in the impotent group, confirming that autonomic neuropathy is the likeliest cause of impotence in the diabetic man. The apparent selectivity of the autonomic nerve lesion may be due to the relative insensitivity of clinical testing. Peripheral nerve conduction studies have always shown greater abnormality than clinical studies.

► [Hope springs eternal for a more effective means of treating the impotent diabetic. With the development of effective prostheses, one would predict a less frantic search. — W.G.R.] ◄

Cigarette Smoking and Diabetic Retinopathy. The impressions that many diabetics with proliferative retinopathy are heavy smokers and that a number of long-term diabetics with minimal retinopathy are nonsmokers led to the postulate that smoking may be related to deterioration of diabetic retinopathy to the proliferative state. Margaret E. Paetkau, T. A. S. Boyd, Bruce Winship and Michael Grace[3] (Univ. of Alberta) tested this hypothesis by analyzing the clinical records of 181 diabetics (85 males and 96 females) seen consecutively in 21 months, including 97 with nonproliferative and 84 with proliferative retinopathy. A cigarette smoker was considered to be a patient who was smoking one or more cigarettes daily or had done so within 7 years of the study.

Lipid plaques were found at the macula in 30 adult-onset diabetics and 1 juvenile-onset diabetic; only 19% of these 31

---

(3) Diabetes 26:46–49, January, 1977.

patients were cigarette smokers. Younger diabetics were more likely than older ones to have been smokers. Proliferative retinopathy tended to increase in frequency with cigarette consumption, and among smokers the proportion of patients with proliferative changes tended to increase with duration of diabetes. Smoking was significantly related to the frequency of proliferative retinopathy in patients who had had diabetes for 20 years or longer. Proliferation was unrelated to age in both smokers and nonsmokers, and no relation with the age at onset of diabetes was apparent in either group.

Animal and human studies have suggested that carbon monoxide causes a separation of arterial endothelial cells and edema, and such an effect could aggravate diabetic retinopathy. Patients with retinopathy have an increased tendency to platelet aggregation; this could be due to nicotine. If the present findings are confirmed, diabetics should be strongly urged to avoid smoking.

► [I would change the last sentence to read, "Regardless of whether or not the present findings are confirmed, diabetics (if not everyone) should be strongly urged to avoid smoking." — W.G.R.] ◄

Subcutaneous Fat in Newborn Infants of Diabetic Mothers: Indication of Quality of Diabetic Control. Infants of diabetic mothers tend to have more adipose tissue than normal at birth, presumably because of fetal hyperglycemia and hyperinsulinism. Andrew Whitelaw[4] (Univ. of London) sought to determine whether maternal blood glucose concentrations are related to subcutaneous fat in newborns as measured by skin-fold thickness and adipose cell size. Forty infants of mothers with established diabetes or gestational diabetes were studied within 72 hours of birth. Fourteen mothers had not required insulin in pregnancy. Adipose tissue was aspirated from the lateral gluteal area of 31 infants.

All infants of mothers with a mean blood glucose value above 6 mM/L had skin-fold measurements exceeding 1 SD above the normal mean, whereas 16 of 30 infants of mothers with lower glucose values had measurements within 1 SD of the normal mean. Neonatal skin-fold thickness percentage was significantly correlated with mean maternal blood glu-

---

(4)   Lancet 1:15–18, Jan. 1, 1977.

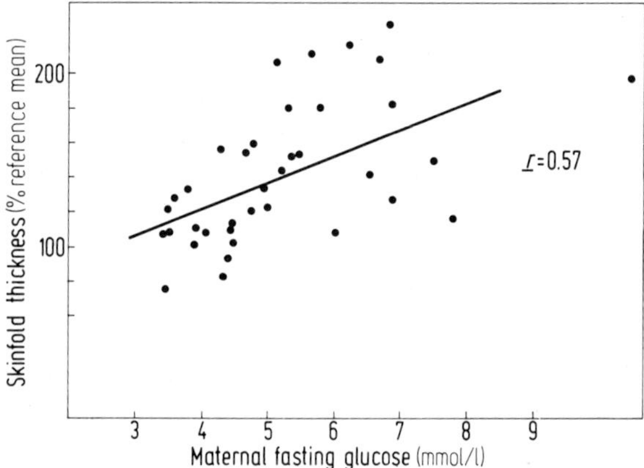

Fig 62. — Sum of skin-fold thickness at eight sites in 37 infants expressed as percentage of reference mean for gestational age, plotted against fasting blood glucose values of their mothers. (Courtesy of Whitelaw, A.: Lancet 1:15–18, Jan. 1, 1977.)

cose concentration and with maternal fasting blood glucose values (Fig 62). Skin-fold thickness was particularly high in infants of mothers who were hyperglycemic while fasting. Most infants of diabetic mothers had larger adipose cells than reference babies, and adipose cell diameter was significantly correlated with the maternal fasting blood glucose value. The most obese infants had the largest adipose cells, and correlation was close between mean adipose cell diameter and skin-fold thickness.

The findings support the hypothesis that in diabetic pregnancy fetal hyperglycemia and hyperinsulinism stimulate increased triglyceride synthesis in and enlargement of adipose cells and lead to an increase in subcutaneous fat. The most obese infant in this sample had a mean adipose cell volume about 4 times that of reference infants of the same gestational age. It seems unlikely that there was a large increase in adipose cell numbers.

▶ [Quantitation of something generally suspected was done by this author. This reminds me of the adage, "To measure is to know."—W.G.R.]

Studies on Etiology of "Brittle Diabetes": Relationship between Diabetic Instability and Insulinogenic Reserve. Kenji Shima, Ryoichi Tanaka, Suzue Morishita,

Seiichiro Tarui, Yuichi Kumahara and Mitsuo Nishikawa[5] (Osaka Univ.), with the technical assistance of Norio Sawazaki, studied the relation between diabetic instability and insulinogenic reserve or plasma IgG insulin-binding capacity in 46 insulin-treated diabetic outpatients to clarify possible etiologic mechanisms for brittle diabetic control. Evaluation of insulinogenic reserve was based on elevations of plasma C peptide immunoreactivity (CPR) during the oral glucose tolerance test (OGTT). Degree of instability of control was quantified by the SD of 10 fasting blood glucose values determined in the prior 6 months of outpatient attendance. The patients represented a broad spectrum of diabetes stability. None had renal insufficiency. Plasma CPR was determined by radioimmunoassay.

Fig 63. – Correlation between SD of 10 values of fasting blood glucose and maximum difference among them in insulin-treated diabetics. Blood specimens for determination of these blood glucose values were obtained most recently during 6-month period before OGTT, while subjects were attending hospital as outpatients. Open circles represent patient with plasma CPR response to oral glucose (ΔCPR > 0.2 ng/ml). Crosses and solid circles represent patients showing no discernible plasma CPR rise (ΔCPR $\leq$ 0.2 ng/ml) during OGTT from basal level of higher *(crosses)* or lower *(solid circles)* than 1 ng/ml. (Courtesy of Shima, K., et al.: Diabetes 26:717–725, August, 1977.)

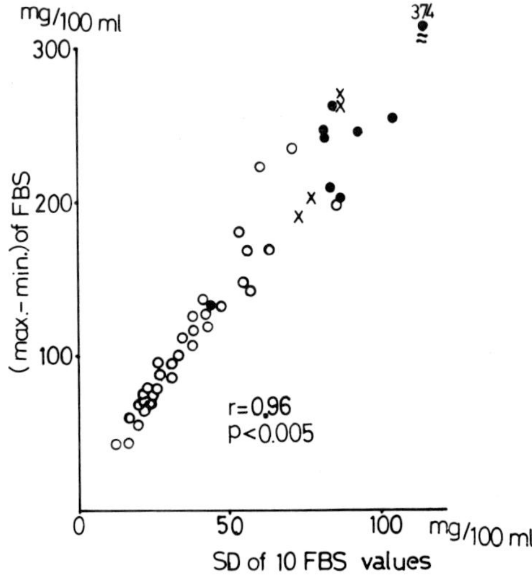

(5)   Diabetes 26:717–725, August, 1977.

The SD of 10 fasting blood sugar values correlated well with the maximum difference among the values (Fig 63). A negative correlation was evident between insulin secretory ability and blood glucose regulatory instability. Insulin-binding capacity of plasma IgG was not correlated with the SD value. Although immunoreactive glucagon (IRG) responses to arginine infusion were observed in 7 unstable diabetics, plasma IRG did not increase during insulin-induced hypoglycemia, in which condition IRG rose significantly in 7 stable diabetics. Plasma cortisol responses to insulin-induced hypoglycemia were demonstrated in both these groups. Plasma CPR did not decrease in unstable diabetics, but it did fall in stable patients after insulin injection. The unstable and stable groups did not differ significantly in age, duration of diabetes or of insulin therapy or dose of insulin.

Total lack of insulinogenic reserve results in loss of automatic regulation of circulating insulin, and this seems to be essential for causing hyperlability of diabetic control. Pancreatic A cell dysfunction is also attributable in part to metabolic variability in brittle diabetes. Inappropriate glucagon secretion may also be responsible for diabetic instability.

► [The ability to measure C peptide as an index of residual beta cell function has produced a number of studies like this and, not surprisingly, as we suspected before our ability to quantitate it, residual beta cell function seems to favor better diabetic control. — W.G.R.] ◄

Glucosyltransferase Activity and Diabetic Microangiopathy. Thickening of the basement membrane and deposit of collagen-like substances in vascular lesions are well-known findings in diabetes, suggesting altered glycoprotein metabolism. J. Duhault and M. Lonchampt[6] (Suresnes, France) measured renal glucosyltransferase activity in rats made diabetic with alloxan or streptozotocin injection and also in the renal cortex of genetically diabetic mice. Male albino rats received two subcutaneous injections of 100 mg alloxan per kg 48 hours apart or one intravenous injection of 65 or 80 mg streptozotocin per kg. The diabetes was not controlled for at least 4 weeks. Some rats received daily injections of slow-release protamine zinc insulin for 3 weeks before they were killed.

---

(6)   Biomedicine 27:127–131, April, 1977.

The only significant observed modification was in endogenous enzyme activity, which was lower in diabetic than in control rats. Specific glucosyltransferase activity was practically unchanged in alloxan-treated and streptozotocin-treated animals. Results were the same in spontaneously diabetic mice. Return to normal endogenous activity occurred in diabetic rats treated with insulin. No correlation was found between specific glucosyltransferase activity and blood sugar at the moment the rats were killed.

It is not possible to conclude that the glucosyltransferases play a prominent role in basement membrane thickening in diabetics. Other possibilities, such as an excess of peptides rich in hydroxylysine or slow catabolism, must be considered as explanations for the basement membrane thickening.

► [I have been teaching our medical students the "gospel" that increased glucosyltransferase activity is responsible for basement membrane thickening, and then I run across this! Is nothing sacred?

Speaking of "sacred" reminds me of my childhood days when I thought the local Catholic school was named the "Scared Heart School." — W.G.R.]

Three-Year Controlled Follow-up Study of Persons Identified in a Mass Screening Program for Diabetes. Mass screening programs for diabetes have been popular for many years, but serious questions have been raised about whether such programs can identify diabetes. Harold B. Houser, Wilma Mackay, Narendra Verma and Saul Genuth[7] (Case Western Reserve Univ.) reviewed experience with a program in Cleveland, which has screened over 600,000 persons since 1964. The effectiveness of the program 3–5 years after testing in the area of patient interaction with the medical care system was assessed by a questionnaire survey of screened persons. Each of 529 persons identified as positive in the industrial screening program was matched with a negative screenee for sex, race, age and place of employment. Of the positive screenees, 204 were confirmed by retesting, 141 were not confirmed and 184 were not retested by glucose tolerance study. The confirmed group was slightly older than the other two groups.

A 3-year follow-up by mail questionnaire showed that deaths were more frequent in confirmed positives (7%). The self-perceived current health status was poorer for this

---

(7)   Diabetes 26:619–627, July, 1977.

group than for their controls. Significant weight loss occurred in the confirmed and not-retested positives. A positive screening test resulted in increased early contact with physicians, but only confirmed positives had evidence of continued increased contact. Oral antidiabetes drugs were currently used by 28% of the confirmed positives, 17% of those not retested and 1% of those not confirmed.

With no clear evidence of modification of behavior toward continued medical care, and considering the potential harm of improper or early exhibition of oral drugs or incorrect labeling of persons as diabetic, the possible benefits of early physician intervention and weight loss do not appear to offset the potential nonbenefit of mass screening for diabetes. Recognition of the "indiscriminate" nature of mass screening, the difficulty in demonstrating benefit to many positive screenees or to the community and the transiency of some positive tests has resulted in a change in the authors' screening program to one of discriminate screening. More-conservative criteria are now used in interpretation of blood glucose values.

▶ [. . . And one of the propaganda messages from the American Diabetes Association is, "Early detection means better control," whatever that means. — W.G.R.] ◀

End-Stage Renal Failure in Juvenile Diabetes Mellitus: A 5-Year Follow-up of Treatment. John C. Mitchell[8] (Mayo Clinic and Found.) carried out a follow-up study of a group of 43 juvenile-onset diabetic patients accepted for renal transplantation for up to 5 years. The 26 men and 17 women had an average age of 36 years when presenting in terminal renal failure and had had clinical diabetes for an average of 21 years. All had an onset of diabetes at or before age 30 years. Complications of microvascular and macrovascular disease were present at the onset of pretransplantation dialysis, and most patients had neuropathy, retinopathy, symptomatic ischemic heart disease and hypertension. Thirty-four patients received renal transplants, whereas 3 remained on dialysis and 6 died while awaiting initial transplantation.

After 5 years, 15% of the men and 23.5% of the women had died while on dialysis. Six of the 20 men who had transplan-

---

(8) Mayo Clin. Proc. 52:281–288, May, 1977.

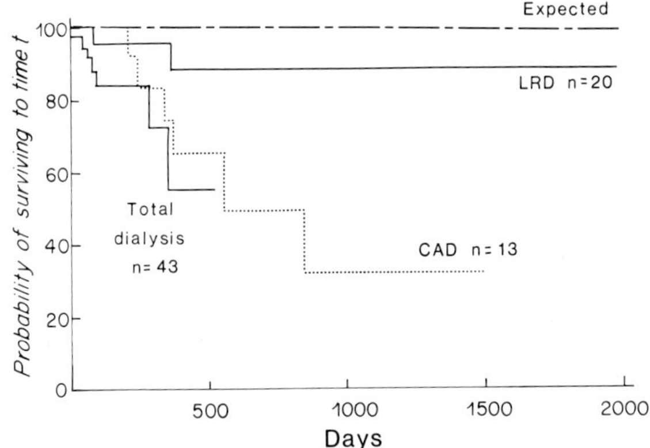

Fig 64. — Cumulative survival by mode of treatment (actuarial method of Kaplan, E. L., and Meier, P.: J. Am. Stat. Assoc. 53:457, 1958) compared with survival of an age- and sex-matched normal population. *LRD,* living related donor; *CAD,* cadaver donor. (Courtesy of Mitchell, J. C.: Mayo Clin. Proc. 52:281–288, May, 1977.)

tation died. One woman died 2 weeks after transplantation. Cardiovascular and cerebrovascular events accounted for over half the total deaths. Four of 15 deaths occurred after nephrectomy. The 1-year survival was 55% in patients on chronic dialysis and 65% after cadaver kidney transplantation (Fig 64), compared with 88% after living related donor transplantation. The cumulative survival for the living related donor group was nearly 82%. Diabetic blindness appeared to stabilize after transplantation. Neuropathy improved in several patients after transplantation. Only 3 of 16 men who survived were working, and only 6 of 12 women could function as housewives or at outside work.

In addition to early transplantation, the use of chronic peritoneal dialysis may be of major benefit to patients awaiting transplantation of a cadaver kidney. Pretreatment of cadaver organs with cyclophosphamide and methylprednisolone may be associated with better graft survival in the recipient. Rehabilitative efforts should be increased for patients who are neurologically stable and have useful vision and relatively little peripheral vascular disease. The 5-year survival of juvenile-onset diabetics who are vigorously treated for renal failure is now approaching 70%.

▶ [Some bright spots are shown in an otherwise dismal situation. —W.G.R.] ◀

Peripheral and Autonomic Nerve Function in Newly Diagnosed Diabetes Mellitus. A delay in peripheral nerve motor-conduction velocity (MCV) in diabetics can be demonstrated before symptoms of peripheral neuropathy develop, and subclinical autonomic neuropathy may be detected in patients with established diabetes by several simple techniques. D. M. Fraser, I. W. Campbell, D. J. Ewing, A. Murray, J. M. M. Neilson and B. F. Clarke[9] (Royal Infirm., Edinburgh) attempted to determine if abnormal autonomic nerve function is present in newly diagnosed diabetics and if it responds to treatment. Ten newly diagnosed male diabetics were studied. Six patients aged 18–40 years received insulin and 4 aged 46–58 years received sulfonylurea (chlorpropamide). The respective mean durations of symptoms were 8 and 12 weeks. The MCV was estimated in the right common peroneal, ulnar and median nerves. Autonomic nerve function was assessed with the Valsalva maneuver, the sustained handgrip test, the R-R interval variation in resting heart rate and the postural fall in blood pressure.

Blood glucose levels fell satisfactorily on treatment in both groups of patients. The mean MCV was delayed at diagnosis in both groups and improved significantly in the insulin-treated group. Terminal latency was slightly prolonged in the insulin-treated patients and improved somewhat after treatment. Abnormalities were most apparent in the common peroneal nerve. One sulfonylurea-treated patient had an abnormal Valsalva response at the outset and on follow-up at 6 months. All patients had normal handgrip responses and no postural hypotension. Two insulin-treated patients and all sulfonylurea-treated patients had abnormal R-R findings at the outset. One of the latter patients improved after the institution of treatment.

Abnormalities of autonomic nerve function are discernible at the time of diagnosis of diabetes. Improvement in autonomic function cannot necessarily be expected even if sat-

(9)   Diabetes 26:546–550, June, 1977.

isfactory diabetic control is achieved. Although symptomatic autonomic neuropathy is a late manifestation of diabetes, cumulative damage may occur from the time of diagnosis.

▶ [I include this mainly for the description of means of assessing autonomic dysfunction. It would appear that this, too, can be detected before it is clinically apparent from the symptoms. — W.G.R.] ◀

On the Cause of Raised Serum Amylase in Diabetic Ketoacidosis. The serum amylase level is abnormally elevated in over 60% of patients with diabetic ketoacidosis, and upper abdominal pain suggestive of pancreatitis often occurs. Both pancreatitis and liver injury have been suggested as explanations. Andrew L. Warshaw, Edward R. Feller and Kang-Hyun Lee[1] (Boston) studied changes in circulating amylase isoenzymes during diabetic ketoacidosis in 13 patients with marked hyperglycemia, ketoacidosis and elevated serum creatinine levels. Seven had elevated serum amylase levels. For comparison, blood was also obtained from 15 nondiabetic patients with acute pancreatitis and from 15 normal subjects.

The 7 patients with amylase elevations had a return to normal levels in the first 2 days of treatment. Five of these patients had epigastric pain, as did 3 of the 6 with normal amylase levels. Three of those with pain were thought to have pancreatitis. Two of the 7 patients had slightly increased alkaline phosphatase levels, but there was no other evidence of liver dysfunction. Amylase-creatinine clearance ratios and serum lipase levels were normal in the 3 hyperamylasemic patients studied. Six of the 7 ketoacidotic patients with hyperamylasemia had distinct increases in salivary-type isoamylases and normal concentrations of pancreatic amylases. In the seventh patient, only pancreatic isoamylases were increased. In the patients with acute pancreatitis, only pancreatic amylases were increased.

Salivary-type hyperamylasemia in diabetics with ketoacidosis excludes the pancreas as being responsible for the increase in serum amylase. No evidence of liver involvement was obtained. Any pancreatic contribution to hyperamylasemia must be very small in most cases of diabetic ketoacidosis. It is suggested that hyperamylasemia in this setting

---

(1)   Lancet 1:929–931, Apr. 30, 1977.

is most often caused by a systemic derangement of carbohydrate metabolism.

► [I wonder if the dehydration accompanying diabetic acidosis could lead to salivary gland dysfunction and thus the hyperamylasemia.— W.G.R.] ◄

Prolonged Follow-up in Diabetic Retinopathy Treated by Sectioning the Pituitary Stalk. Interest in pituitary ablation has increased with the realization that the results of photocoagulation may be less successful than expected and with improvement in surgical techniques. Bruce R. Zimmerman and George D. Molnar[2] reviewed the records of all 40 patients who underwent pituitary ablation for diabetic retinopathy at the Mayo Clinic in 1961–68. Patients with more than minimal renal impairment were excluded from the series, but about half the patients had other diabetic complications, most often mild peripheral neuropathy. The 24 men and 16 women had a mean age of 35 years. Mean duration of diabetes at operation was 20 years. Only 1 patient was not insulin dependent at the time of surgery. All patients received cortisone preoperatively.

One patient died postoperatively of meningitis. The 27 patients who died during follow-up were followed for a mean of 63 months. Complications included 1 case of blindness immediately after operation, 3 minor flap infections, 22 cases of diabetes insipidus, 14 cases of hyponatremia and 3 cases of seizures unrelated to hypoglycemia or hyponatremia. Two patients had transient organic brain syndrome unrelated to hyponatremia. One optic nerve had to be sectioned for optimum exposure in each of 6 patients, and in 7 an olfactory nerve was sectioned. Pituitary ablation was successful by endocrine criteria in 85% of cases. Visual acuity was stable or improved in 79% of patients at 1 year, and retinopathy was stable or improved in 68%. At last follow-up, visual acuity was stable or improved in 77% and retinopathy in 62%. Nine of 13 patients over age 40 at operation had stable or improved acuity at last follow-up. Five of 9 patients with unsuccessful ablation had stable or improved visual acuity at last follow-up.

Young, well-motivated diabetic patients with florid retinopathy have the best chance of improving or maintaining

---

(2)   Mayo Clin. Proc. 52:233–237, April, 1977.

vision when pituitary ablation is done before fibrosis has begun to develop, and this is a reasonable recommendation for such patients.

▶ [I guess old procedures, like old soldiers, never die, they just fade away. This retrospective, uncontrolled study is unlikely to bring about a resurrection. — W.G.R.] ◀

Plasma Glucose Levels: Long-Term Effect of Diet in the Chicago Coronary Prevention Evaluation Program. The fat-modified diets being widely recommended to reduce serum cholesterol and lower the risk of premature atherosclerotic disease often involve a decreased total fat intake, and the total carbohydrate intake may be increased. Eduardo Farinaro, Jeremiah Stamler, Melissa Upton, Louise Mojonnier, Yolanda Hall, Dorothy Moss and David M. Berkson[3] (Chicago) evaluated the effects of such diets on carbohydrate metabolism in 150 men prone to coronary disease who participated in a coronary prevention program. The men were aged 40–59 years at entry and were followed for at least 4 years. Forty-three subjects had glucose tolerance tests both initially and at 2 years. The general dietary plan was intended to reduce total fat intake to about 30% of total calories and to restrict the caloric intake moderately to produce weight loss of 1 lb per week.

A favorable effect on fasting glycemia and glucose tolerance was found. The diet was low in cholesterol and saturated fat and moderate in polyunsaturated and total fat; some fat was replaced by carbohydrate. Decreased weight and serum cholesterol values at 2 years were accompanied by a modest but significant fall in fasting and postload glycemia. At 4 years, fasting glycemia levels remained slightly below baseline in normoglycemic men. In men with suspected fasting hyperglycemia at baseline, a sustained fall in weight and serum cholesterol was associated with sizable reductions in fasting glycemia and improved glucose tolerance. The decrease in plasma glucose was significantly related to the decrease in weight. There was no evidence of impaired glucose tolerance with long-term use of the diet. Improved glucose tolerance was observed at 2 years, even in men with findings indicative of impaired tolerance at baseline.

---

(3) Ann. Intern. Med. 86:147–154, February, 1977.

Diets of this type are effective in reducing elevated lipid values and weight and in maintaining and enhancing prognostically favorable plasma glucose concentrations. The dietary approach may already be playing a role in the current reduction in United States mortality rates from coronary heart disease and from all causes.

► [We know that weight loss in diabetics will generally improve blood glucose levels. Here it is well shown that this applies to subjects with lesser degrees of glucose intolerance. To the last sentence we could add, "or perhaps increased exercise." – W.G.R.] ◄

Control of Juvenile Diabetes Mellitus and Its Relationship to Endogenous Insulin Secretion as Measured by C Peptide Immunoreactivity. Sequential studies of beta cell function in diabetics who require insulin have been complicated by the development of circulating antibodies to exogenous insulin, which interfere with the conventional radioimmunoassay for insulin. Luiz A. Grajwer, Rosita S. Pildes, David L. Horwitz and Arthur H. Rubenstein[4] (Chicago) used an immunoassay for human C peptide to determine whether residual pancreatic beta cell secretory capacity is present in juvenile diabetics and thus influences the ability to control their diabetes. Thirty-five insulin-requiring diabetics aged 5–20 years and 11 healthy children aged 4–11 years were studied. After a 12-hour fast, glucose and C peptide immunoreactivity (CPR) were measured before and 1 hour after administration of 1 gm glucose per kg orally to a maximum dose of 50 gm. Among the 19 male and 16 female diabetics, 14 patients had had diabetes for over 5 years. Control was poor in 10 at the time of the study.

Residual beta cell function, defined as a CPR above 0.5 ng/ml, was present in 71% of the patients; 10 patients had no detectable beta cell function. No correlation with the age at onset of diabetes, insulin dose, fasting glucose values or growth hormone concentrations was observed, but significantly more patients with diabetes of less than 5 years' duration had CPR concentrations above 0.5 ng/ml. All patients with CPR values above 2 ng/ml were adequately controlled. Significantly more poorly controlled patients had fasting growth hormone concentrations above 10 ng/ml. Growth hormone concentrations averaged 13.7 ng/ml in the

---

(4) J. Pediatr. 90:42–48, January, 1977.

group with absent beta cell function and 7.6 ng/ml in those with residual function; the difference was not significant.

Residual insulin secretion in diabetics may facilitate good control, but absent beta cell reserve is not always associated with poor diabetic control. Measurement of total CPR is technically much easier than measurement of free C peptide, and the former may be a more sensitive measure of continuing beta cell function when levels of free C peptide are too low to be detected by immunoassay.

▶ [Several articles assessing residual beta cell function have appeared. Since C peptide is secreted in equimolar quantities with insulin from the beta cell, its measurement allows the estimation of insulin in the blood of the insulin-treated patient, which is actually coming from the beta cell. — W.G.R.] ◀

Proliferative Diabetic Retinopathy: Treatment with Xenon Arc Photocoagulation; Interim Report of Multicenter Randomized Controlled Trial. For the British Multicentre Photocoagulation Trial, the coordinating committee consisted of D. W. Hill, R. K. Blach, H. Cheng, E. M. Kohner, H. Keen, P. Armitage, J. Bailey and A. M. Hamilton and other participants were Magnus Odland, G. Lovatt, E. W. G. Davies, G. Paterson, D. A. Pyke, P. K. Watkins, A. Chignell, T. J. Ffytche, C. Lowy, P. H. Sonksen, N. R. Galloway, M. V. Wells and D. S. J. Maw.[5] Patients presenting at diabetic clinics with visual symptoms and those found on screening to have proliferative diabetic retinopathy were entered into the trial if both eyes were similarly affected and if survival for at least 1 year was expected. None had more than minimal fibrous retinitis proliferans in the fundus or macular scarring. Treated eyes underwent xenon arc photocoagulation, mostly under retrobulbar anesthesia. An attempt was made to coagulate all flat retinal vessels except those too near the macula or over the papillomacular bundle. Treatment was given as often as new vessels were detected. More recently, large areas of nonperfused retina were treated diffusely in eyes with new vessels on the disc.

Of the 100 patients, 58 were followed for 2 years and 23 of these for at least 3 years. Most patients had been insulin dependent from the outset; mean duration of diabetes was

---

(5) Br. Med. J. 1:739–741, Mar. 19, 1977.

16.3 years. The difference in deterioration of treated and untreated eyes with respect to visual acuity was significant after 3 years. The difference was significant only for patients with new disc vessels. Eighteen patients became blind in one or both eyes by the last follow-up; 13 were blind only in the untreated eye and 1 only in the treated eye. The most common cause of blindness was vitreous hemorrhage. More treated than untreated eyes with new disc vessels showed improved clinical ratings, and more untreated eyes became unassessable because of unclear media. Of 45 patients without new disc vessels initially who were followed for 1 year, 3 developed new vessels on both discs, 3 developed them in the treated eye and 6 developed them in the untreated eye only.

These and previous findings emphasize the need for early diagnosis and evaluation of diabetic retinopathy. Treatment should be timely and adequate, with systematic follow-up and further treatment where indicated. Inadequate treatment or delay in its application may prejudice the prognosis for an eye that may pass quickly from a treatable state to one with irreversible retinopathy.

► [A similar study done here in the United States was interrupted before the expected 5 years of study because the differences in treated versus nontreated eyes were so dramatic (See Am. J. Ophthalmol. 81:383, 1976). The message is that we should get diabetic eyes with neovascularization to the ophthalmologist for photocoagulation treatment promptly. — W.G.R.] ◄

Treatment of Insulin-Induced Lipoatrophy. The cause of insulin-induced lipoatrophy, a rather common and disfiguring complication of insulin therapy, is unknown. S. G. Th. Hulst[6] (Utrecht, The Netherlands) reports the results of treatment of 20 children having lipoatrophy with monocomponent and less purified insulins. The patients were among 167 children admitted with diabetes. Fourteen of the 20 were girls. The mean age was 11.2 and the mean duration of diabetes and insulin therapy was 4.1 years. Ten children were given monocomponent insulins, whereas 10 received the insulins they had used previously. Several preparations were used. Insulin was injected with size 18 disposable needles in both groups (Fig 65).

The 10 children who used monocomponent insulins

---

(6) Diabetes 25:1052–1054, November, 1976.

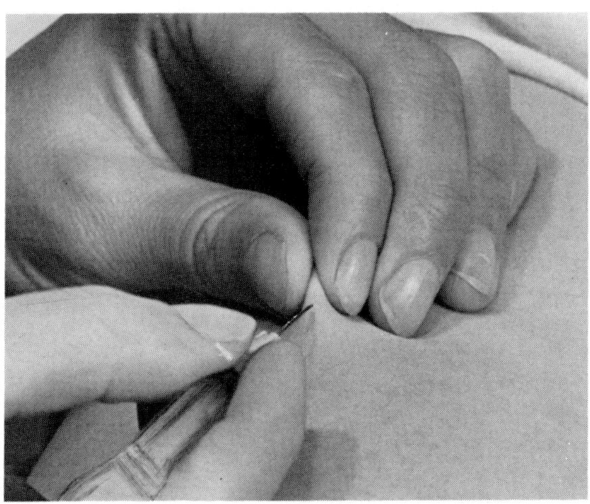

Fig 65.—Injection of insulin into the lipoatrophic area (note the thin skin fold). (Courtesy of Hulst, S. G. Th.: Diabetes 25:1052–1054, November, 1976.)

showed marked disappearance of the lipoatrophy after 2 months of treatment. Thickness at the sites of lipoatrophy disappeared completely and no abnormalities were detected after 6 months of treatment. The 10 children who used their previous insulins showed essentially the same mode of recovery, but some lipoatrophy was still evident after 2 months of treatment. The lipoatrophy had disappeared completely after 6 months of treatment.

The primary factor in treating insulin-induced lipoatrophy appears to be careful injection of insulin into the atrophic area. It does not seem worthwhile to change the insulin regimen in a well-controlled young diabetic in order to treat insulin-induced lipoatrophy. It may be advisable to begin insulin treatment with monocomponent insulins in young diabetics.

► [I included this article primarily for Figure 65. This method of treatment, by the way, was described first in 1949.—W.G.R.] ◄

Phenytoin in Treatment of Diabetic Symmetric Polyneuropathy. Christopher D. Saudek, Steven Werns and Marcus M. Reidenberg[7] (Cornell Univ.) tested the hypothe-

____

(7) Clin. Pharmacol. Ther. 22:196–199, August, 1977.

sis that short-term phenytoin administration relieves the symptoms of symmetric diabetic polyneuropathy in a double-blind, controlled, crossover study in which symptoms were quantified objectively. Subjects with known clinical diabetes and approximately symmetric symptoms of neuropathy in the distal extremities, with absent ankle jerks and reduced vibratory sensation, were included in the trial. Symptoms of more advanced polyneuropathy were present variably, but no patient had findings consistent with other diabetic neuropathies. Patients received placebo or 100 mg phenytoin 3 times daily for 1 week, after an initial dose of 600 mg the 1st day of the week, and were then crossed over for 3 weeks. The dosage was adjusted to achieve plasma concentrations of 5 – 20 mg/L.

Twelve patients were studied for 23 weeks on phenytoin and 23 weeks on placebo. All were insulin-dependent diabetics, with known diabetes for a mean of 15 years. Mean age was 55 years. All but 3 patients had other complications of diabetes. Plasma phenytoin concentrations above 5 mg/L were documented in 16 patients. No difference in total symptoms was seen with and without phenytoin therapy, and no effect of phenytoin on pain, analyzed as a single symptom, was demonstrated. The blood glucose concentration after a meal was significantly higher during phenytoin administration; the mean increase was 44.6 mg/dl. Side effects were more frequent during phenytoin therapy. In 2 patients toxicity led to discontinuance of phenytoin therapy.

Phenytoin has no role in the treatment of symmetric diabetic polyneuropathy. The effect of giving the drug for a longer period is unknown. A hyperglycemic effect of phenytoin was clearly demonstrated in these insulin-dependent diabetics, but insulin dosage adjustment would presumably overcome this response if phenytoin were indicated, as for instance to control a seizure disorder.

► [My own small experience agrees with this report. I have generally had better luck with carbamazepine (Tegretol). – W.G.R.] ◄

Glucose Tolerance and Insulin Secretion in Hyperthyroidism. O. Ortved Andersen, Th. Friis and B. Ottesen[8] (Copenhagen) evaluated glucose tolerance and insulin se-

---

(8)   Acta Endocrinol. (Kbh.) 84:576 – 587, March, 1977.

cretion during oral and intravenous glucose tolerance tests and intravenous tolbutamide tests in 42 patients with hyperthyroidism. The mean patient age was 52. Twenty-eight patients had a diffuse goiter, 7 a multinodular goiter and 7 a toxic adenoma. Eight patients had all three tests, whereas 12 had only oral glucose and tolbutamide tests, 19 had only intravenous glucose and tolbutamide tests, 1 had only intravenous glucose and 2 had only intravenous tolbutamide tests. All 22 control subjects were of normal weight; their mean age was 47. Fifty-four normal-weight controls with a mean age of 38 had previously had intravenous glucose tests. Of the 42 patients, 24 were studied during or after treatment with antithyroid drugs; they had been euthyroid for a mean of 9 months at the second examination.

Serum glucose and insulin concentrations were significantly elevated in study patients compared with controls. The serum glucose became normal during or after treatment, but the serum insulin remained elevated. Hyperthyroid patients had a more marked rise in serum glucose on oral testing than did controls and had a higher and more rapid insulin response. The serum insulin 2 hours after the glucose load was lower than in controls. Treatment resulted in a reduced response of serum glucose levels compared with untreated subjects. The insulin response to a glucose load was unchanged. On intravenous glucose testing, patients had lower K values than controls; 18% had diabetic values. All but 4 of 23 patients had increased K values during treatment. The insulin response remained unchanged. The serum glucose response to intravenous tolbutamide was greater in patients than in controls, decreasing by 44% as against 33% in controls, and the insulin response was greater in hyperthyroid patients as compared with controls. Treatment resulted in a further fall in serum glucose. The insulin response was unchanged in treated patients compared with untreated patients but was significantly enhanced compared with normal subjects.

These findings indicate enhanced sensitivity or an increase in mass of the beta cells in hyperthyroidism. Results of glucose tolerance tests point to increased peripheral insulin resistance. The normalized glucose tolerance and persistently enhanced insulin secretion during treatment support the assumption that hyperthyroidism causes an increase in the beta cell mass.

► [. . . or as likely, perhaps, as hypermetabolic and hyperfunctional.— W.G.R.] ◄

Metabolic Effects of Somatostatin in Maturity-Onset Diabetes. Somatostatin, a potent inhibitor of insulin and glucagon secretion, has been suggested as a therapeutic agent in diabetes mellitus on the basis of its hypoglycemic effects in normal and diabetic man, but the effects of prolonged infusions have been transitory in normal man. William V. Tamborlane, Robert S. Sherwin, Rosa Hendler and Philip Felig[9] (Yale Univ.) studied the effects of prolonged somatostatin infusions in non-insulin-dependent patients with maturity-onset diabetes. Five men and 3 women, aged 33–65 years and with fasting plasma glucose concentrations of 130–295 mg/100 ml, were studied. All were managed by diet alone. Five patients were obese. Subjects were studied in the postabsorptive state after an overnight fast. Somatostatin was infused in a dose of 5 μg/sq m per minute for 5 hours.

The findings are illustrated in Figure 66. Plasma insulin values were reduced by 50–55% during somatostatin infusion and plasma glucagon concentrations were reduced by 45–50%. Somatostatin produced an early fall in plasma glucose concentration, followed by a progressive increase. The infusion resulted in an increment in β-hydroxybutyrate fivefold greater than that seen when saline was given. Total branched-chain amino acids increased by 43% after somatostatin but were unchanged after saline. Responses of plasma glucose, insulin, glucagon, ketones and amino acids to somatostatin were identical in obese and nonobese diabetic patients.

The results are similar to previous findings in normal subjects. Accentuation of hyperglycemia and hyperketonemia by somatostatin in maturity-onset diabetes argues against its use in patients with this condition. Recent evidence that somatostatin interferes with carbohydrate absorption may explain its failure to aggravate postprandial hyperglycemia consistently, despite suppression of insulin. Use of somatostatin might also be associated with worsened diabetic con-

---

(9)   N. Engl. J. Med. 297:181–183, July 28, 1977.

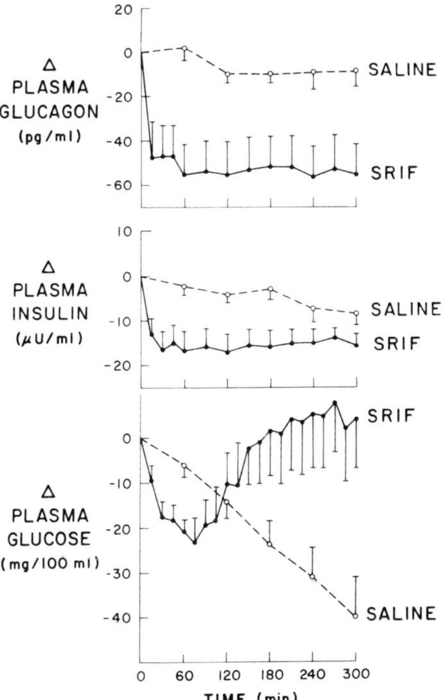

Fig 66.—Effect of somatostatin *(SRIF)* administration on plasma glucagon, insulin and glucose values in maturity-onset diabetes. Means ± SEM are shown. Plasma glucagon and insulin values were significantly reduced on SRIF infusion compared with saline infusion (P < 0.05 to 0.025). Plasma glucose concentrations were significantly reduced during SRIF infusion at 60 minutes (P < 0.001) and were significantly greater than during saline control infusion at 180–300 minutes (P < 0.025 to 0.001). (Courtesy of Tamborlane, W. V., et al.: N. Engl. J. Med. 297: 181–183, July 28, 1977.)

trol in patients with juvenile-onset diabetes, in whom residual insulin secretion has been demonstrated.

▶ [Oh well, maybe it will be helpful in the treatment of tall young girls who are concerned about their eventual height. — W.G.R.] ◀

Induction of Glycosuria and Hyperglycemia by Topical Corticosteroid Therapy. Edward C. Gomez and Phillip Frost[1] (Mount Sinai Med. Center, Miami Beach, Fla.), in the course of studying the effects of percutaneous absorption

(1)   Arch. Dermatol. 112:1559–1562, November, 1976.

of two topical steroid preparations, observed evidence of altered glucose metabolism in 2 psoriatic patients who had abnormal glucose tolerance but no overt diabetes. One patient had an abnormal response to glucose tolerance testing and then developed postprandial hyperglycemia and glycosuria during topical administration of 0.1% halcinonide cream under occlusion. The second patient with similar glucose tolerance test findings exhibited postprandial hyperglycemia when treated similarly with 0.1% betamethasone valerate cream. Two other patients with mildly abnormal glucose tolerance showed no evidence of altered glucose metabolism when similarly treated with halcinonide cream. In each instance the contents of a 15-gm tube of steroid cream was applied to the torso and proximal parts of the extremities at 12-hour intervals for 5 days, and the areas were occluded with plastic film. The film was removed 2 hours before the next application.

Plasma cortisol declined during treatment in these patients, indicating significant systemic absorption of the topically applied steroid. Abnormal glucose metabolism was present before treatment and was temporarily aggravated during treatment. The effects did not appear to be related to a specific steroid preparation. This induction of glycosuria and hyperglycemia is probably a rare occurrence, requiring preexistent impairment of glucose metabolism, use of large amounts of a potent steroid and alteration of the epidermal barrier. Because of the increasing potency of topical steroid preparations, it appears likely that topical steroid therapy will require careful attention to side effects now associated with the use of systemic corticosteroids.

► [This is a predictable happening as topical steroids become more potent. – W.G.R.] ◄

Metoclopramide Stimulation of Gastric Motility and Emptying in Diabetic Gastroparesis. Patients with diabetes occasionally have a syndrome of episodic nausea, vomiting and gastric retention of food. Its pathogenesis is unknown but autonomic parasympathetic neuropathy may play an important role. Conventional antiemetic therapy is often ineffective, and gastric surgery to promote drainage has failed to produce long-lasting relief. George F. Longstreth, Juan-R. Malagelada and Keith A. Kelly[2] (Mayo Clinic

---

(2) Ann. Intern. Med. 86:195–196, February, 1977.

and Found.) studied the effects of metoclopramide, a drug that enhances gastric emptying, in a young diabetic patient with severe gastroparesis.

Woman, 19, had recurrent vomiting and poor control of diabetes, which had been diagnosed at age 9. Episodes of vomiting had begun at age 18 and had increased in frequency and failed to respond to conventional antiemetic therapy. Gastrointestinal studies showed only reduced gastric peristalsis and retained food particles. The patient improved markedly when given 15 mg metoclopramide 4 times daily, orally. The vomiting stopped, 9 kg of weight were gained and the diabetes became easier to control. The patient continues to improve after 6 months of follow-up.

Metoclopramide was injected intragastrically in this patient just before she took a solid-liquid meal incorporating a polyethylene glycol marker. The drug markedly increased the rate of type II gastric contractions and strikingly increased the rate of gastric emptying.

The mechanism of action of metoclopramide has not been clearly elucidated, but it increases the frequency and amplitude of type II gastric contractions both in health and after vagotomy and enhances gastric emptying in patients having gastric stasis after surgery. More information is needed on the physiologic and therapeutic roles of metoclopramide in diabetic gastroparesis but the current data are encouraging.

▶ [This drug is phonetically similar to another drug used in the treatment of diabetes. — W.G.R.] ◀

Sexual Aspects of the Female Diabetic. Little is documented about the effects of diabetes on female sexuality. Max Ellenberg[3] evaluated sexuality in 54 consecutive female diabetics with clinical neuropathy, as evidenced by absent deep reflexes and by sensory impairment in the feet and toes. Forty-six female diabetics without demonstrable neuropathy were matched with those who had neuropathy for age and duration of diabetes. Most patients were aged 30–60 years, and the vast majority had had diabetes for over 10 years.

There was no difference between the two groups in libido or orgasm. All but 10 patients with neuropathy had libido and orgasmic reaction, as did 38 of the 48 patients without neuropathy. Only 3 patients with neuropathy reported absent libido and orgasm. No patient reported persistence of

---

(3)   Mt. Sinai J. Med. N.Y. 44:495–500, July–Aug., 1977.

libido with loss of orgasmic reaction. The entire spectrum of neuropathic complications was seen in the group with neuropathy, including complications associated with impotence in male diabetics. Other complications such as severe retinopathy, nephropathy including significant azotemia, peripheral vascular disease and severe necrobiosis lipoidica diabeticorum had no apparent effect on sexual performance in the female diabetics.

There is no anatomical, neurologic or physiologic basis to explain observed sexual differences in diabetic females. The emotional attitude toward the partner is of greater importance for female sexual responses than for male responses. An objective measurement of female sexual responsiveness would be helpful in assessment of any effects of diabetes on sexuality in females.

▶ [One wonders if lack of the necessity of having an erection in order for intercourse to occur accounts for this difference between male and female diabetics—i.e., women don't have to "rise to the occasion."—W.G.R.]

Surgical Treatment of Necrobiosis Lipoidica Diabeticorum is outlined by Bruce J. Dubin and Ernest N. Kaplan[4] (Stanford Univ.). Necrobiosis lipoidica diabeticorum (NLD) is a histologically specific degeneration of connective tissue that is usually managed medically, but the plastic surgeon may be called upon to treat patients with refractory cases. Women are predominantly affected, usually between the 3d and 4th decades of life. Most patients present with bilateral involvement of the pretibial regions or ankles. The typical established lesion is an irregular, round or elliptic, well-demarcated plaque with an atrophic, waxy-appearing center. The earliest lesion is often a round, red, firm papule. The lesions are usually asymptomatic. The natural history is variable, but the usual course is of slow, gradual extension over many years, with periods of relative remission. Areas of necrobiosis and an infiltrate of lymphocytes, plasma cells, histiocytes, epithelioid cells and giant cells are found in the corium. Vascular changes are prominent. Lipid deposits are found in the areas of necrobiosis.

Medical management has been largely unsuccessful. Most workers recommend excision and skin grafting for extensively ulcerated lesions. Deep excision in 7 patients led to

---

(4) Plast. Reconstr. Surg. 60:421–428, September, 1977.

freedom from recurrent disease within the treated areas. In the 1 failure the excisions were done at the level of healthy-appearing subcutaneous tissue. In all cases in which deep excision was performed, prominent perforating vessels were found that seemed to underlie the center of each lesion. These vessels may be related in a specific pathogenetic manner to development of the skin lesions. Adequate surgery must include excision of the lesion at the level of the muscular fascia, even if the subcutaneous tissue appears grossly to be free from disease. The indications for surgical treatment should be broadened, and operation should be performed earlier. Severe ulceration was the indication in only 4 of these patients. Two patients had severe pruritus without ulceration, and 1 had severe pain without ulceration. Results were successful in all these patients.

► [Deep excision down to underlying fascia seems to be the key to success here. — W.G.R.] ◄

Abdominal Pain Caused by Diabetic Radiculopathy. Abdominal pain secondary to radiculopathy has been recognized in diabetics, but this relation is poorly documented in the literature. George F. Longstreth and Albert D. Newcomer[5] (Mayo Clinic and Found.) encountered 4 diabetics with significant abdominal pain secondary to radiculopathy in the past few years. In each case the diagnosis was not considered until after an extensive investigation for malignancy, which frequently included invasive procedures, yielded normal results. One patient had abdominal pain of a changing nature, weight loss and preceding thigh pain strongly suggestive of "femoral neuropathy." Diffuse neuropathy and decreased gastrointestinal motility were also present. The second patient had pain that disappeared within several months but also had persistent electromyographic abnormality in the paraspinal muscles. One patient underwent laparotomy before the cause of his pain was discovered; he had subtle neurologic signs reflecting radiculopathy. The fourth patient had extensive investigation for pancreatic malignancy because of abdominal pain and weight loss; he also had a distal sensory and autonomic neuropathy.

Significant abdominal pain secondary to thoracic radiculopathy can develop in diabetics. All these 4 patients had

(5) Ann. Intern. Med. 86:166–168, February, 1977.

adult-onset diabetes. Onset of pain was gradual and initially intermittent, but later pain became more frequent or constant. It was described as a pressure discomfort or sharp pain in the upper abdomen and sometimes in the lower chest and the region of the thoracic spine. Only 2 patients described paresthesia. Anorexia and weight loss were prominent in 3 cases. Neurologic clues to radiculopathy were subtle in the 2 patients who manifested them. Electromyography showed evidence of involvement of many thoracic or lumbar nerve roots, or both, in all cases. Pancreatic carcinoma was a major consideration in some cases. The differential diagnosis includes pain from varicella-zoster. Radiculopathy should be considered in the diabetic with abdominal pain of obscure origin, and if radiculopathy is suspected, electromyography should be performed.

► [This is getting radiculous! – W.G.R.] ◄

The following review articles are recommended to the reader:

Bar, R. S., and Roth, J.: Insulin receptor status in disease states of man, Arch. Intern. Med. 137:474, 1977.

Chuchinov, R. H., and Daughaday, W. H.: Current concepts of somatomedin and other biologically related growth factors, Diabetes 25:994, 1976.

Felig, P., et al.: Amino acid and protein metabolism in diabetes mellitus, Arch. Intern. Med. 137:507, 1977.

────── Insulin, glucagon and somatostatin in normal physiology and diabetes mellitus, Diabetes 25:1091, 1976.

Ganda, O. P., and Soeldner, S.: Genetic, acquired and related factors in the etiology of diabetes mellitus, Arch. Intern. Med. 137:461, 1977.

Herberg, L., and Coleman, D. L.: Laboratory animals exhibiting obesity and diabetes syndromes, Metabolism 26:59, 1977.

Kitabchi, A.: Proinsulin and C peptide: A review, Metabolism 26:547, 1977.

McGarry, J. D., and Foster, D. W.: Hormonal control of ketogenesis, Arch. Intern. Med. 137:495, 1977.

Marble, A.: Late complications of diabetes: A continuing challenge, Diabetologica 12:193, 1976.

Rubenstein, A. H., et al.: Clinical significance of circulating C peptide in diabetes mellitus and hypoglycemic disorders, Arch. Intern, Med. 137:625, 1977.

Schade, D. S., and Eaton R. P.: The controversy concerning counterregulatory hormone secretion: A hypothesis for the prevention of diabetic ketoacidosis? Diabetes 26:596, 1977.

Shen, S.-W., and Bressler, R.: Clinical pharmacology of oral antidiabetic agents: Part I, N. Engl. J. Med. 296:493, 1977.

———— Part II, N. Engl. J. Med. 296:787, 1977.

Unger, R. H., and Orci, L.: Role of glucagon in diabetes, Arch. Intern. Med. 137:482, 1977.

Williamson, J. R., and Kilo, C.: Current status of capillary basement membrane disease in diabetes mellitus, Diabetes 26:65, 1977.

Winegrad, A. I., and Greene, D. A.: Diabetic polyneuropathy: The importance of insulin deficiency, hyperglycemia and alterations in myoinositol metabolism in its pathogenesis, N. Engl. J. Med. 295:1416, 1976.

Hypoglycemia and Glucagon

Familial Hyperglucagonemia: Autosomal Dominant Disorder. All cases of hyperglucagonemia reported to date have been sporadic. Guenther Boden and Oliver E. Owen[6] (Temple Univ.) report a hereditary form of hyperglucagonemia, discovered in the family of a patient with the clinical glucagonoma syndrome. Four relatives of the patient had elevated plasma levels of immunoreactive glucagon that persisted throughout observation periods of 22–25 hours, as well as over several weeks during which levels were measured sporadically. The subjects also exhibited distinct abnormalities in the release and suppression of immunoreactive glucagon.

The family's pedigree is shown in Figure 67. Glucagon levels remained elevated throughout observations in all 5 subjects; 3 had several major peaks, some clearly related to food intake. No major declines in glucagon followed intravenous glucose infusion. Subnormal responses to intravenous arginine were noted in most subjects. One patient had supranormal basal insulin levels, no immunoreactive insulin response to intravenous glucose and diabetic glucose tolerance. About two thirds of immunoreactive glucagon in fasting plasma from the symptomatic subject eluted with the glucagon marker on gel filtration of the plasma. Most activity from the asymptomatic subjects eluted between the proinsulin marker and void volume and within the void volume, and less than 15% eluted in the region of the glucagon marker.

The finding of hyperglucagonemia in 5 of 10 members of this family suggests a familial disorder. The data are most compatible with autosomal dominant mode of inheritance. The prevalence of familial hyperglucagonemia is not known. In view of the long, benign course of the disease in the propositus and since no tumor was found in any asymp-

---

(6) N. Engl. J. Med. 296:534–538, Mar. 10, 1977.

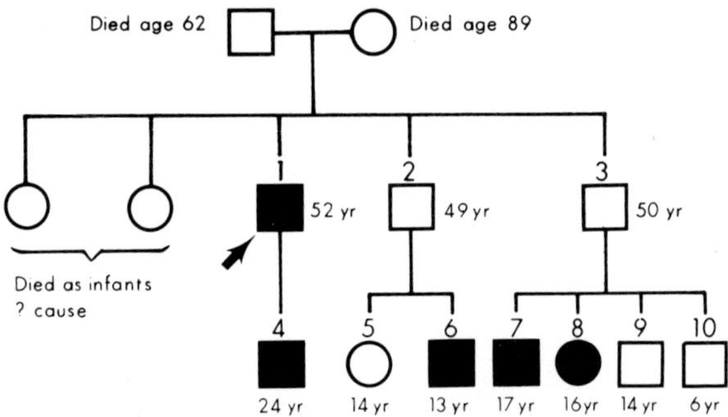

Fig 67. – Pedigree of a family with hyperglucagonemia. The propositus is indicated by the arrow. Subjects with hyperglucagonemia are indicated by the closed symbols and those with normal immunoreactive glucagon values by the open symbols. (Courtesy of Boden, G., and Owen, O. E.: N. Engl. J. Med. 296:534–538, Mar. 10, 1977.)

tomatic subject, it was decided not to carry out surgical exploration but rather to follow all subjects semiannually.

► [Perhaps this is a forme fruste of multiple endocrine neoplasia, type I? –W.G.R.] ◄

Salivary Gland Hyperglycemic Factor: Extrapancreatic Source of Glucagon-like Material. There is considerable molecular heterogeneity among, and several sources of, circulating immunoreactive glucagons, and "pancreatic-specific" antiserums raised to pancreatic glucagon can cross-react with some nonislet glucagons. A. M. Lawrence, S. Tan, S. Hojvat and L. Kirsteins[7] (VA Hosp., Hines, Ill.) have found a significant amount of a large immunoreactive glucagon-like material in the submaxillary salivary glands of rabbits, rats and mice and a measurable amount in the submaxillary glands of human beings. Insignificant amounts are present in the parotid and sublingual glands of rodents and man. The material, which is urea stable, shows identical immunoassay dilution curves when measured with the highly specific K-30 glucagon antiserum. Low concentrations of glucose stimulate and high concentrations suppress release of the material. Arginine promotes its brisk release in vitro. Somatostatin does not influence arginine-stimulated secretion and insignificantly suppresses basal release in vitro. Injections of immunoequivalent amounts of

---

(7)   Science 195:70–72, Aug. 6, 1976.

the glucagon from rat gland elicited a hyperglycemic effect comparable with that obtained with porcine pancreatic glucagon.

The findings support speculations that the salivary glands may possess endocrine as well as exocrine functions. Salivary gland glucagon may be the source of the circulating glucagon reported in pancreatectomized and eviscerated rats. It seems likely that the extremely high levels of pancreatic glucagon found in poorly controlled diabetics may contribute to early acceleration of ketogenesis and hepatic glycogenolysis and gluconeogenesis. It is also possible that in the severely insulinopenic diabetic, glucagons of extra-pancreatic sources contribute to measurements of total circulating glucagon. Further study is needed to determine the biologic significance of the release of a large glucagon-like material, possibly a proglucagon, from the submaxillary gland.

▶ [There is a chap in Chicago, who shall remain nameless, who claims that extirpation of submaxillary glands helps diabetic retinopathy. Most of us think this is quackery, but I accused Doctor Lawrence of exonerating him with this study. — W.G.R.] ◄

Hypoglycemia in Man: Pathologic and Physiologic Variants. Thomas J. Merimee and John E. Tyson[8] determined whether an effective means exists to distinguish the physiologic hypoglycemia of fasting from pathologic hypoglycemia. Fasts were conducted for 72 hours in 60 women and 20 men of normal weight, 16 obese subjects and 6 of 11 patients with proved insulinoma. The obese patients exceeded ideal body weight by 25–45%. Subjects fasted after receiving a 150 to 200-gm carbohydrate diet for 2 weeks. Activity was similar after admission for all subjects. Two of the 6 insulinoma patients exceeded ideal body weight by 10–20%.

Only the pattern of change of the immunoreactive insulin-to-glucose ratio (I/G) ratio calculated at major intervals of the fast provided a clear distinction between the groups. Plasma glucose values alone did not make the distinction. In no instance did the mean I/G ratio during fasting equal or exceed the control value in a subject of normal weight. Ratios rose dramatically during fasting in all insulinoma pa-

---

(8)   Diabetes 26:161–165, March, 1977.

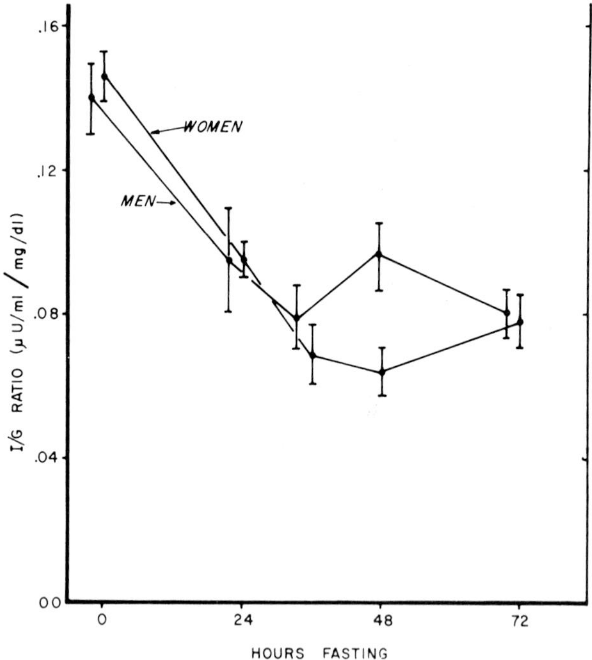

Fig 68.—Insulin-glucose ratios are shown at 0, 24, 48 and 72 hours of fasting for 60 women and 20 men of normal weight. All points are $\bar{X} \pm$ SEM. The I/G ratio of men differed from that of women only at the 48-hour sampling period (P < 0.05). (Courtesy of Merimee, T. J., and Tyson, J. E.: Diabetes 26:161–165, March, 1977.)

tients. Normal obese patients did not exhibit glucose values below 55 mg/dl. The findings in normal subjects are shown in Figure 68. The basal I/G ratio alone was potentially misleading because of overlap between subjects with simple obesity and insulinoma patients. Change in the I/G ratio was independent of the techniques used to measure glucose and insulin.

Although plasma glucose values often decrease to 40 mg/dl or less in women during a short-term fast, I/G ratios decline in a characteristic manner. When the I/G ratio increases during a fast, hypoglycemia secondary to an insulin-producing tumor can be predicted. A consistent increase in the I/G ratio, rather than an arbitrary, absolute figure for the basal ratio, is the primary diagnostic feature.

▶ [Doctor Merimee's interesting observations on the hypoglycemia of fasting were included in the 1976 YEAR BOOK (p. 221), and it was surprising to see the low blood sugar levels (<35 mg/dl) achieved with fasting in some normal women. This follow-up study shows that the change in the I/G ratio with fasting distinguishes the normal subject from the patient with an islet cell adenoma. — W.G.R.] ◀

Nonautonomous Function of a Pancreatic Insulinoma. Elliot J. Rayfield, Marie Pulini, Avrum Golub, Arthur H. Rubenstein and David L. Horwitz[9] report data on a patient with a pancreatic beta cell tumor who did not become significantly hypoglycemic during a 72-hour fast and who exhibited almost complete suppression of C peptide reactivity (CPR) after an infusion of exogenous insulin.

Woman, 56, presented with weakness, visual blurring and sweating of 7 years' duration, not triggered by fasting or exercise and occurring at any time of the day. She had a 1-year history of hypertension, treated with 50 mg hydrochlorothiazide daily and 5 mg diazepam 3 times daily. A thyroid nodule was detected. Fasting hypoglycemia was never documented during two hospitalizations or on three glucose tolerance tests done on an outpatient basis. The lowest fasting plasma glucose recorded was 56 mg/dl. Symptoms occurred during hypoglycemic phases of tolbutamide and glucose tolerance tests and an insulin suppression test. Laparotomy revealed a pancreatic adenoma, which was removed and found to be a beta cell lesion. No recurrence of hypoglycemic episodes had been noted 6 months postoperatively, when an oral glucose tolerance test was normal.

Plasma glucose remained above 50 mg/dl during a 72-hour fast. The tumor contained 23.8 units immunoreactive insulin per gm, a level compatible with insulinoma. Stimulation tests with tolbutamide and glucose were more helpful in making a diagnosis than were suppression tests in this case. The tumor may have retained a capacity to respond normally to both decreases and increases in plasma glucose. The overall release of insulin was presumably larger than normal because of the larger number of beta cells in the tumor.

Pancreatic beta cell tumors, like other endocrine tumors, may exhibit a spectrum from autonomous to nonautonomous function.

▶ [Since pseudohypoglycemia is so prevalent in our population, separating the "wheat from the chaff," so to speak, is an exercise we have been

---

(9) J. Clin. Endocrinol. Metab. 43:1307–1311, December, 1976.

called on to do not infrequently. The existence of patients such as this one certainly doesn't make the job any easier. — W.G.R.] ◄

Insulin, Proinsulin, Glucagon and Gastrin in Pancreatic Tumors and in Plasma of Patients with Organic Hyperinsulinism. Few studies have compared basal and stimulated plasma insulin and proinsulin concentrations with the contents in islet neoplasms. Masaki Hayashi, John C. Floyd, Jr., Sumer Pek and Stefan S. Fajans[1] (Univ. of Michigan) quantitated various hormones in extracts of tumors from 27 patients with pancreatic islet cell neoplasms, in 1 patient with nesidioblastosis, in extracts of uninvolved pancreas from 11 tumor patients and in 15 control pancreata. Eighteen patients had solitary adenomas, 6 had adenomatosis and 3 had carcinomas. Twenty-two patients had received diazoxide orally or by infusion.

Mean insulin concentrations in solitary adenomas and adenomas of patients with adenomatosis were higher than in control organs, but in all patients except 1 the concentration was lower than in islet tissue of control pancreas, assuming that islet volume is 1% of the pancreas. Percentage proinsulin was elevated in 52% of tumors. Adenoma insulin content correlated with increments in plasma insulin after tolbutamide administration. Insulin and proinsulin were not suppressed in uninvolved pancreas. Fasting plasma glucagon concentration was elevated in patients with islet cell adenomatosis and with islet cell carcinoma. The mean concentration of glucagon in tumors was lower than that in control pancreata. Some adenomas had elevated concentrations of gastrin.

Insulin-secreting islet cell tumors have a decreased storage capacity for insulin. Elevated tumor amounts of proinsulin may be due to decreased insulin storage capacity and in some cases to decreased conversion to insulin also. Solitary adenomas may also contain excess amounts of pancreatic hormones other than insulin. Elevated plasma glucagon concentrations in patients with organic hyperinsulinism may indicate malignancy, microadenomatosis or multiple endocrine adenoma syndrome. Hypergastrinemia may have the same significance in patients presenting with fasting hypoglycemia and hyperinsulinemia. Chronic hyperin-

---

(1)   J. Clin. Endocrinol. Metab. 44:681–694, April, 1977.

sulinism and hypoglycemia due to adenoma do not suppress the insulin and proinsulin contents of uninvolved pancreas.

► [The most interesting aspect of this study for me is the finding of multiple hormones within a single adenoma. — W.G.R.] ◄

Hypoglycemia Secondary to Metastases to the Liver: Case Report and Review of the Literature. Only 8 cases of hypoglycemia resulting from metastatic liver disease have been reported. Syed Younus, J. Soterakis, A. J. Sossi, S. K. Chawla and P. A. LoPresti[2] (Queens Hosp. Center, Jamaica, N. Y.) describe a patient who had hypoglycemia as a result of prostatic carcinoma metastatic to the liver.

Man, 76, presented in coma 7 years after surgery for prostatic carcinoma. He had had hematuria for the past 4 years, and bladder metastases had been documented and treated by cobalt therapy and a permanent cystostomy. A nodular liver was felt 6 cm below the costal margin. The patient regained consciousness when given 50 ml of 50% dextrose; the initial serum glucose concentration was 36 mg/100 ml. A liver scan showed multiple filling defects consistent with metastatic disease (Fig 69) and a biopsy showed carcinoma consistent with prostatic tumor. The serum immunoreactive insulin value was below 1μU/ml at a serum glucose concentration of 39 mg/100 ml. Constant intravenous and oral glucose administration was necessary to prevent severe hypoglycemia. The patient

Fig 69 (left). — Liver scan before chemotherapy.
Fig 70 (right). — Liver scan after chemotherapy.
(Courtesy of Younus, S., et al.: Gastroenterology 72:334–337, February, 1977.)

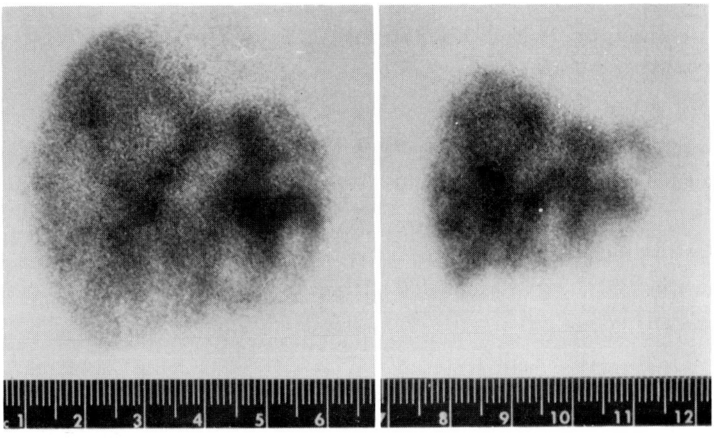

(2)   Gastroenterology 72:334–337, February, 1977.

was treated with Cytoxan and 5-fluorouracil for 3 weeks, with some decrease in glucose requirements, but marrow suppression occurred and chemotherapy was stopped. Reinstitution of treatment, with diethylstilbestrol added, further reduced the glucose requirement, and the liver became smaller (Fig 70). The patient had no hypoglycemic symptoms a year after admission. He has since been lost to follow-up.

The rarity of hypoglycemia associated with diffuse liver disease reflects the great reserve capacity of the liver to maintain normal glucose levels. A humoral hypoglycemic factor seems unlikely in this case, since immunoreactive insulin was not elevated. Chemotherapy appeared to reduce the size of the metastases, which were probably consuming excessive amounts of glucose; a decreased glucose requirement resulted. Symptomatic hypoglycemia in a patient with metastatic liver disease can be alleviated by chemotherapy, through a reduction in the size and number of metastatic nodules in the liver.

► [One wonders if a humoral substance such as nonsuppressible insulin-like activity soluble in ethanol (NSILA-S), as reported by Roth et al. in patients with non-insulin-producing mesenchymal tumors, was present. – W.G.R.] ◄

Hypoglycemia of Infancy and Nesidioblastosis: Studies with Somatostatin. Harry J. Hirsch, Sherry Loo, Nancy Evans, John F. Crigler, Jr., Robert M. Filler and Kenneth H. Gabbay[3] (Boston) used somatostatin to investigate the pancreatic endocrine dysfunction in an infant with severe intractable hypoglycemia, inappropriately elevated insulin levels and nesidioblastosis. Nesidioblastosis is characterized by beta cells and small islets arising from the pancreatic ductules.

Female infant, admitted to Children's Hospital, Boston, at age 2 months, had been noted at age 2 hours to be hypoglycemic and to have seizures despite prednisone and diazoxide therapy. The patient was hypotonic and responded minimally to auditory or visual stimuli. After somatostatin studies, an 80% pancreatectomy was performed at age 4 months, with some improvement in glucose homeostasis. Half of the remaining pancreatic tissue was resected at age 9 months, with considerable improvement. Neurologic and developmental evaluations at age 1 year were normal. The pancreatic pathology was consistent with nesidioblastosis. A glucose infusion of 0.75 gm per kg of body weight per hour was needed to main-

---

(3) N. Engl. J. Med. 296:1323 – 1326, June 9, 1977.

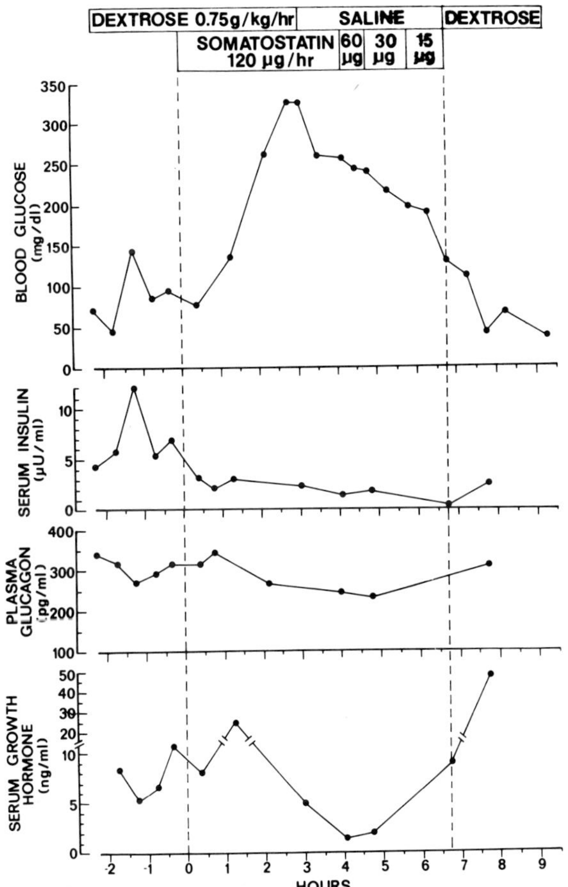

Fig 71.—Effect of somatostatin infusion on blood glucose and immunoreactive insulin, glucagon and growth hormone levels. (Courtesy of Hirsch, H. J., et al.: N. Engl. J. Med. 296:1323–1326, June 9, 1977.)

tain a mean preprandial blood glucose of 37 mg/dl. The effects of somatostatin infusion are shown in Figure 71. Insulin was suppressed within 20 minutes of the start of the infusion and preceded the rise in blood glucose by about 1 hour. Subcutaneous injections of protamine zinc somatostatin produced higher preprandial blood glucose levels for 4–5 days. Better maintenance of the blood glucose was observed on withdrawal of the infusion after a 50-µg injection of protamine zinc somatostatin.

Idiopathic hypoglycemia of infancy has been associated with pancreatic nesidioblastosis, and the association was striking in the present patient. The presence of nests of pure beta cells within the pancreas, unassociated with other cell types, may explain the apparent defect in basal and, perhaps, stimulated insulin secretion. Idiopathic hypoglycemia of infancy appears to be a disorder of basal insulin regulation secondary to the histologic features of nesidioblastosis. Subtotal pancreatectomy remains the main effective treatment of this condition.

► [Not only is somatostatin useful in hyperglycemic states, here it was of short-term use in the management of hypoglycemia. — W.G.R.] ◄

Lunchtime Gin and Tonic a Cause of Reactive Hypoglycemia. Reactive hypoglycemia occurs in a large proportion of normal subjects ingesting pure glucose solutions on an empty stomach, but only a few manifest neuroglycopenic symptoms. Relatively large amounts of sugar are taken on an empty stomach in the form of soft drinks used as mixers to dilute alcohol, and alcohol can itself cause hypoglycemia under certain conditions. Stephen J. D. O'Keefe and Vincent Marks[4] (Guildford, England) studied the combined effects of alcohol and glucose on the production of reactive hypoglycemia in 10 normal subjects, none of them heavy drinkers. A dose of 50 gm ethanol was given in 143 ml water plus 730 ml of either Schweppes tonic water containing 61.4 gm carbohydrate, mainly as sucrose, or Slimline Schweppes tonic containing 0.5 gm carbohydrate. Drinks were taken in 145-ml volumes at about 10-minute intervals in the 1st hour.

In no subject did the blood glucose fall below 2.5 mmol/L with Slimline tonic, and plasma insulin remained below the limit of accurate measurement. Addition of alcohol to the carbohydrate solution increased the maximal plasma insulin response by about 100%, and the plasma insulin remained higher for a longer time than after tonic water alone (Fig 72). There was a significantly greater hypoglycemic rebound after the gin and tonic than after tonic alone. Blood alcohol levels rose similarly after both alcoholic drinks. Less mood change occurred with the low-carbohydrate drink, and neuroglycopenia did not occur.

A combination of sucrose and alcohol results in a more

(4) Lancet 1:1286–1288, June 18, 1977.

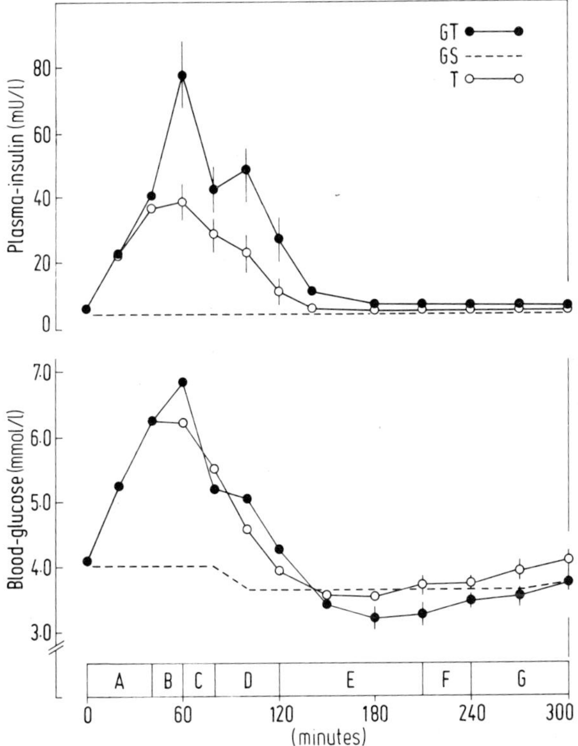

Fig 72.—Mean plasma insulin and blood glucose levels in 10 healthy subjects given gin and tonic *(GT)*, gin and Slimline tonic *(GS)* or tonic alone *(T)* on three different occasions. Significant differences between GT and T are indicated by insertion of the SEM. *A*, normal and hungry. *B*, mild intoxication, cheerful, talkative, progressive loss of inhibitions, loss of hunger. *C*, mild ataxia, minor speech disturbances, less cheerful, less drunk. *D*, mood change (depressed), becoming sleepy. *E*, very sleepy, feeling chilled (neuroglycopenic stage). *F*, recovery, awake. *G*, very hungry, occasional headache. Drinks consumed during first 60 minutes. (Courtesy of O'Keefe, S. J. D., and Marks, V.: Lancet 1:1286–1288, June 18, 1977.)

profound hypoglycemic "overswing" than does sugar alone, apparently due to a greater insulin response to gin and tonic than to tonic alone. Since neuroglycopenia, like alcohol intoxication, can seriously impair intellectual activity and judgment, this effect is of social and economic importance. Ingesting the same amount of alcohol without added sugar or going without food altogether is not associated with the same risk of acquiring hypoglycemia. Very few persons know the alcohol content of their drinks, let alone their carbohydrate content, and the observations are of concern, particularly to those involved with automobiles and other aspects of safety.

► [No wonder the British are in economic trouble! Their businessmen need to switch to the three-martini tax-deductible lunch to avoid the hypoglycemic mental impairment. — W.G.R.] ◄

Hepatic Glycogen Synthetase Deficiency: Definition of Syndrome from Metabolic and Enzyme Studies on Nine-Year-Old Girl. Hepatic glycogen synthetase deficiency leading to inability to synthesize glycogen is a rare cause of hypoglycemia in childhood. Identical twins with the defect were described by Lewis et al. in 1963, but no further cases have been detected. A. Aynsley-Green, D. H. Williamson and R. Gitzelmann[5] report metabolic and enzyme studies on a girl that prove the existence of the enzyme defect.

Girl, 9, had exhibited behavior changes and drowsiness in the morning in infancy when daytime feeding was established, which were reversed by food. Occasional morning seizures developed at age 7, and at age 7½ the patient was examined and found to be small but not otherwise physically abnormal. She was drowsy and disoriented in the morning, with a fasting blood glucose concentration of 20 mg/100 ml, and the urine gave a strong reaction for ketone bodies. Glycosuria consistently developed during the day after meals. Hyperglycemia and hyperlactatemia followed feeding. After 18 months the liver was palpable at 1 cm. The IQ was normal. Metabolic studies and liver and abdominal wall muscle biopsies confirmed hepatic glycogen synthetase deficiency. The patient was told to take protein-rich meals every 4 hours during the day and night. She had not had any seizures 6 months later and was alert on waking. Her height velocity increased from 4.8 cm per year before treatment to 8.8 cm per year during this period.

Metabolic profiles showed fasting hypoglycemia and hyperketonemia but normal lactate in this patient and hyperglycemia and hyperlactatemia after meals. Glucagon caused a rise in glucose 3 hours after a meal, with a fall in lactate and alanine; no such effect was seen after a 12-hour fast. Normal increments in glucose followed oral galactose or alanine. Biopsies showed subnormal hepatic glycogen con-

___

(5) Arch. Dis. Child. 52:573–579, July, 1977.

tent but normal muscle content. Glycogen synthetase was virtually absent from liver but fully active in muscle.

It is postulated that some children with "ketotic hypoglycemia" may have hepatic glycogen synthetase deficiency. A feature of this syndrome is failure of gluconeogenesis to maintain the blood glucose concentration in the fasting state. Failure to release alanine from peripheral muscle probably contributes to the fasting hypoglycemia. Periods of starvation must be prevented; glucose alone is unsatisfactory. Small meals rich in protein, given at 3- or 4-hour intervals, led to dramatic improvement in this patient.

► [This is another unusual cause of hypoglycemia. — W.G.R.] ◄

A Test of Hypothesis That Rate of Fall in Glucose Concentration Triggers Counterregulatory Hormonal Responses in Man. There is clinical evidence, largely anecdotal, that hypoglycemic symptoms can occur in response to a falling glucose concentration before absolute hypoglycemia is present. Ralph A. DeFronzo, Reubin Andres, Turner A. Bledsoe, Gunther Boden, Gerald A. Faloona and Jordan D. Tobin[6] tested this hypothesis in 5 normal young male volunteers within 20% of desirable body weight, evaluated after a 12-hour fast. The arterial blood glucose was acutely raised 200 mg/100 ml above the basal level for 1 hour by a continuous glucose infusion and was then allowed to fall spontaneously.

No increases in plasma growth hormone, cortisol, glucagon or catecholamines occurred while the blood glucose remained above fasting levels, despite a rapid fall in the glucose level. Growth hormone, cortisol and catecholamines were released when the mean blood glucose reached 28 mg/100 ml, 39 mg/100 ml and 39 mg/100 ml, respectively, below the fasting level. Plasma glucagon was suppressed during hyperglycemia and increased as the blood glucose fell below basal levels; it returned to fasting values when the nadir in blood glucose was reached. The plasma insulin response to a rapid fall in blood glucose lagged behind the fall in blood glucose. By the time the fasting glucose level was reached, the plasma insulin was still nearly three times the basal level.

The most important determinant of blood glucose in this

---

(6) Diabetes 26:445–452, May, 1977.

study appeared to be the plasma insulin concentration. In a sense, the hypoglycemia observed is a result of the time course of the fall in insulin being too slow to prevent hypoglycemia from occurring, and of the counterregulatory hormones being ineffective until hypoglycemia occurs. Hypoglycemia is a prerequisite to the release of the counterregulatory hormones. The findings may not be applicable to diabetics with long-standing hyperglycemia, in whom counterregulatory hormones may be released at a different level.

► [I never believed the hypothesis, and this study supports that bias. —W.G.R.] ◄

Pancreatic Calcifications in Malignant Islet Cell Tumors. Calcification in islet cell tumors of the pancreas is infrequent. H. Imhof and P. Frank[7] (Univ. of Chicago) reviewed 623 malignant pancreatic tumors encountered in 1945–75, 23 of which were islet cell tumors, and found 2 with calcifications. None of the 71 benign islet cell tumors seen in 1962–75 had radiologically visible calcifications.

Man, 42, presented with diarrhea and bulky stools. He had a history of partial thyroidectomy for nodular goiter. Pancreatic insufficiency was diagnosed, and a duodenal bulb ulcer was found, as well as a malabsorption pattern and calcification in the tail of the pancreas. Gastric hypersecretion was documented. Continuous abdominal pain and increasing diarrhea developed about 2 years after presentation, and there was upper gastrointestinal bleeding. Penetrating ulcers were found in the pylorus and 3d part of the duodenum. Laparotomy showed two metastatic nodules in the liver, which were found on biopsy to be islet cell tumors. Vagotomy and pyloroplasty were performed. Several gastric and duodenal ulcers were documented in the next year, with calcification in the pancreatic tail (Fig 73). Operation revealed a tumor with calcification in the pancreatic tail, and total gastrectomy, esophagojejunostomy and left hepatectomy were performed. The patient was lost to follow-up 3 years postoperatively.

Eight other cases of calcification in islet cell tumor have been reported. Calcification in pancreatic adenocarcinoma is rare, though mucin-producing lesions may calcify and produce calcified metastases. The calcification in islet cell tumors is focal, coarse and nodular. Many patients have had a long history; the rate of tumor growth was slow in all cases

---

(7)   Radiology 122:333–337, February, 1977.

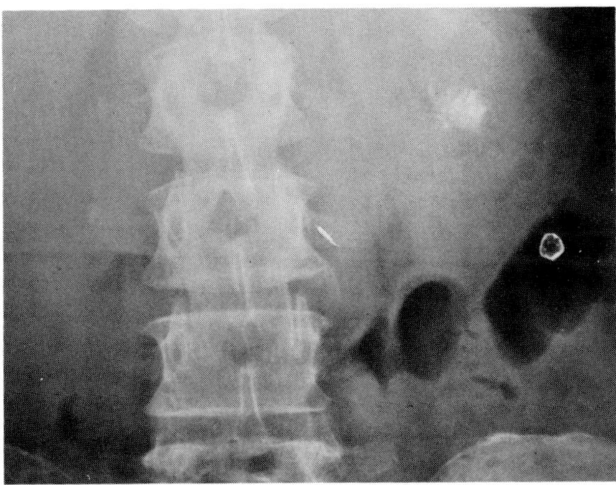

Fig 73.—Abdominal film showing calcifications in tail of pancreas. Calcifications to left of T12, L1 and L2 represent calcifications in abdominal aorta. (Courtesy of Imhof, H., and Frank, P.: Radiology 122:333–337, February, 1977.)

but 1. The pattern of calcification can usually be distinguished from that of chronic pancreatitis. Seven of 10 cases of calcified islet cell tumor have been malignant.

▶ [This is an unusual finding, but if it is present it strongly suggests malignancy. — W.G.R.] ◀

Insulin Receptors in Patients with Insulinomas: Changes in Receptor Affinity and Concentration. The insulin receptor appears to be a major site for the regulation of target cell responsiveness, and insulin is capable of directly modulating the concentration of insulin receptors. Robert S. Bar, Phillip Gorden, Jesse Roth and Carolyn W. Siebert[8] (Natl. Inst. of Health) found an inverse relationship between insulin receptor concentration and the basal level of circulating insulin in 5 patients with insulinomas. Substantial changes in affinity of insulin receptors were detected in 3 of the patients. The patients received 2,500 to 3,500-calorie diets with 45% carbohydrate for at least 3 days before insulin receptor studies.

The concentration of insulin receptors was inversely related to the circulating insulin level in these patients, as was previously observed in obese patients and in thin dia-

---

(8)   J. Clin. Endocrinol. Metab. 44:1210–1213, June, 1977.

betics. The 1 patient with normal circulating insulin had a normal receptor concentration. Receptor affinities were entirely normal in 2 patients, supranormal in 2 and subnormal in 1. Up to fivefold elevations in receptor affinity were observed in 1 patient, but normal receptor affinity and receptor concentration were noted after removal of the tumor, along with a return to normal of insulin and glucose metabolism.

Correlations with the clinical state in patients with insulinoma are clearer when receptor concentration, and especially receptor affinity, are considered in addition to the circulating insulin and proinsulin levels. The decrease in receptor concentration in patients with insulinoma appears to be a direct result of the hyperinsulinemia, but the molecular mechanisms responsible for the changes in receptor affinity are unknown. The fact that several clinical states are characterized by elevated affinities and others by depressed affinities suggests that multiple mediators of receptor affinity exist, providing rapid and sensitive adjustments of the insulin receptor.

► [Further evidence is presented that what I like to call the "feed-forward" mechanism is operative in controlling hormonal action and, in this case, in helping to protect against hypoglycemia. — W.G.R.] ◄

Lipid Metabolism and Obesity

Triglyceride Storage Disease: Defect in Activation of Lipolysis in Adipose Tissue. Triglyceride storage disease is an uncommon group of disorders with excessive or abnormal accumulation of extralysosomal triglyceride, associated with a metabolic defect in the paths of triglyceride mobilization (lipolysis). David J. Galton, Christine H. Gilbert, James J. Lucey and John A. Walker-Smith[9] (St. Bartholomew's Hosp., London) report autopsy and metabolic findings in a child with failure of activation of adenyl cyclase by catecholamines and abnormal triglyceride deposits in peripheral adipose tissue.

Microcephalic girl, weighing 2.4 kg at birth, had soft tissue swellings over the extremities and markedly impaired motor and social development. Severe feeding difficulties and infections led to emaciation by age 9 months, but the limb deposits persisted. At age 5 years the child was grossly emaciated, weighing 8.2 kg (Fig 74). She died at age 6 years 3 months of extensive bronchopneumonia. Examination at age 4 had shown severe limb spasticity, blindness with nystagmus and deafness. Optic atrophy and hepatomegaly were present. Serum triglyceride concentration was 182 mg/100 ml. Lipoprotein electrophoresis, plasma proteins and fasting glucose were normal. Skin biopsy showed increased focal extension of adipose tissue into the dermis.

Autopsy showed a microcephalic brain, with gross ventricular dilatation, bronchopneumonia and abnormal subcutaneous fat deposits (Fig 75). In the brain the normal layering of cortical neurons was lost and abnormal aggregates of neurons were seen in many areas. Many neurons were poorly developed, and the white matter exhibited areas of spongiosis and demyelination. Hepatic fat deposits were present mainly in the centrilobular zones and also in the Kupffer cells. The triglyceride content of isolated adipocytes was reduced. Basal levels of cyclic adenosine monophosphate were greater than in adult adipose tissue, but no stimulation was seen after isoprenaline incubation.

---

(9) Pediatrics 59:442–447, March, 1977.

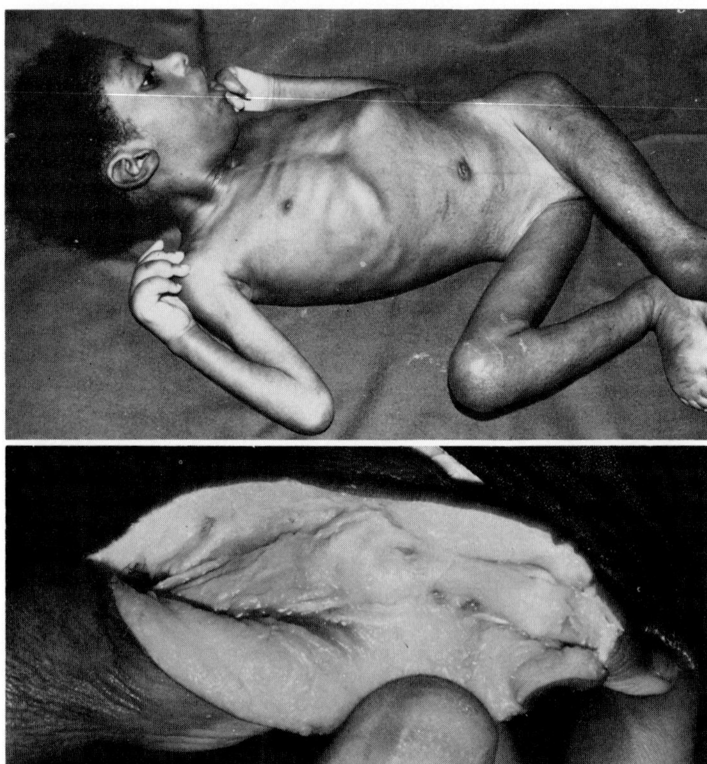

Fig 74 (top). — Appearance at age 5 years 3 months.
Fig 75 (bottom). — Appearance of right 2d finger at autopsy, showing deposits of adipose tissue despite gross emaciation.
(Courtesy of Galton, D. J., et al.: Pediatrics 59:442–447, March, 1977.)

The effects of profound emaciation on lipolysis are unknown. The finding of severe cachexia with peripheral triglyceride deposits in adipose tissue is good evidence for a storage disorder. The only metabolic defect found in the abnormal tissue in this patient was a defect in lipolysis. It is possible that the metabolic defect contributed to the storage disorder, and that a defect of adenyl cyclase in the brain contributed to the neuron abnormalities.

► [I included this article primarily because the only triglyceride storage disease of which I was previously aware is simple obesity. — W.G.R.] ◄

Chorionic Gonadotropin in Weight Control: Double-Blind Crossover Study. The efficacy of human chorionic gonadotropin (hCG) in weight reduction programs has been controversial. Previous controlled studies have involved small numbers of patients or have deviated from the injection schedule originally proposed by Simeons. Robert L. Young, Robert J. Fuchs and Myron J. Woltjen[1] performed a double-blind, controlled, crossover study of 202 patients treated with hCG and a saline placebo in a weight reduction program. Serial measurements of weight and skin-fold thickness were made, and subjective patient responses were assessed. The dietary program was designed to follow that of Simeons, involving a 500-calorie diet, begun after the first 2 days of injections. Patients received injections of 120 units of hCG or placebo 6 days a week. A gradual increase in calories was allowed after 6 weeks of injections, and after a 6-week maintenance period, injections were given for another 6 weeks. All patients had a calculated excess of at least 18.2 kg fat and were aged 18 or over.

No difference in weight loss or change in percentage body fat was found in patients who completed the first series of injections, and changes in the subsequent maintenance phase did not differ between the two groups. No differences in change in skin-fold thickness were observed. Significantly greater weight and body fat losses occurred in the first than in the second treatment phase in both groups. After the crossover phase, the overall mean weight losses were 6.8 kg on hCG and 7 kg on placebo. The respective overall percentage body fat losses were 3.2 and 3.4. Dropout rates were comparable during hCG and placebo administration. No patient missed more than three consecutive injections. No significant differences in subjective response were found during hCG and placebo injections.

No significant difference between hCG and placebo injections was observed in this study of patients participating in a weight reduction program. There was no evidence of better weight loss maintenance as a result of hCG injections. A second course of management was less effective regardless of the injection given during the first course.

▶ [This form of treatment has received attention in previous YEAR BOOKS. One hopes these are the final words on the subject.

---

(1)   J.A.M.A. 236:2495–2497, Nov. 29, 1976.

I was asked by one of the local medical societies last year to review the records of a physician who had an inordinate number of patients with Fröhlich's syndrome in his practice. He said he saw so many because he specialized in obesity, just as a hematologist would expect to see many patients with leukemia. He was treating his patients with a "pituitary extract," which—you guessed it—turned out to be hCG. Needless to say, his patients had likely examples of pseudo-Fröhlich's syndrome.—W.G.R.] ◄

Spontaneous and Experimental Human Obesity: Effects of Diet and Adipose Cell Size on Lipolysis and Lipogenesis. The mechanisms by which caloric imbalance occurs in the obese have not been completely elucidated. If the adipocyte is the site for signals about caloric stores, studies of adipose tissue from lean subjects before and after weight gain and from obese subjects before and after weight loss might show differences that would persist after correcting for the number of adipocytes. G. A. Bray, J. A. Glennon, L. B. Salans, E. S. Horton, E. Danforth, Jr., and E. A. H. Sims[2] evaluated this hypothesis in 8 normal subjects and 7 obese patients. Five normal subjects completed the weight-gain part of the study, eating increased amounts of food to gain weight. The obese patients lost weight by caloric restriction until the size of their fat cells was nearly normal. A diet of 1800 kcal/sq m/day was given, with either 100 or 300 gm carbohydrate/sq m/day. Lipogenesis was evaluated with use of C-pyruvate-3.[14]

The small fat cells from obese patients showed no significant stimulation of lipogenesis by glucose and no effect of dietary carbohydrate intake. In studies on lypolysis there was a positive and significant correlation between release of glycerol and fat cell size. With large fat cells the response to isoproterenol was stimulated two- to fourfold in the presence of 1 μg/ml, especially during the high-carbohydrate diet, but small fat cells showed little stimulatory effect of isoproterenol on glycerol release. Glycerol release in response to dibutyryl cyclic adenosine monophosphate (AMP) was similar in large fat cells from nonobese subjects and obese subjects on the high-carbohydrate diet, but the small cells of obese subjects showed a reduced basal release of glycerol and a reduced response to dibutyryl cyclic AMP. Significant enzyme differences were noted after weight gain in the small

<hr>

(2)   Metabolism 26:739–747, July, 1977.

fat cells from nonobese men, but no enzyme changes were associated with the change in diet in obese subjects.

These studies showed enhanced basal lipolysis and augmented lipolytic responses to isoproterenol by large fat cells. The findings support the possibility that adipose tissue is the site for generation of signals for the amount of fat stored in the adipose tissue. Changes in adipose tissue, if they occur, are however only one component of any control system for food intake. The central or peripheral receptors that recognize the signals, if any, generated from adipose tissue are an equally important part of the system.

▶ [In this and related studies it appears that the size of the fat cell generates signals to determine satiety. Where the signal(s) originates and what it is remain problematic. – W.G.R.] ◀

Effects of Diabetes Mellitus on Cholesterol Metabolism in Man. The increased rate of atherosclerosis in diabetic patients and their alleged increase in cholesterol gallstones suggested that cholesterol metabolism may be altered in this disease. Lynn J. Bennion and Scott M. Grundy[3] (Natl. Inst. of Health, Phoenix, Ariz.) investigated cholesterol metabolism in Pima Indians with maturity-onset diabetes and no appreciable ketosis. Pima Indians have a high degree of genetic homogeneity and a high prevalence of diabetes, with a distinct increase in atherosclerosis as in white populations. Six subjects were investigated on a metabolic ward, before and during subcutaneous administration of regular and isophane insulins. Cholesterol balance studies were performed with ^{14}C-cholic acid.

All subjects had marked hyperglycemia and glycosuria before treatment. Serum cholesterol and triglyceride concentrations were significantly higher during untreated hyperglycemia. Fecal neutral steroid excretion was greater before treatment in each subject. In each, cholesterol balance was greater during the time when insulin was not given. In all subjects the bile acid pool was larger during the untreated period than during insulin therapy. All the major species of bile acids were increased proportionately in the untreated hyperglycemic state. A decrease in gallbladder bile saturation by cholesterol was observed in the untreated

---

(3)   N. Engl. J. Med. 296:1365–1371, June 16, 1977.

state, with an increase in bile saturation by cholesterol on insulin treatment.

The findings are consistent with the hypothesis that when maturity-onset diabetes is poorly controlled, there is a generalized increase in hepatic lipid production, reflected by greater excretion of neutral and acidic steroids and by an elevation of plasma cholesterol and triglyceride concentrations. Insulin therapy appears to reverse this accelerated lipid synthesis. Improved control reduces plasma lipid values, but it appears to enhance the risk of supersaturated bile and cholesterol gallstones by decreasing bile acid synthesis.

► [Here's how to take cholesterol out of your arteries and put it in your gallbladder! — W.G.R.] ◄

Type III Hyperlipoproteinemia ("Remnant Removal Disease"): Insight into Pathogenetic Mechanism. Although uncommon, type III hyperlipoproteinemia is important because it is often associated with accelerated peripheral and possibly coronary atherosclerosis and because the arterial lesions may be reversible by treatment of the hyperlipidemia. Broad-β disease has been explained by both overproduction of apoprotein B, saturating the normal metabolic path responsible for converting remnants to low-density lipoproteins (LDL), and by a primary defect of remnant removal, i.e., impaired catabolism of remnants to LDL. Alan Chait, John D. Brunzell, John J. Albers and William R. Hazzard[4] (Seattle) report findings in a case of type III hyperlipoproteinemia, which suggest that impaired remnant removal is the major pathogenetic mechanism.

A woman, aged 57, with palmar-planar xanthomas but no evidence of ischemic heart or peripheral vascular disease, was studied. Biochemical features were characteristic of type III hyperlipoproteinemia. Metabolic studies were done with ^{125}I-labeled very-low-density lipoprotein (VLDL) from a patient with a type IV pattern. Clearance of activity from the apoprotein B moiety of VLDL was slow after the injection, and appearance of activity in LDL was delayed. Despite a 60% increase in the rate of VLDL production, treatment with 1 μg ethinyl estradiol per kg daily resulted in decreased plasma lipid concentrations, return toward normal of lipoprotein composition and correction of the defect in

(4) Lancet 1:1176–1178, June 4, 1977.

VLDL catabolism, with increased conversion to LDL. The VLDL-apoprotein B half-life was 5.5 hours during estrogen therapy, compared to 17.8 hours in the untreated state. The respective VLDL-apoprotein B turnover rates were 0.563 and 0.301 mg/kg/per hour.

The primary defect in type III hyperlipoproteinemia appears to be impaired catabolism of VLDL. The hypolipidemic effect of estrogen seems to be unique to this type of hyperlipoproteinemia. The hypolipidemic response to estrogen observed in this and other patients seems to result from partial correction of an abnormality in the removal of VLDL and its remnants.

▶ [This disorder also responds well to clofibrate, which at one time, I believe, was thought to have estrogenic activity. One may speculate that the effect of estrogen on transport proteins is operative here. — W.G.R.] ◀

Effect of a Protein-Sparing Diet and Brief Fast on Nitrogen Metabolism in Mildly Obese Subjects. Body nitrogen is spared when a total fast is modified by small amounts of dietary protein, and nitrogen balance has been maintained in obese patients given a protein-sparing modified fast (PSMF). Bruce R. Bistrian, Joerg Winterer, George L. Blackburn, Vernon Young and Mindy Sherman[5] determined whether nitrogen equilibrium can be achieved in minimally obese patients by the use of a protein source free from fat and thus significantly lower in calories. Five young, mildly obese women were used in the study. A formula diet providing total calories at 1.2 times basal energy expenditure was initially taken, followed by a PSMF with 1.5 gm egg white per kg. The egg white was then withdrawn for 1 week, and a PSMF with meat protein was then given for 1 week.

The diets were well tolerated. Bowel movements were more frequent and sometimes loose when egg white was consumed. Nitrogen balance was slightly negative initially, improving in each succeeding week of the PSMF. Nitrogen balance was negative during the total fast, but significantly positive during consumption of the PSMF with meat protein; it differed from initial values although protein intake was identical in both periods.

These findings confirm the nitrogen-sparing effect of

---

(5)   J. Lab. Clin. Med. 89:1030–1035, May, 1977.

small amounts of dietary protein as a modification to a fast. A larger role for the PSMF in the management of the semi-starved state is suggested. Although nitrogen equilibrium may not always be achievable in those with smaller fat reserves, significantly better nitrogen sparing over that found with isocaloric amounts of other nutrients can be anticipated. Suggested applications include not only weight reduction in the obese, but also use in the common clinical situation of hospitalized ill patients, especially those with sepsis or infection or those receiving therapeutic corticosteroids.

► [These findings are not surprising. The enthusiasm for the PSMF has cooled considerably since the associated deaths have been reported. One of the preparations I saw on the shelf of my local drug store was made of hydrolyzed collagen, a notoriously low-quality protein relative to essential amino acid content. —W.G.R.] ◄

Abnormalities of Circulating 25-OH-Vitamin D after Jejunal-Ileal Bypass for Obesity: Evidence of an Adaptive Response. Steven L. Teitelbaum, John D. Halverson, Margaret Bates, Leslie Wise and John G. Haddad[6] (St. Louis) measured circulating levels of 25-OH-vitamin D in 44 patients who had had small bowel bypass for obesity. The 35 women and 9 men had a mean age of 33.8. They had had end-to-end anastomosis of the jejunum and ileum 4–40 months before this study; 35 cm of proximal jejunum and 10 cm of distal ileum were left in continuity. Patients had lost a mean of 48.2 kg at the time of study. Only 1 patient had vitamin D supplementation for 6 months before the study. Repeat measurements of serum 25-OH-vitamin D levels were made in 8 patients after a mean time of 18.5 months. Two patients were studied after the oral administration of 5 μg 25-OH-vitamin D_3 per kg. Six patients had iliac crest biopsies after intestinal bypass.

Abnormally low levels of circulating 25-OH-vitamin D were found in 61% of patients. A more rapid rate of weight loss was associated with lower levels of the metabolite, but the levels rose progressively with time after surgery. Most low levels were found within 15 months after surgery. Metabolite levels were directly related to the levels of total serum calcium, which were low in 43% of patients. No correlation with circulating magnesium was noted, although this component was abnormally low in 52% of the group. There

---

(6)   Ann. Intern. Med. 86:289–293, March, 1977.

was little evidence of densitometric osteopenia in the study group. Oral administration of 25-OH-vitamin D_3 resulted in subnormal elevations of serum metabolite levels. Half the bone biopsy specimens were histologically normal.

Despite apparent abnormalities of mineral metabolism in this group of patients, there was less evidence of densitometrically evaluated bone disease. Small bowel bypass appears to result in at least transient deficits in circulating 25-OH-vitamin D. Clinically significant skeletal disease may become apparent on long-term follow-up of these patients. Prolonged observation may be necessary because vagaries in calcium and phosphorus ingestion may theoretically influence long-term mineral metabolism.

► [These findings are not surprising, because these patients have a severe malabsorption state immediately postoperatively that improves generally over the following year. − W.G.R.] ◄

Lipoprotein Abnormality in Tangier Disease: Quantitation of A Apoproteins. Tangier disease is a rare disorder of plasma lipid transport characterized by the absence of normal high-density lipoproteins (HDL) and storage of cholesteryl esters in foam cells in many tissues. The 21 patients described represent 15 kindred. There is an absolute decrease in the amounts of the major apoproteins of HDL, apolipoprotein A-I (Apo A-I) and apolipoprotein A-II (Apo A-II) in plasma in Tangier disease. G. Assmann, E. Smootz, K. Adler, A. Capurso and K. Oette[7] (Univ. of Cologne) used a double-antibody radioimmunoassay technique and double immunoelectrophoresis to further characterize the distribution and quantities of these apoproteins in Tangier plasma. Three patients homozygous for Tangier disease contributed Tangier plasma for study.

Compared with normal plasma, the total amounts of labeled apoproteins A-I and A-II in Tangier plasma were less than 1% and 5−7%, respectively. About 90% of the Apo A-I sedimented when ultracentrifugations of plasma were done at density 1.21 gm/ml KBr. Over 95% of Apo A-II floated under these conditions. In normal plasma, about 90% of both apoproteins is found in the 1.063 to 1.21-gm/ml potassium bromide density fraction. Dissociation of the A apoproteins was confirmed by double immunoelectrophoresis with mono-

---

(7)   J. Clin. Invest. 59:565−575, March, 1977.

specific antiserums. Immunochemical and electrophoretic studies did not provide evidence of a structural abnormality of apoprotein A-I.

These findings strongly suggest that normal high-density lipoproteins are absent from Tangier plasma. Further study is needed to determine whether the defect in Tangier disease resides in a structural apoprotein abnormality or in a regulatory gene mutation affecting the synthesis of A apoproteins. Elucidation of the nature of protein-protein and protein-lipid interactions in normal HDL will promote understanding of the origin of the dissociation of the A apoproteins in Tangier plasma.

▶ [The A apoproteins, the protein portion of HDL, apparently function primarily to transport cholesterol from peripheral tissues to the liver. The observation that the level of HDL cholesterol is inversely related to the incidence of coronary heart disease will likely stimulate further interest in their control. — W.G.R.] ◀

The following review article is recommended to the reader:

Brady, R. O.: Heritable catabolic and anabolic disorders of lipid metabolism, Metabolism 26:329, 1977.

Gastrointestinal Hormones

Effect of Chronic Antacid Ingestion on Serum Gastrin and Gastric Secretion. Incomplete inhibition of gastrin release by acid has been suggested in patients with duodenal ulcer, possibly due to secondary hyperplasia of the gastrin cell population from frequent feedings and antacid therapy. James H. Caldwell, Charles T. Cline, Arthur W. Fox and Samuel Cataland[8] (Ohio State Univ.) studied the effects of chronic antacid ingestion on fasting serum gastrin and basal and stimulated acid secretion in 25 healthy subjects, 12 men and 13 women aged 21–35 years. Ten subjects were studied before and after 6 weeks of ingestion of 30 ml aluminum-magnesium hydroxide suspension (Maalox) 4 times daily. Ten were studied before and after use of 15 ml aluminum-magnesium hydroxide plus calcium carbonate (Camalox) 4 times daily for 6 weeks. Augmented histamine tests were performed, and serum gastrin was measured by radioimmunoassay. Five subjects underwent identical studies 6 weeks apart.

Neither experimental group showed significant changes in basal acid secretion or gastric secretory responses to histamine or to a test meal after 6 weeks of antacid therapy. No significant change in fasting serum gastrin was observed. No group showed significant changes in fasting serum calcium or magnesium values.

These data do not exclude the possibility that antacid therapy produces an augmented serum gastrin response to food, but such treatment appears not to alter the functional parietal cell mass or functional gastrin activity. It is impossible to extrapolate the data directly to patients predisposed to peptic ulcer, but the ubiquity of antacid consumption makes it unlikely that ulcer patients who are naive with regard to antacid use could be found for such study. The resistance of gastrin to acid inhibition that is characteristic of

(8)   Am. J. Dig. Dis. 21:863–866, October, 1976.

duodenal ulcer patients is unlikely to result from simple quantitative changes in serum or tissue gastrin.

► [Well, let's have another rousing round of "Tums for the tummy."— W.G.R.] ◄

Motilin: Spectrum and Mode of Gastrointestinal Actions are discussed by Wolfram Domschke[9] (Univ. of Erlangen-Nuremberg). Motilin has now taken the first steps out of the candidate hormone reserve toward recognition as a gastrointestinal hormone. Brown et al. suggested that the increased motor activity of canine fundic pouches observed on alkalinization of the duodenum could be due to inhibition of release of an inhibitory agent or release of a stimulatory agent from the duodenal mucosa. Subsequently a gastric motor-stimulating property was isolated from duodenal extracts and termed "motilin." The first synthesis of a norleucine analogue of motilin was achieved by Wünsch et al., in 1973. Recently, synthesis of the docosapeptide corresponding to 13-methionine-motilin was reported by Yajima et al. A population of enterochromaffin cells in the dog, pig, baboon and human intestine contain, and presumably synthesize, store and secrete, motilin. Motilin appears to cause contractions by stimulating receptors on or in the muscle cell. Susceptibility is greatest in gastric and duodenal muscle strips, and nonintestinal smooth muscle does not respond to the polypeptide.

A specific, sensitive radioimmunoassay was recently established for human plasma motilin by Bloom et al. Synthetic 13-norleucine-motilin has been reported to increase gastric acid and pepsin secretion and pancreatic bicarbonate and protein output in dogs. Stimulation of gastric pepsin output has been described in man. Dose-dependent increases in lower esophageal sphincter pressure have been described in man. Gastric emptying in man is slowed by infused 13-norleucine-motilin, and the small bowel transit of a barium meal is reduced. Motilin appears not to induce gallbladder contractions. No instance of induction or facilitation of hormone release by motilin has been described. Motilin reduces leucine incorporation into gastric mucosa protein and may act as a functional antagonist of pentagastrin. No

---

(9) Am. J. Dig. Dis. 22:454–461, May, 1977.

cardiovascular effects of infused 13-norleucine-motilin have been observed in man.

▶ [This gastrointestinal endocrinology gets more complex by the year. — W.G.R.] ◀

Response of Gastric Inhibitory Polypeptide (GIP) to Test Meal in Chronic Pancreatitis: Relationship to Endocrine and Exocrine Insufficiency. It has been suggested that GIP is an obvious incretin candidate, and patients with chronic pancreatitis have been reported to release more GIP after a test meal or an oral glucose load than normal subjects. R. Ebert, W. Creutzfeldt, J. C. Brown, H. Frerichs and R. Arnold[1] (Univ. of Göttingen) investigated 29 patients with chronic pancreatitis with respect to the interdependence of the immunoreactive GIP (IR-GIP) response to a test meal and the degree of exocrine pancreatic insufficiency and changes in serum immunoreactive insulin (IRI), immunoreactive gastrin (IRG) and glucose. Fifteen healthy subjects were also studied. Twelve patients had pancreatic calcifications. Eight patients had overt diabetes and 14 were subclinical diabetics. A mixed meal of 1,031 calories was ingested within 10 minutes.

Serum IR-GIP levels rose sharply after the test meal and remained elevated for at least 5 hours. Serum levels of IRG, IRI and glucose rose less sharply and began to fall after 3 hours, without reaching fasting values at 5 hours. Integrated IR-GIP and glucose responses were significantly greater in the patients with pancreatitis than in controls. The IRI response in patients was significantly smaller, whereas the IRG response did not differ from that of controls. The IR-GIP and IRG responses were similar in patients with mild and severe maldigestion, but the latter had a much smaller IRI response and a much greater glucose response. The IR-GIP rise in patients with a moderately impaired IRI response was significantly greater than the increase in patients with nearly normal or severely impaired IRI responses.

The IR-GIP response to a test meal is determined by at least two factors: (1) feedback control via insulin secretion and (2) assimilation of fat. In chronic pancreatitis, endocrine insufficiency may induce an exaggerated GIP re-

(1)   Diabetologia 12:609–612, December, 1976.

sponse, and severe exocrine insufficiency may prevent fat-induced GIP release. Gastrin is not involved in the different GIP response of patients with chronic pancreatitis. Further studies are needed to determine whether hypersecretion of glucagon can inhibit IR-GIP release.

▶ [Speaking of acronyms! – W.G.R.] ◀

Localization of Gastric Inhibitory Polypeptide Release by Intestinal Glucose Perfusion in Man. No studies have been reported comparing the effectiveness of different parts of the small bowel in the endogenous release of gastric inhibitory polypeptide (GIP). Fred B. Thomas, Don F. Shook, Thomas M. O'Dorisio, Samuel Cataland, Hagop S. Mekhjian, James H. Caldwell and Ernest L. Mazzaferri[2] (Ohio State Univ.) localized GIP release in man by carrying out segmental glucose perfusions of the small bowel in 19 healthy subjects, 12 women and 7 men aged 19–35 years. All subjects were within 10% of ideal body weight and had normal carbohydrate tolerance. All took a 100-gm carbohydrate diet for at least 3 days before study. Perfusion studies were carried out at midduodenum, proximal jejunum, midjejunum and ileum after a 12-hour fast. A solution of glucose with polyethylene glycol was used. Immunoreactive GIP was measured by using a highly purified porcine GIP labeled with ^{125}I.

Preperfusion GIP concentrations were below assay sensitivity (125 pg/ml) in all subjects. After glucose perfusion, maximal serum GIP concentrations were 1,383, 904, 545 and 305 pg/ml in the duodenum, proximal jejunum, midjejunum and ileum, respectively. Integrated GIP secretion was significantly greater with duodenal and proximal jejunal perfusion than with more distal perfusion. Peak serum insulin concentrations and integrated insulin secretion were also significantly greater with perfusion of the duodenum or proximal jejunum. Serum glucose concentrations, integrated serum glucose and glucose absorption were similar for the four areas perfused.

The findings indicate that the proximal small intestine is the primary site of endogenous GIP release in man, but that smaller amounts of GIP are also released by the distal small bowel. Differences in serum GIP concentration and integrat-

(2)   Gastroenterology 72:49–54, January, 1977.

ed GIP secretion between the uppermost small bowel and the midjejunum may be due to a decrease in tissue GIP beyond the midjejunum.

► [All these studies on GIP make one GASP! – W.G.R.] ◄

Streptozocin-Treated Verner-Morrison Syndrome: Plasma Vasoactive Intestinal Peptide and Tumor Responses. Robert F. Gagel, Mary E. Costanza, Ronald A. DeLellis, Richard A. Norton, Stephen R. Bloom, Harry H. Miller, Angelo Ucci and Larry Nathanson[3] followed a patient with the Verner-Morrison syndrome with elevated plasma vasoactive intestinal peptide (VIP) levels and a nonbeta islet cell carcinoma of the pancreas, who responded dramatically to streptozocin therapy.

Woman, 53, had had watery diarrhea of increasing severity for 5 months. Thyroid hormone had been given for a nodular goiter a year previously. The initial serum potassium level was 2.4 mEq/L and fulminant diarrhea was present. Up to 10 L intravenous isotonic saline as well as 150 – 250 mEq potassium were required to maintain normal hydration and electrolyte balance. A thyroid scan showed a cold nodule in the left lobe and a liver scan showed two nodular defects consistent with metastatic disease. Hepatic angiography showed multiple foci of metastatic tumor in the liver. Plasma secretin, pancreatic glucagon, plasma gastric inhibitory peptide and serum gastrin levels were normal. The plasma VIP was 250 pg/ml by radioimmunoassay. Laparotomy revealed a pancreatic tumor which had occluded the splenic vein and spread to the right lobe of the liver; several liver biopsy specimens showed a nonbeta islet cell carcinoma that was positive for VIP by immunohistochemical techniques.

The patient was given 500 mg streptozocin per sq m daily, intravenously, for 5 days and then prednisone was added. By the 12th day diarrhea decreased, and, every 6 weeks, courses of streptozocin were repeated; by day 60 bowel movements had returned to normal. The plasma VIP fell gradually to normal within 5 months of the start of treatment. Most measurable disease disappeared on treatment. Glycosuria appeared after the 9th course of therapy and streptozocin was temporarily discontinued. The patient is asymptomatic at present and the most recent VIP value was normal.

The mechanism of the Verner-Morrison syndrome is thought to be hypersecretion by the small bowel and secondary inhibition of acid secretion by the stomach. The evidence that VIP is the etiologic agent for the diarrhea is im-

____

(3) Arch. Intern. Med. 136:1429 – 1435, December, 1976.

pressive but circumstantial. Levels of VIP correlated well with symptom and tumor regression in the present case but there is disagreement concerning its ultimate specificity as a tumor marker in diarrheal patients.

► [In the 1977 YEAR BOOK (p. 243) we included a report on the use of streptozocin in the Zollinger-Ellison syndrome. Here is an extension to its use in a closely related malady. — W.G.R.] ◄

The following review articles are recommended to the reader:

Carter D. C.: Inhibitors of gastric secretion: Current progress, Br. J. Surg. 63:788, 1976.

Pearse, A. G. E., et al.: The newer gut hormones, Gastroenterology 72:746, 1977.

Rayford, P. L., Miller, T. A., and Thompson, J. C.: Secretin, cholecystokinin and newer gastrointestinal hormones: Part I, N. Engl. J. Med. 294:1093, 1976.

——— Part II, N. Engl. J. Med. 294:1157, 1976.

——— and Thompson, J. C.: Gastrin, Surg. Gynecol. Obstet. 145:257, 1977.

Welbourn, R. B.: Apudomas of the gut, Am. J. Surg. 133:13, 1977.

Adrenal Medulla

Attempted Treatment of Inoperable Pheochromocytoma with Streptozocin. Streptozocin is a nitrosourea antibiotic that has been used with varying success to treat patients with islet cell tumors and is on trial for medullary thyroid carcinoma. Bruce P. M. Hamilton, Issam E. Cheikh and Luis E. Rivera[4] (Univ. of Maryland) submitted 2 patients who had inoperable pheochromocytoma to an adequate trial of streptozocin and followed the responses closely with urinary catecholamine determinations. No improvement was documented in either patient.

CASE 1.—Man, 41, who presented with neurofibromatosis and weight loss, was found to have two left lung masses and osteolytic lesions and a right adrenal mass. Spinal cord decompression was necessary for metastatic pheochromocytoma. The patient was given 1.54 mg streptozocin by infusion weekly, with phenoxybenzamine, but no urinary vanillylmandelic acid response was seen, and the metastases continued to enlarge before the patient died. No response was obtained with doxorubicin.

CASE 2.—Woman, 28, with an unresectable tumor, received 1.5 gm streptozocin weekly for 4 weeks, with no apparent response. Subsequently pulmonary metastases appeared.

Pheochromocytoma was confirmed histologically in both these patients. The tumors showed no response to streptozocin, either biochemically or by a reduction in mass, although both patients received enough drug to produce an antitumor effect, if this were going to occur, by Schein's criteria. Possibly intra-arterial infusion of the drug should have been tried, but no strong data indicate the superiority of this technique over the routine intravenous route.

► [Here is another therapeutic maneuver that gets "no cigar." Streptozocin has been found useful in the management of metastatic pancreatic islet cell tumors producing hypoglycemia, Zollinger-Ellison syndrome and pancreatic cholera, as well as malignant carcinoid. —W.G.R.] ◄

(4)   Arch. Intern. Med. 137:762–765, June, 1977

Single-Voided Urine Metanephrine Assays in Screening for Pheochromocytoma. The metanephrine test has proved to be the best urinary catecholamine assay for routine screening for pheochromocytoma, but 24-hour urine collections have been necessary. Norman M. Kaplan, Norman J. Kramer, O. Bryan Holland, Sheldon G. Sheps and Celso Gomez-Sanchez[5] evaluated the use of random urine samples in 100 hypertensive patients without and 7 patients with pheochromocytoma. Controls had pressures above 160/95 mm Hg and were receiving no antihypertensive drugs. All the pheochromocytomas were proved solitary lesions. Six patients had adrenal tumors, and 1 patient had multiple extra-adrenal sympathetic tissue tumors. Metanephrine was eluted from 20-ml aliquots of urine on an Amberlite resin column and quantitated by spectrophotometry.

Metanephrine excretion tended to be higher during the day and lower late at night in control hypertensive patients, but the maximal variation between 4-hour periods was only 35%, and the value never approached 1 μg/mg creatinine. The 7 pheochromocytoma patients had distinctly high metanephrine concentrations throughout 24 hours; at no time did the values fall near 1 μg/mg creatinine. Excretion of metanephrine in simultaneously collected 24-hour and single-voided urine specimens was strongly correlated, particularly when both values were expressed as micrograms per milligram of creatinine. The mean metanephrine level in single-voided urine specimens from 500 consecutive patients with a diagnosis of essential hypertension was 0.351 ± 0.356 (2 SD), with a range of $0.06 - 1.18$ μg/mg creatinine.

More experience is needed to determine that false negatives do not occur with this approach. If there is clinical evidence of pheochromocytoma and the single-voided specimen contains less than 1 μg metanephrine per mg creatinine, a 4- to 8-hour specimen should be collected from the onset of a spell of anxiety, headache, sweating or tachycardia. If the single-voided specimen contains over 1 μg metanephrine per mg creatinine, a 24-hour specimen should be collected and analyzed for metanephrines, total catecholamines and

(5)   Arch. Intern. Med. 137:190–193, February, 1977.

vanillylmandelic acid. Normal children under age 15 excrete larger amounts of metanephrine than do adults.

▶ [A practical approach to screening for pheochromocytoma is presented. The big question is, "Is the yield high enough to warrant screening all hypertensive patients for it?" I suppose as the cost comes down with approaches like this, the benefit ratio will go up. –W.G.R.] ◀

Preliminary Report: Radioimmunoscan of Sympathetic Ganglia and Adrenal Medulla is described by Gregorio Skromne-Kadlubik, Eduardo Gamez Valdez, Antonio Férez, M. Medina and César Celis.[6] Nerve growth factor is a polypeptide, found in mouse sarcomas, snake venom and the salivary glands of certain mammals, which is necessary for the growth and development of the nervous system, especially the autonomic system. Injection of antiserum to the factor in newborn animals leads to near-total destruction of the sympathetic ganglia. Antiserum labeled with ^{131}I was injected to determine whether scans could be obtained of the sympathetic nervous system in mammals. Nerve growth factor from the submaxillary glands of mice and antibodies labeled with radioiodine were used in the study. The antiserum was injected intravenously into groups of rats, and the rats were killed after 2–24 hours. Rectilinear scans were made of the whole body 4 hours after injection.

About 2% of the administered dose of ^{131}I-antinerve growth factor concentrated in the sympathetic ganglia. Scans obtained at 4 hours showed preferential deposit of activity on both sides of the spinal cord, including both adrenal ganglia (medulla). No rat exhibited intolerance or radiotoxicity.

The use of ^{131}I-antinerve growth factor appears to provide a safe diagnostic tool for the sympathetic chain and adrenal medulla. No stimulation of the sympathetic nervous system was observed. The technique might be of use in human subjects. Sympathetic ganglia might be destroyed by a single dose of radiation, with the use of an appropriate dose of ^{131}I-antinerve growth factor.

▶ [An ingenious technique is offered here. I could surely use something like it in a patient with recurrent pheochromocytoma who I am following. Five paragangliomas were removed last summer and she still has elevated levels of urinary vanillylmandelic acid and catecholamines. –W.G.R.] ◀

---

(6) J. Urol. 117:225–226, February, 1977.

Hypoglycemia as Complication of Removal of a Pheochromocytoma. Hyperglycemia is a common associated disorder in patients with pheochromocytoma. C. T. B. Allen and D. Imrie[7] (Victoria Genl. Hosp., Halifax, N.S.) report a case of potentially fatal hypoglycemia that followed successful excision of a pheochromocytoma, a condition not previously described in the literature.

Man, 60, presented with "nervous" episodes, occurring for 12 years, and blood pressure of 180/100 mm Hg, documented for at least 2 years. Ischemic ECG changes had been found. Urinary values for catecholamines and vanillylmandelic acid were greatly increased, and a solitary right adrenal tumor was visualized. After preparation of the patient with phenoxybenzamine and propranolol, the tumor was removed; a hypertensive episode occurred when it was manipulated at operation. Positive fluid balance was maintained during surgery. The patient became normotensive without hypotensive episodes after removal of the tumor, but 2 hours postoperatively he gradually became comatose and areflexic. A blood glucose concentration of 35 mg/dl was reported. Consciousness returned rapidly when intravenous 50% dextrose was given, and an infusion of 15% dextrose in Ringer's lactate maintained the blood glucose concentrations at 90–130 mg/dl for the next 24 hours. Subsequently the sugar requirement appeared to return to within normal limits, and an infusion of 5% dextrose at a rate of 100 ml per hour maintained a normal blood glucose value.

A reactive rise in insulin after removal of exposure to epinephrine and propranolol therapy may both have contributed to postoperative hypoglycemia in this case, as may phentolamine administration. Preoperative assessment of glucose homeostasis before and after adrenergic blockade and careful monitoring of the blood glucose concentration in the early postoperative period are strongly recommended for patients with pheochromocytoma. Intraoperative and postoperative administration of dextrose solution of adequate concentration is also recommended.

► [This is an interesting observation. One wonders if a transient cortisol deficiency may have been operative. – W.G.R.] ◄

► [At last, the traditional final comment (the Editor says with a sigh of relief; the reader hears with some trepidation)! During the past year, the Editor underwent an extraordinary sequence of experiences that seems worth summarizing. He got sick. We pick up the narrative about 2 years ago when he and his wife attended a meeting held in a lovely Hawaiian hotel.

(7)   Can. Med. Assoc. J. 116:363–364, Feb. 19, 1977.

He worked hard (honest!) during the meeting, but immediately afterward became ill with an all-too-familiar attack characterized by severe unremitting cough, headache and temperatures to 104 F. He was attended by high-class colleagues whose efforts were unsurprisingly ineffectual. His emotional response to this illness ran true to form; his face turned to the wall with bristling at any human contact. His wife kept her usual devoted vigil. They returned home as soon as he was semimobile. He continued to feel "run down." Each morning he coughed up large amounts of white mucoid sputum and his nose ran like a spring freshet.

This sorry state of affairs persisted for several months and finally, in desperation, he gave up one of his oldest and most cherished vices, pipe smoking. The symptoms were exacerbated rather than relieved. Once a day he would suddenly begin a coughing bout that progressing with increasing intensity, would, at last, culminate in the flow of much white mucopurulent sputum. The coughing was disruptive and increasingly painful, and paper tissue consumption rose to the point where his wife developed a sharp eye for "Kleenex sales." It became clear that the attacks were most likely to occur between the hours of 3 and 5 A.M. He would rise wearily from bed, unable to lie flat, and take himself to the study where, between coughs, he would work on projects, such as the completion of the YEAR BOOK. He would be awakened from his sleep, he noted, if he permitted an arm to emerge from beneath the bedcovers, and attacks could be precipitated by exposure to the lightest stirring of air. (He felt like a doddering old man when he demanded of his family that they close windows and doors to protect him from a refreshing breeze.) He also found that attacks could be precipitated by physical activity (a real nuisance on the handball court).

He knew that there were no psychologic precipitating factors because by this time his unvarying emotional stance was one of barely suppressed fury. While his symptoms could be perceived as truly threatening to his health, if not his life, he felt no fear or anxiety. There was no emotional room for anything except for an abiding, deep anger. He had atavistic fantasies in which his chest was possessed by demons, demons whom he dared to emerge for a frontal fight to the finish.

He reviewed some diagnostic possibilities. Carcinoma of the lung and bronchiectasis were considered but, on only one or two occasions after protracted coughing, did he ever note bloody sputum. He thought an allergic disease most likely because allergies ran in his family. His older brother had suffered from asthma in childhood, a fact that added to the stock of favorite family stories. Several years ago, his brother, his mother and he were discussing his brother's childhood attacks and his mother insisted that her ancient and honorable treatment was very effective. When his brother and an attack, he was forced to swallow some kerosene. He would promptly and predictably become nauseated, vomit and the attack would abate. His brother sat quietly through this narrative, and, when it was completed, he said, "And, do you know, to this day I can't stand the taste of kerosene!"

The family history also included the 2 oldest (of the Editor's 6) sons, who had typical asthma that almost completely remitted with the onset of puberty. The second oldest son also had mild atopic dermatitis. Because the Editor frequently was aware of rhonchi but had never noticed classic wheezing, he decided that he was suffering from "asthmatic bronchitis."

Finally, in desperation, he sought the advice of a bright, young allergist who took a careful history and asked, during the course of the physical examination, that his patient expire deeply and forcefully. This precipitated not only a dramatic coughing attack, but classic expiratory wheezes obvious to both examiner and examinee. The diagnosis of asthma was established.

The patient promised (but not faithfully) to be cooperative and a workup proceeded. He had increased residual air, and a microscopic examination of his sputum was bright with the scintillating granules of eosinophils. Terbutaline and aminophylline therapy was instituted, but with little effect. The patient went off to the family summer cottage in Michigan hoping for improvement with the environmental change, but he was again disappointed. By this time sympathetic friends and family were tiptoeing around a glowering animal. Finally, in a telephone conversation he discussed with his allergist the possibility of instituting beclomethasone inhalation therapy. Agreement was reached and after about 5 days of increasing despair and unmitigated rancor, the miracle happened. A remission occurred.

This illness taught him a good deal. He recognized that, in part, his unfocused anger was an effective device to fortify a flagging sense of invulnerability. He learned that one had to acquire some expertise as a bombardier to deliver the beclomethasone inhalant directly to the posterior pharynx rather than to direct it ineffectually at the palate or tongue with the possibility of providing a fertile field for local *Candida* organisms. He learned that exhaling the steroid through the nose rather than through the mouth will ameliorate some of the nasal symptoms.

With the remission, his old behavior returned. He lapsed in his role as patient and did not contact the allergist to undergo skin tests as promised. He thought it possible that the illness in Hawaii had established a "vicious cycle," poorly defined, but which, if broken, would lead to a cure. He discontinued therapy without consulting anyone. He promptly relapsed and then reinstituted treatment, remaining, up to the present, almost asymptomatic.

Ever the educator, he thought it worthwhile to have himself presented at Grand Rounds, a function at which he usually presides. He introduced the Rounds in a characteristic fashion. "Today we have a rather special patient. He is an individual for whom I have the warmest regard and a respect verging on adulation . . . ."—T.B.S.] ◄

The following review article is recommended to the reader:

Axelrod, J.: Catecholamines and hypertension, Clin. Sci. Mol. Med. 51:415s, 1976.

T

Index to Authors